Geigy Scientific Tables

Geigy Scientific Tables

Volume 6

Bacteria
Fungi
Protozoa
Helminths

Edited by C. Lentner

Eighth, revised and enlarged edition
Published by CIBA–GEIGY

ISBN 0-914168-55-X
Library of Congress Catalogue No. 81-70045

ISBN 3-905298-02-3

CIBA-GEIGY Limited, Basel,
Medical and Pharmaceutical Information

Editor: Cornelius Lentner
Associate editor: Charlotte Lentner

American edition published by
CIBA-GEIGY Corporation,
Medical Education Division,
West Caldwell, New Jersey 07006

Printed in Switzerland

By way of explanation

This completely revised and expanded 8th edition of the *Geigy Scientific Tables* represents the continuation of a work that has stood the test of time. Its aim is to provide scientists and, in particular, doctors with a concise compendium of scientific data backed by literature references and thus to spare them much laborious searching.

The vast increase in the amount of subject matter to be included has meant that the *Geigy Scientific Tables* have had to be steadily extended, with the result that they are becoming too voluminous to be published in a single book. Dividing the book up into several separate volumes has made it possible to incorporate a number of additional chapters and has also helped to ensure that the data on the various branches of knowledge are more up-to-date than they could have been in a single-volume work.

The volumes so far published are: 'Units of Measurement, Body Fluids, Composition of the Body, Nutrition' (Volume 1), 'Introduction to Statistics, Statistical Tables, Mathematical Formulae' (Volume 2), 'Physical Chemistry, Composition of Blood, Hematology, Somatometric Data' (Volume 3), 'Biochemistry, Metabolism of Xenobiotics, Inborn Errors of Metabolism, Pharmacogenetics and Ecogenetics' (Volume 4), 'Heart and Circulation' (Volume 5). At present no further volumes are in preparation; Volume 6 completes the 8th edition.

CIBA-GEIGY Limited, Basel

Editors' note

This tabular synopsis of about 500 important pathogenic organisms is arranged under the following taxonomic headings: bacteria (including Rickettsiae), fungi (Eumycetes), protozoa and helminths (worms). Since virology has become a most complex discipline in its own right, viruses are not included here. Some of the organisms listed in this volume have been reported to cause disease only in single cases, whereas others give rise to morbidity in millions of cases: it has been estimated that 1000 million persons are infected with *Mycobacterium tuberculosis* and that 1–3 million deaths occur annually from tuberculosis[1]; some vector-borne diseases, such as malaria and schistosomiasis, also exact a heavy toll in human life and suffering (Table 1).

Table 1 *Incidence of some vector-borne diseases*[2]

Disease	Estimated number of infected persons	Number of persons at risk
Malaria	280 million	2100 million
Schistosomiasis	200 million	500 to 600 million
Lymphatic filariasis	90 million	905 million
Onchocerciasis	18 million	90 million
Chagas' disease	16 to 18 million	90 million
Leishmaniasis	12 million	350 million

Several diseases have been associated with newly recognized pathogens, e.g. *Borrelia burgdorferi*, *Legionella pneumophila*, *Helicobacter pyloris*, *Ehrlichia* species, *Chlamydia pneumoniae*, and Microsporidia. At the same time, some well-known organisms are now causing previously unknown syndromes: for example, *Escherichia coli* strains that acquire special virulence plasmids cause diarrheal disease, *Clostridium botulinum* can produce the syndrome of the hypotonic infant, *Staphylococcus aureus* and *Streptococcus pyogenes* the toxic shock syndrome.

Despite advances in chemotherapy and large-scale international disease-control measures, infectious diseases are still a worldwide problem. With increasing travel and migration, the use of immunosuppresive drugs, and the spread of acquired immunodeficiency syndrome, physicians anywhere may see infections caused by previously unfamiliar pathogens. Malnutrition, crowded living conditions, and poor sanitation are factors known to promote the spread of pathogenic organisms, but even in highly developed countries infectious diseases are a threat (Table 2).

Table 2 *Notifiable infectious diseases in the USA, 1991*[3]

Disease	Number of registered cases
Gonorrhea	602577
AIDS	43389
Syphilis	
– primary and secondary	41006
– congenital	1703
Tuberculosis	23543
Measles	9488
Lyme disease	8884
Haemophilus influenzae (invasive disease)	2582
Rocky Mountain spotted fever	635
Typhoid fever	456
Toxic shock syndrome	274
Tularemia	188
Leprosy	140
Brucellosis	89
Psittacosis	87
Encephalitis	76
Botulism	
– food-borne	22
– infant	70
Trichinosis	61
Leptospirosis	59
Tetanus	49
Plague	10
Diphtheria	2
Anthrax	0

The editors would like to extend their thanks to all those who have offered their help and advice in compiling this volume of the *Geigy Scientific Tables*, in particular the authors of the various sections: Dr. H. BRODHAGE (bacteria), Prof. H. P. R. SEELIGER (fungi), and Prof. G. S. NELSON (protozoa, helminths). We are indebted to Dr. T. HEYMER for contributing the drawings in the section on fungi.

A key to the pathogens possibly associated with a particular illness, or to the diseases that may be caused by a particular pathogen, is provided in the index at the end of the volume.

Basel, July 1992

C. LENTNER
CH. LENTNER

References

[1] Report of a Joint IVAT/WHO Study Group on Tuberculosis Control, *Wld Hlth Org. techn. Rep. Ser.*, No. 671 (1982).
[2] KNUDSEN and SLOFF, *Bull. Wld Hlth Org.*, **70**, 1 (1992).
[3] *Morb. Mort. wkly Rep.*, **40**, No. 52, 898 (1991).

Acknowledgments

The publishers and editors are indebted to the following for their contributions and assistance in compiling this volume of the Geigy Scientific Tables:

Dr. H. Brodhage
Splendidhalde 15
CH–6045 Meggen, Switzerland
(Bacteria)

Dr. T. Heymer
Siefenfeldchen 39
D–5303 Bornheim 1, Federal Republic of Germany
(Fungi)

Dr. S. Lal
Chest Unit
Bury General Hospital
Walmersley Road
Bury BL9 6PG
Lancashire, UK
(Tuberculosis)

Prof. G. S. Nelson
Liverpool School of Tropical Medicine
Pembroke Place
Liverpool L3 5QA, UK
(Protozoa, Helminths)

Prof. H. P. R. Seeliger
Department of Hygiene and Microbiology
University of Würzburg
Josef-Schneider-Strasse 2
D–8700 Würzburg, Federal Republic of Germany
(Listeriosis, Fungi)

Prof. S. J. Yawalkar
Medical Department
CIBA–GEIGY Limited
CH–4002 Basel, Switzerland
(Leprosy)

The publishers and editors wish to thank the following scientific bodies, and publishing houses for permission to reproduce data or illustrations:

Churchill Livingstone, Edinburgh
(page 18)

Mosby-Year Book, Inc., Chicago, IL
(page 25)

U.S. Department of Health and Human Services,
Centers for Disease Control, Atlanta, GA
(pages 55, 67, 119)

World Health Organization, Geneva
(pages 117, 118, 120, 125, 126, 135)

Contents

Notes for the guidance of users

As a rule, all symbols, abbreviations, etc. used are defined or explained at the place where they occur. The Commonwealth of Independent States has been abbreviated to CIS throughout this volume. For 'Bacterial Toxins' and 'Mode of Action of Antibiotics', the reader is referred to *Geigy Scientific Tables*, Volume 4.

The abbreviations used in the literature references are those recommended by UNESCO (*World Medical Periodicals*, 1961 and 1968)[1].

Greek alphabet

Greek character		Greek name	Roman equivalent
Upright	Italics		
Α α	*Α α*	alpha	A a
Β β	*Β β*	beta	B b
Γ γ	*Γ γ*	gamma	G g
Δ δ	*Δ δ*	delta	D d
Ε ε, ∈	*Ε ε, ∈*	epsilon	Ĕ ĕ
Ζ ζ	*Ζ ζ*	zeta	Z z
Η η	*Η η*	eta	Ē ē
Θ ϑ, θ	*Θ ϑ, θ*	theta	Th th
Ι ι	*Ι ι*	iota	I i
Κ ϰ, κ	*Κ ϰ, κ*	kappa	K k
Λ λ	*Λ λ*	lambda	L l
Μ μ	*Μ μ*	mu	M m
Ν ν	*Ν ν*	nu	N n
Ξ ξ	*Ξ ξ*	xi	X x
Ο ο	*Ο ο*	omicron	Ŏ ŏ
Π π, ϖ	*Π π, ϖ*	pi	P p
Ρ ϱ	*Ρ ϱ*	rho	R r
Σ σ, ς	*Σ σ, ς*	sigma	S s
Τ τ	*Τ τ*	tau	T t
Υ υ	*Υ υ*	upsilon	Y y
Φ φ, ϕ	*Φ φ, ϕ*	phi	Ph ph
Χ χ	*Χ χ*	chi	Ch ch
Ψ ψ	*Ψ ψ*	psi	Ps ps
Ω ω	*Ω ω*	omega	Ō ō

Reference

[1] CLEGG, H. A. (Ed.), *World Medical Periodicals*, 3rd ed., World Medical Association, New York, 1961, and WARE, M. (Ed.), supplement to the 3rd edition, New York, 1968.

Introduction

All organisms can be divided into 2 major kingdoms, the Procaryotae, which comprise the bacteria and cyanophytes (blue-green algae), and the Eucaryotae, which include all other organisms whether protists, plants or animals[1] (Table 1). Divisions, classes, orders, families, genera and species are progressively smaller, non-overlapping subsets of the kingdom. As discussed by STALEY and KRIEG[3], the basic taxonomic group in bacterial systematics is the species. A bacterial species may be regarded as a collection of strains that have certain features in common and differ considerably from other strains. One strain of a species is designated as the type strain: this strain serves as the name-bearer strain of the species – and is the reference specimen for the name. A species consists of the type strain and all other strains that are considered to be sufficiently similar to it to warrant inclusion with it in the species. This concept of species involves making subjective judgements; therefore some bacterial species have greater phenotypic and genetic diversity than others. A more rigorous species definition, e.g. defining a species at the level of DNA structures, would be desirable; however, classification schemes based on genetic relatedness may be questioned when the impact of transposable elements on the procaryotic genome is taken into account.

A species may be divided into two or more subspecies based on minor but consistent phenotypic variations within the species or on genetically determined clusters of strains within the species. The subspecies is the lowest taxonomic rank that has official standing in nomenclature. Ranks below subspecies (infrasubspecific ranks, Table 2) have no official standing in nomenclature but often have great practical usefulness.

With a few exceptions, the arrangement and the nomenclature in the tables on pages 11–73 are in accordance with *Bergey's Manual of Systematic Bacteriology*[4]. For classification of bacteria, see next page.

References

[1] GIBBONS and MURRAY, *Int. J. system. Bact.*, **28**, 1 (1978).
[2] MURRAY et al., *Medical Microbiology*, Wolfe, London, 1990, page 5.
[3] STALEY and KRIEG, in WILLIAMS et al. (Eds.), *Bergey's Manual of Systematic Bacteriology*, Volume 4, Williams & Wilkins, Baltimore, 1989, page 2299.
[4] KRIEG and HOLT (Eds.), *Bergey's Manual of Systematic Bacteriology*, Volume 1, Williams & Wilkins, Baltimore, 1984; SNEATH et al. (Eds.), *Bergey's Manual of Systematic Bacteriology*, Volume 2, Williams & Wilkins, Baltimore, 1986; STALEY et al. (Eds.), *Bergey's Manual of Systematic Bacteriology*, Volume 3, Williams & Wilkins, Baltimore, 1989; WILLIAMS et al. (Eds.), *Bergey's Manual of Systematic Bacteriology*, Volume 4, Williams & Wilkins, Baltimore, 1989.

Table 1 *Procaryotic and eucaryotic cell structure*[2]

	Procaryotae	Eucaryotae
Nuclear structure		
– DNA	Single, naked, ring-formed chromosome	Multiple chromosomes associated with histones
– Nuclear membrane	Absent	Present
Cytoplasmic structures		
– Endoplasmic reticulum	Absent	Present
– Mitochondria	Absent	Present
– Ribosomes	70 S (M_r 2.6×10^6)	80 S (M_r 4.3×10^6)
– Lysosomes	Absent	Present
– Plasma membrane	Present; no sterols except in *Mycoplasma*	Present; contains sterols
Cell wall	Complex structure with peptidoglycan layer, protein and lipids	Absent or composed of cellulose or chitin
Capsule	Frequently present	Absent

S: sedimentation coefficient
M_r: relative molecular mass

* GRAM-positive bacteria have a relatively simple cell wall, with a thick peptidoglycan layer surrounded by a polysaccharide capsule. The cell envelope of GRAM-negative bacteria is more complex, with a thin peptidoglycan layer sandwiched between an inner and an outer membrane, the latter containing phospholipids. The space between the membranes is called the periplasmic space

Table 2 *Infrasubspecific ranks*[3]

Preferred name	Synonym	Applied to strains with specific properties
Biovar	Biotype	Special biochemical or physiological properties
Serovar	Serotype	Distinctive antigenic properties
Pathovar	Pathotype	Pathogenic properties for certain hosts
Phagovar	Phagotype	Ability to be lysed by certain bacteriophages
Morphovar	Morphotype	Special morphological features

Classification of bacteria pathogenic in man
(abridged from *Bergey's Manual of Systematic Bacteriology*, Volumes 1–4)

The italic numbers are the serial numbers appearing in column 1 of the tables.

Spirochetes

Order	Spirochaetales Buchanan	
Family	Spirochaetaceae Swellengrebel	
Genus	*Treponema*	*1–5a*
Genus	*Borrelia*	*6–9*
Family	Leptospiraceae Hovind-Hougen	
Genus	*Leptospira*	*10, 11*

Aerobic or microaerophilic, motile, helical and vibrioid Gram-negative bacteria

Genus	*Spirillum*	*12*
Genus	*Campylobacter*	*13–15*

Gram-negative aerobic rods and cocci

Family	Pseudomonadaceae Winslow et al.	
Genus	*Pseudomonas*	*16–21*
Genus	*Xanthomonas*	*22*
Family	Rhizobiaceae Conn	
Genus	*Agrobacterium*	*23*
Family	Legionellaceae Brenner et al.	
Genus	*Legionella*	*24, 25*
Family	Neisseriaceae Prévot	
Genus	*Neisseria*	*26–28*
Genus	*Moraxella*	*29–31*
Genus	*Acinetobacter*	*32*
Genus	*Kingella*	*33*
Other genera		
Genus	*Flavobacterium*	*34*
Genus	*Alcaligenes*	*35*
Genus	*Brucella*	*36–38a*
Genus	*Bordetella*	*39–41*
Genus	*Francisella*	*42*

Facultatively anaerobic Gram-negative rods

Family	Enterobacteriaceae (Rahn) Ewing et al.	
Genus	*Escherichia*	*43*
Genus	*Shigella*	*44–47*
Genus	*Salmonella*	*48–63*
Genus	*Citrobacter*	*64, 65*
Genus	*Klebsiella*	*66–70*
Genus	*Enterobacter*	*71–73*
Genus	*Serratia*	*74, 75*
Genus	*Edwardsiella*	*76*
Genus	*Proteus*	*77, 78*
Genus	*Providencia*	*79, 80*
Genus	*Morganella*	*81*
Genus	*Yersinia*	*82–84*
Genus	*Kluyvera*	*85*
Not recorded		
Genus	*Ewingella*	*86*
Family	Vibrionaceae Veron	
Genus	*Vibrio*	*87–90*
Genus	*Aeromonas*	*91, 92*
Genus	*Plesiomonas*	*93*
Family	Pasteurellaceae Pohl	
Genus	*Pasteurella*	*94*
Genus	*Haemophilus*	*95–98a*
Genus	*Actinobacillus*	*99, 100*
Other genera		
Genus	*Chromobacterium*	*101*
Genus	*Cardiobacterium*	*102*
Genus	*Calymmatobacterium*	*103*
Genus	*Gardnerella*	*104*
Genus	*Eikenella*	*105*
Genus	*Streptobacillus*	*106*

Anaerobic Gram-negative straight, curved and helical rods

Family	Bacteroidaceae Pribram	
Genus	*Bacteroides*	*107–113*
Genus	*Fusobacterium*	*114–116*
Genus	*Leptotrichia*	*117*
Not recorded		
Genus	*Mobiluncus*	*117a*
Genus	*Helicobacter*	*117b*

Anaerobic Gram-negative cocci

Family	Veillonellaceae Rogosa	
Genus	*Veillonella*	*118*

Rickettsias

Order	Rickettsiales Gieszczykiewicz	
Family	Rickettsiaceae Pinkerton	
Tribe	Rickettsieae Philip	
Genus	*Rickettsia*	*119–126*
Genus	*Rochalimaea*	*127*
Genus	*Coxiella*	*128*
Tribe	Ehrlichieae Philip	
Genus	*Ehrlichia*	*129, 131*
Family	Bartonellaceae Gieszczykiewicz	
Genus	*Bartonella*	*130*
Not recorded		
	Agent of bacillary angiomatosis	*131a*
	Agent of cat-scratch disease	*131b*

Chlamydias

Order	Chlamydiales Storz and Page	
Family	Chlamydiaceae Rake	
Genus	*Chlamydia*	*132–134*

Mycoplasmas

Class	Mollicutes Edward and Freundt	
Order	Mycoplasmatales Freundt	
Family	Mycoplasmataceae Freundt	
Genus	*Mycoplasma*	*135, 135a*
Genus	*Ureaplasma*	*136*

Gram-positive cocci

Family	Micrococcaceae	
Genus	*Stomatococcus*	*136a*
Genus	*Staphylococcus*	*137–139a*
Other genera		
Genus	*Streptococcus*	*140–151*
Genus	*Leuconostoc*	*152, 153*
Genus	*Aerococcus*	*154*
Genus	*Peptostreptococcus*	*155, 156*

Endospore-forming Gram-positive rods and cocci

Genus	*Bacillus*	*157–161*
Genus	*Clostridium*	*162–170d*

Regular, nonsporing Gram-positive rods

Genus	*Lactobacillus*	*171*
Genus	*Listeria*	*172, 173a*
Genus	*Erysipelothrix*	*174*

Irregular, nonsporing Gram-positive rods

Genus	*Corynebacterium*	*175–177*
Genus	*Arcanobacterium*	*178*
Genus	*Arachnia*	*179*
Genus	*Propionibacterium*	*180*
Genus	*Eubacterium*	*180a*
Genus	*Actinomyces*	*181–183*
Genus	*Bifidobacterium*	*184*

Mycobacteria

Family	Mycobacteriaceae Chester	
Genus	*Mycobacterium*	*185–195*

Nocardiform actinomycetes

Genus	*Nocardia*	*196, 197*
Genus	*Rhodococcus*	*198*
Genus	*Oerskovia*	*199*

Nonphotosynthetic, nonfruiting gliding bacteria

Order	Cytophagales Leadbetter	
Family	Cytophagaceae Stanier	
Genus	*Capnocytophaga*	*200, 200a*

Streptomycetes

Genus	*Streptomyces*	*201*

Maduromycetes

Genus	*Actinomadura*	*202, 203*

No.	**Bacterium** *Synonyms* Common names	Characteristics	Habitat Host Transmission	Associated disease
1	**Treponema pallidum** subsp. **pallidum** (SCHAUDINN and HOFFMAN) SCHAUDINN Syphilis spirochete	Very fine spirochete, 0.1–0.2 µm wide and 6–20 µm long, with 6–24 regular coils of almost equal length. Difficult to stain (best with GIEMSA); demonstration by dark-field or phase-contrast microscopy preferable. Motile. Attempts at culture on artificial media have so far been unsuccessful	Man. Transmission mainly by sexual intercourse, but also possible by extragenital contacts or transfusion of infected blood. Passage of organism through the placenta (congenital syphilis)[1]	Syphilis. Synonyms: venereal syphilis, lues. See table below and text on next page
2	**Treponema pallidum** subsp. **pertenue** (CASTELLANI) *Spirochaeta pertenuis*	Morphologically indistinguishable from *T. pallidum* subsp. *pallidum*. Cannot be cultured on artificial media	Man. Transmission by contact with infected skin	Yaws. Synonyms: frambesia, pian; also patek (Malaya), parangi (Ceylon), tonga (New Caledonia), coco (Fiji Islands), dubi (Ghana), buba (Zanzibar, East Africa, Antilles, Brazil), aboukoué (Gabon). See also table below
3	**Treponema pallidum** subsp. **endemicum**	Morphologically similar to *T. pallidum* subsp. *pallidum*. Cannot be cultured on artificial media	Man. Transmission by contact with infected mucous membranes, frequently via eating and drinking vessels, tobacco pipes. Child-to-mother transmission is not uncommon[2]	Bejel. Synonyms: endemic syphilis; also dichuchwa (South Africa), skerljevo (Bosnia). See also table below
4	**Treponema carateum** (ex BRUMPT)	Morphologically similar to *T. pallidum* subsp. *pallidum*. Cannot be cultured on artificial media	Man. Transmission by contact with infected skin	Pinta. Synonyms: carate, azul, boussarole, mal del pinto. See also table below
5	**Treponema vincentii** (ex BRUMPT)	Morphologically similar to *T. pallidum* subsp. *pallidum*. Motile, with 4–6 periplasmatic flagella. Grows well in peptone–yeast-extract–serum medium	Human oropharynx	Pathogen of VINCENT's angina, together with *Leptotrichia buccalis*
5a	**Treponema denticola** (ex BRUMPT)	Morphologically similar to *T. pallidum* subsp. *pallidum*. Motile, with 2–3 periplasmatic flagella. Grows well in peptone–yeast-extract–serum medium	Found in the oral cavity of man and chimpanzees	Associated with peridontal disease[3]

[1] TRAMONT, E.C., in MANDELL et al. (Eds.), *Principles and Practice of Infectious Diseases*, 3rd ed., Churchill Livingstone, New York, 1990, page 1794.
[2] MOODIE, P.M., in BRAUDE et al. (Eds.), *Infectious Diseases and Medical Microbiology*, 2nd ed., Saunders, Philadelphia, 1986, page 1361.
[3] Editorial, *Lancet*, **338**, 1177 (1991).

Treponematoses

The pathogenic *Treponema* species are identical in electron micrographs, and it is thought that all the diseases they cause are variations of the same disease entity resulting from differences in environmental factors like climate and sociological conditions. Because the pathogens that cause treponematosis in man cannot be continuously cultivated in vitro, their classification rests on differences in host species susceptibility and in the disease manifestations produced in these hosts.

Characteristics of treponematoses[1, 2]

	Syphilis	Yaws	Pinta	Bejel
Causative organism	*T. pallidum* subsp. *pallidum*	*T. pallidum* subsp. *pertenue*	*T. carateum*	*T. pallidum* subsp. *endemicum*
Geographical distribution	Worldwide	Hot humid regions: tropical areas of Africa, South America, India, Indonesia and the Pacific Islands	Hot humid regions: tropical areas of Central and South America, West Indies, Cuba	Hot dry regions: desert areas of the Middle East, Africa and Southeast Asia; certain areas of Yugoslavia
Age groups	Adults	Children and adolescents	Children and adolescents	Children and adults
Transmission	Sexual intercourse; congenital	Contact with infected skin	Contact with infected skin	Contact with infected mucous membranes; via utensils
Urogenital infection	Yes	No	No	Rare
Incubation period	10–90 days	2–4 weeks	1–3 weeks	Not known
Tissues affected	Almost every body tissue	Skin, bones, soft tissues	Skin	Mucous membranes, skin, muscles, bones
Destructive lesions	Yes	Yes	No	Yes
Condyloma latum	Yes	Yes	No	Yes

Syphilis

Epidemiological data on the incidence of syphilis are available for many countries[3–5, 12]. Detailed information on the incidence for subpopulations in the USA is given in a review from the Centers for Disease Control, Atlanta, GA (see illustration below)[6].

Diagnosis. Diagnosis of the primary infection is based on clinical features and direct demonstration of the treponema (dark-field or phase-contrast microscopy). The main serological tests[4, 5, 7, 8] in use today are:

- VDRL (venereal disease research laboratories slide test) – a non-treponemal test with high incidence of false-positive reactions. Recently a *T. pallidum* Western immunoblot assay for confirmation of syphilis has been discussed[13]
- AMHA-TP (automated microhemagglutination *Treponema pallidum* test)
- FTA-ABS (fluorescent treponemal antibody absorption test)

T. pallidum subspp. *pallidum* and *pertenue*, as well as *T. carateum*, cannot be isolated and cultured on or in artificial media, whereas the other *Treponema* species can be cultured. To be isolated, they require strictly anaerobic conditions, which can be done most easily by the membrane filter method. Amongst others, the following *Treponema* species can be cultured: *T. denticola*, *T. vincentii*, *T. scoliodontum*, *T. phagedenis*.

Remarks. Parenteral benzylpenicillin remains the drug of choice for treating all stages of syphilis[4, 5, 9]. In patients with intolerance to penicillin, a tetracycline, a cephalosporin or erythromycin may be used. Information on dosage regimens is given in appropriate reviews[4, 5, 9–11].

Patients (USA) with positive serology in untreated syphilis[7]

Stage of disease	Test		
	VDRL	AMHA-TP	FTA-ABS
Primary syphilis	70%	50–60%	85%
Secondary syphilis	99%	100%	100%
Latent or late syphilis	70%	98%	98%

References

[1] FITZGERALD, T. J., in BARON, S. (Ed.), *Medical Microbiology*, 2nd ed., Addison-Wesley, Menlo Park, CA, 1986, page 593.
[2] CHULAY, J. D., in MANDELL et al. (Eds.), *Principles and Practice of Infectious Diseases*, 3rd ed., Churchill Livingstone, New York, 1990, page 1808.
[3] ARAL and HOLMES, in HOLMES et al. (Eds.), *Sexually Transmitted Diseases*, 2nd ed., McGraw-Hill, New York, 1990, page 19.
[4] WHO Scientific Group on Treponemal Infections, *Wld Hlth Org. techn. Rep. Ser.*, No. 674 (1982).
[5] WHO Expert Committee on Venereal Diseases and Treponematoses, *Wld Hlth Org. techn. Rep. Ser.*, No. 736 (1986).
[6] ROLFS and NAKASHIMA, *J. Amer. med. Ass.*, **264**, 1432 (1990).
[7] LEE and SPARLING, *J. Amer. med. Ass.*, **242**, 1187 (1979).
[8] ADLER, M. W., *Brit. med. J.*, **288**, 551 (1984).
[9] *Med. Lett. Drug. Ther.*, **33**, No. 860 (1991).
[10] MUSHER, D. M., *Ann. intern. Med.*, **109**, 849 (1988).
[11] ZENKER and ROLFS, *Rev. infect. Dis.*, **12**, Suppl. 6, S 590 (1990).
[12] DE SCHRYVER and MEHEUS, *Bull. Wld Hlth Org.*, **68**, 639 (1990).
[13] BYRNE et al., *J. clin. Microbiol.*, **30**, 115 (1992).

Trends in race- and gender-specific incidence of primary and secondary syphilis in the USA, 1981–1989[6]

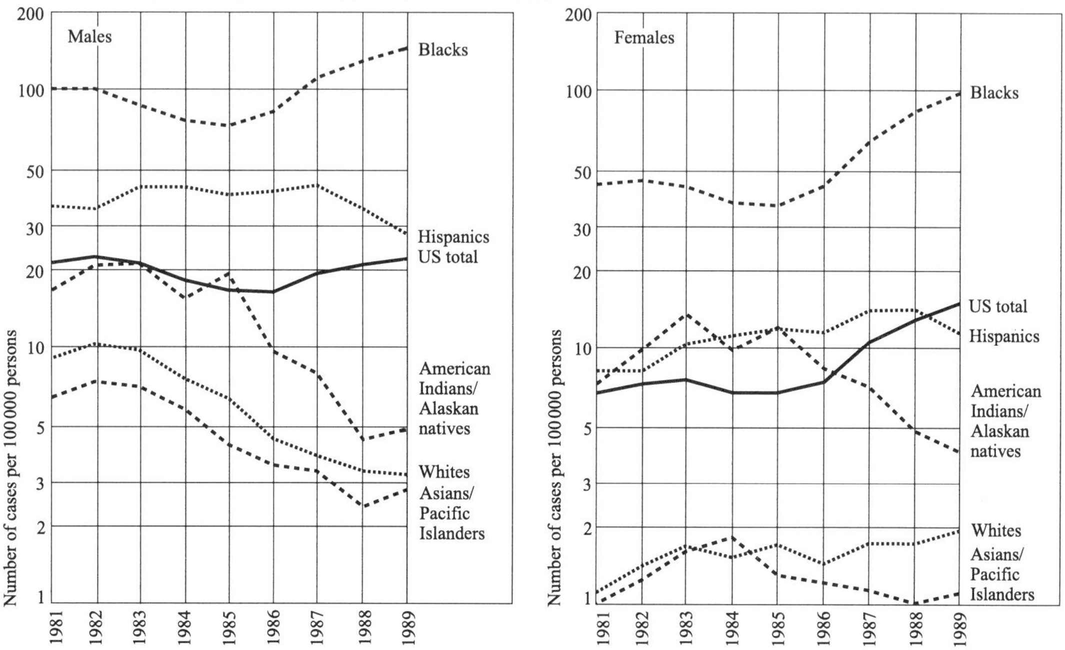

No.	Bacterium *Synonyms* Common names	Characteristics	Habitat Host Transmission	Associated disease
6	**Borrelia burgdorferi** (BURGDORFER) Agent of Lyme disease	GRAM-negative spirochete, 0.2 to 0.3 µm wide and 20–30 µm long, loosely coiled, with 7–11 flagella. As for other *Borrelia*, the cell is made up of a protoplasmic cylinder surrounded by a cytoplasmic membrane, then by flagella and finally by an outer membrane. Growth in BARBOUR-STOENNER-KELLY medium[1,2]. Indirect fluorescence (IFA) and enzyme-linked immunosorbent assay (ELISA) for the detection of antibodies to *B. burgdorferi*[2–4]	Host: wild and domestic animals, including birds. Transmission through the bite of hard-shelled ticks[5–7]: *Ixodes dammini* (northeastern and midwestern parts of USA) *Ixodes pacificus* (western parts of USA) *Ixodes ricinus* (Europe, CIS) *Ixodes persulcatus* (Asia) Transmission also by flies and flying insects[8]. Passage of organisms through the placenta (gestational Lyme borreliosis)[9]	Lyme disease, lyme borreliosis[4–6, 10–12] (previously an unrecognized arthropathy confined to regions around Lyme, Connecticut) Stage 1: localized infection (erythema chronicum migrans), usually within 30 days of exposure to the tick vector Stage 2: disseminated infection (involvement of CNS, heart and musculosceletal system), weeks or months after stage 1 Stage 3: persistent infection (arthritis, tertiary neuroborreliosis), weeks to years after stage 2 *Remarks.* The organism is generally sensitive to penicillins, tetracyclines and erythromycin, but the relationship between *in vitro* antibiotic susceptibility and clinical activity is not well established[5, 13, 14]
7	**Borrelia recurrentis** (LEBERT) BERGEY et al. *Spirochaeta recurrentis* *Spiroschaudinnia recurrentis*	GRAM-negative spirochete, 0.3 to 0.6 µm wide and 8–18 µm long, with 3–8 coils. Good staining with diluted carbol fuchsine, gentian violet or GIEMSA[15]. Culture possible in rabbit serum with exclusion of O_2 (for production of antigen)	Host: man. Transmission by lice (*Pediculus humanus*) via conjunctival sac and skin lesions	Relapsing fever[16], worldwide. Incubation period 2–10 days *Remark.* For treatment, a tetracycline – with benzylpenicillin as an alternative – has been recommended[17]
8	**Borrelia hispanica** (DE BUEN) STEINHAUS *Spirochaeta hispanica*	Morphologically similar to *B. recurrentis*	Host: rodents, man. Transmission by ticks (*Ornithodoros marocanus*), not lice	Relapsing fever in Spain, Portugal and northwest Africa
9	Other *Borrelia* species: see table below			

[1] BARBOUR et al., *Yale J. Biol. Med.*, **57**, 521 (1984).
[2] BARBOUR, A. G., *Clin. Microbiol. Rev.*, **1**, 399 (1988).
[3] MAGNARELLI et al., *J. Amer. med. Ass.*, **259**, 1147 (1988); MAGNARELLI, L. A., *J. Amer. med. Ass.*, **262**, 3464 (1989).
[4] DATTWYLER and LUFT, *Rheum. Dis. Clin. N. Amer.*, **15**, 727 (1989).
[5] STEERE et al., *Ann. intern. Med.*, **107**, 725 (1987); STEERE, A. C., *New Engl. J. Med.*, **321**, 586 (1989).
[6] HERZER et al., *Klin. Wschr.*, **64**, 206 (1986).
[7] BURGDORFER, W., *Rheum. Dis. Clin. N. Amer.*, **15**, 775 (1989).
[8] PACHNER, A. R., *Trends Neurosci.*, **12**, 177 (1989).
[9] MACDONALD, A. B., *Rheum. Dis. Clin. N. Amer.*, **15**, 657 (1989).
[10] MALAWISTA and STEERE, *Advanc. intern. Med.*, **31**, 147 (1986).
[11] SHAPIRO, E. D., *Curr. Opin. infect. Dis.*, **3**, 638 (1990).
[12] SIGAL, L. H., *Amer. J. Med.*, **88**, 577 (1990).
[13] *Med. Lett. Drug. Ther.*, **31**, No. 794 (1989).
[14] LUFT and DATTWYLER, *Rheum. Dis. Clin. N. Amer.*, **15**, 747 (1989).
[15] SWAIN, R. H. A., in MACKIE and MCCARTNEY (Eds.), *Medical Microbiology*, Churchill Livingstone, Edinburgh, 1978, page 393.
[16] HORTON and BLASER, *Arch. intern. Med.*, **145**, 871 (1985).
[17] *Med. Lett. Drug. Ther.*, **32**, No. 817 (1990).

Borrelia *species associated with human disease*[1]

Borrelia spp.	Disease	Arthropod vector	Geographic distribution of disease
B. hermsii	New World tick-borne relapsing fever	*Ornithodoros hermsi*	Western United States and Canada
B. turicatae	New World tick-borne relapsing fever	*Ornithodoros turicatae*	Southwestern United States and Mexico
B. parkeri	New World tick-borne relapsing fever	*Ornithodoros parkeri*	Western United States and Baja California
B. mazzottii	New World tick-borne relapsing fever	*Ornithodoros talaje*	Mexico and Central America
B. venezuelensis	New World tick-borne relapsing fever	*Ornithodoros rudis*	Central America and northern South America
B. duttonii	Old World tick-borne relapsing fever	*Ornithodoros moubata*	Sub-Saharan Africa
B. crocidurae	Old World tick-borne relapsing fever	*Ornithodoros erraticus*	North Africa, East Africa, Near East, Middle East, and southeast Europe
B. persica	Old World tick-borne relapsing fever	*Ornithodoros tholozani*	Middle East, Greece and Central Asia
B. hispanica	Old World tick-borne relapsing fever	*Ornithodoros marocanus*	Iberian peninsula and northwest Africa
B. latyschewii	Old World tick-borne relapsing fever	*Ornithodoros tartakowskyi*	Iran, Afghanistan, south-central CIS, Iraq and southwestern CIS
B. caucasica	Old World tick-borne relapsing fever	*Ornithodoros asperus*	Iraq and southwestern CIS
B. recurrentis	Louse-borne relapsing fever	*Pediculus humanus*	Worldwide
B. burgdorferi	Lyme disease	*Ixodes dammini*	Eastern United States
		Ixodes ricinus	Europe, western CIS
		Ixodes pacificus	Western United States

Reference [1] BARBOUR and HAYES, *Microbiol. Rev.*, **50**, 381 (1986).

No.	Bacterium *Synonyms* Common names	Characteristics	Habitat Host Transmission	Associated disease
10	**Leptospira interrogans** (STIMSON) WENYON *Spirochaeta interrogans*	Filaments, 6 to over 12 µm long, 0.1 µm wide, tightly coiled, often with hook-like ends. Very motile. Aerobic. Oxidase-positive. Best isolated in the acute stage. Examination of blood using liquid STUART medium or semisolid FLETCHER medium, both of which contain rabbit serum, or EMJH medium which contains albumin and fatty acid in lieu of serum[1]. All cultures are incubated at room temperature or 30°C in the dark for up to 6 weeks[2]. Animal testing may be required	Kidneys and urine of rodents (mainly rats and mice), pigs, cattle, horses and other animals	Anicteric leptospirosis[3,4]: common milder form (fever, headache, myalgia, malaise, seldom vascular collapse) Icteric leptospirosis (WEIL's disease)[3,4]: severe form (jaundice, renal failure, hemorrhage, vascular collapse, disturbance of consciousness) Incubation period 2–26 (average 10) days[5] *Remark*. Intravenous benzylpenicillin or ampicillin has been advocated for the treatment of severe forms of WEIL's disease[6] See also text below
11	**Leptospira biflexa** (WOLBACH and BINGER) NOGUCHI *Spirochaeta biflexa*	Morphologically similar to *L. interrogans*. Laboratory animals not susceptible to infection. Can be cultured at low temperature	Commonly found in natural fresh water, tap water, occasionally in seawater and in animals	No significance in man
12	**Spirillum minus** CARTER *Spirillum minor*	Corkscrew-like rods with 2 to 6 turns, 3–5 µm long, ~0.2 µm wide. Highly motile, with one or more flagella at each pole. GIEMSA or WRIGHT's staining. Demonstration by dark-field microscopy	Carriers: rats, mice, squirrels, cats, dogs, ferrets and weasels. Transmission through bite of these animals	Pathogen of one of the two forms of rat-bite fever[7]. Synonym: sodoku. Worldwide distribution, predominance in the Far East (Japan). Incubation period ca. 2 weeks (rarely up to 2 months). Primary lesion at site of bite, with characteristic dark-red skin eruption; feverish spells of 1–2 days' duration at irregular intervals (3–10 days). Endocarditis. For the other form of rat-bite fever, see *Streptobacillus moniliformis (No. 106)*

[1] ALEXANDER, A. D., in BRAUDE et al. (Eds.), *Infectious Diseases and Medical Microbiology*, 2nd ed., Saunders, Philadelphia, 1986, page 381.
[2] BARON and FINEGOLD (Eds.), *Bailey & Scott's Diagnostic Microbiology*, 8th ed., Mosby, St. Louis, 1990, page 449.
[3] World Health Organization, *Wkly epidem. Rec.*, **60**, 248 (1985).
[4] FARRAR, W. E., in MANDELL et al. (Eds.), *Principles and Practice of Infectious Diseases*, 3rd ed., Churchill Livingstone, New York, 1990, page 1813.
[5] SANFORD, J. P., *New Engl. J. Med.*, **310**, 524 (1984).
[6] WATT et al., *Lancet*, **1**, 433 (1988).
[7] WASHBURN, R. G., in MANDELL et al. (Eds.), *Principles and Practice of Infectious Diseases*, 3rd ed., Churchill Livingstone, New York, 1990, page 1827.

Leptospirosis

Two large groups of organisms are now distinguished within the genus *Leptospira*: the 'pathogenic leptospira' (*Leptospira interrogans*) and the 'apathogenic saprophytic leptospira' (*Leptospira biflexa*). Both groups can be further differentiated on the basis of their antigenic structures. The pathogenic leptospira can be subdivided into 19 different serogroups with about 180 serovars. The apathogenic leptospira can be divided into 38 serogroups with 65 serovars. The serovars found most commonly in human infection include *canicola, icterohaemorragiae, pomona, autumnalis, grippotyphosa, hebdomadis, australis, hardjo*[1].

The various *Leptospira* serovars were formerly associated with specific clinical pictures. It has now become evident that no clinical syndrome is exclusively attributable to a specific serovar and that no serovar invariably causes the same pattern of illness[2]. The term 'WEIL's disease' is a designation for severe leptospirosis, the lethality of which has dropped in recent years from between 25% and 40% to 5% or less[2].

References

[1] World Health Organization, *Wkly epidem. Rec.*, **60**, 237 (1985); FARRAR, W. E., in MANDELL et al. (Eds.), *Principles and Practice of Infectious Diseases*, 3rd ed., Churchill Livingstone, New York, 1990, page 1813.
[2] EDWARDS, G. A., in BRAUDE et al. (Eds.), *Infectious Diseases and Medical Microbiology*, 2nd ed., Saunders, Philadelphia, 1986, page 1543.

No.	Bacterium *Synonyms* Common names	Characteristics	Habitat Host Transmission	Associated disease
13	**Campylobacter fetus** subsp. **fetus** VÉRON and CHATELAIN *Vibrio fetus* var. *intestinalis* *Vibrio fetus-ovis* *Campylobacter fetus* subsp. *intestinalis*	GRAM-negative, slender, comma- and S-shaped rods, 0.2–0.3 µm wide, 1.5–5 µm long. A specific surface protein of the capsule leads to impaired C3b-binding[1]. Motile, with 1 flagellum at one or both poles. Grows at 25 °C, but usually not at 42 °C. For differentiation, see table below	Source of infection: gastrointestinal tract, blood and bile of infected sheep and cattle. Transmitted orally	Pathogen of septicemia (without splenomegaly), meningitis, meningoencephalitis, thrombophlebitis, septic arthritis, enteritis[2,3] *Remark*. Treatment for most infections with gentamicin[3]
14	**Campylobacter jejuni** (JONES et al.) VÉRON and CHATELAIN *Vibrio jejuni* *Vibrio hepaticus* *Campylobacter fetus* subsp. *jejuni*	GRAM-negative, small, comma- and S-shaped, tightly coiled rods. Motile, with 1 flagellum at one or both poles. Grows on special culture media (SKIRROW, BUTZLER) at 42 °C, with 5–10% O_2 and 3–10% CO_2. No enterotoxin yet found, although the organism appears to have invasive capacity. For differentiation, see table below	Source of infection: gastrointestinal tract of domestic and wild animals, especially birds (poultry)[4]. Surface water polluted with fecal material, contaminated drinking water[5] and milk (defective pasteurization)[4]. Origin of *C. jejuni* infections similar to those of genus *Salmonella*; unlike salmonellae, however, *C. jejuni* organisms do not multiply in foodstuffs	Worldwide important pathogen for enteritis, especially in children and young adults[2,6–9,14]. (In England and Wales, more than 32000 cases were reported in 1989[4].) Incubation period 1–7 days, in the majority of cases 2–4 days. After 2–3 days, symptoms (diarrhea and abdominal pain) normally abate. Some patients develop acute colitis requiring treatment. Rare complications are septicemia, meningitis[9] and septic arthritis[10] *Remarks*. Resistance to antimicrobial drugs may be a problem and susceptibility tests should be performed[11]. Usually ciprofloxazin or erythromycin are effective[5,11]
15	Other *Campylobacter* species of clinical importance:			
	Campylobacter laridis	See table below		Diarrhea[12,15]
	Campylobacter upsaliensis	See table below		Diarrhea[13,15]
	Campylobacter coli	See table below		Diarrhea[4,14,15]
	Campylobacter hyointestinalis			Diarrhea[15]
	Campylobacter cinaedi			Diarrhea[15]
	Campylobacter fennelliae			Diarrhea[15]

[1] BLASER et al., *J. clin. Invest.*, **81**, 1434 (1988).
[2] COVER and BLASER, *Ann. Rev. Med.*, **40**, 269 (1989).
[3] MORRISON et al., *Rev. infect. Dis.*, **12**, 387 (1990).
[4] SKIRROW, M. B., *Lancet*, **336**, 921 (1990).
[5] MENTZING, L. O., *Lancet*, **2**, 352 (1981); PALMER et al., *Lancet*, **1**, 287 (1983).
[6] BLASER and RELLER, *New Engl. J. Med.*, **305**, 1444 (1981).
[7] Editorial, *Lancet*, **2**, 1437 (1982).
[8] LEVIN and GOODMAN, *J. Amer. med. Ass.*, **253**, 1303 (1985).
[9] RUEF et al., *Schweiz. med. Wschr.*, **118**, 302 (1988).
[10] EBRIGHT and RYAN, *Amer. J. Med.*, **76**, 321 (1984).
[11] *Med. Lett. Drug. Ther.*, **32**, No. 817 (1990).
[12] BROCZYK et al., *Lancet*, **1**, 164 (1987).
[13] GOOSSENS et al., *Lancet*, **335**, 584 (1990).
[14] BHADRA et al., *J. Infect.*, **24**, 55 (1992).
[15] BLASER, M. J., in MANDELL et al. (Eds.), *Principles and Practice of Infectious Diseases*, 3rd ed., Churchill Livingstone, New York, 1990, page 1649.

Differential characteristics of several species of the genus Campylobacter[1,2]

	C. jejuni	*C. coli*	*C. laridis*	*C. fetus* subsp. *fetus*	*C. upsaliensis*	'*C. pylori*'*
Clinical manifestation	Enteric, extraintestinal	Enteric, extraintestinal	Enteric, extraintestinal	Extraintestinal, seldom enteric	Enteric	Gastric
Catalase activity	+	+	+	+	– (or weak)	+
Urease activity	–	–	–	–	–	+
Oxidase activity	+	+	+	+	+	+
Nitrite reduction	+	+	+	+	+	–
Hippurate hydrolysis	+◊	–	–	–	–	–
C-19 fatty-acid reduction	+	+	–	–	–	+
Growth at 25 °C	–	–	–	+	–	–
Growth at 37 °C	+	+	+	+	+	+
Growth at 42 °C	+	+	+	Variable	+§	Variable

* *Campylobacter pylori* has been renamed *Helicobacter pylori* [*Int. J. system. Bact.*, **39**, 397 (1989)]. See *No. 117b*.
◊ 5–10% of *Campylobacter jejuni* strains are hippurate-negative.
§ Occasional isolates fail to grow at 42 °C.

References

[1] BLASER, M. J., in MANDELL et al. (Eds.), *Principles and Practice of Infectious Diseases*, 3rd ed., Churchill Livingstone, New York, 1990, page 1649.
[2] SMIBERT, R. M., in KRIEG and HOLT (Eds.), *Bergey's Manual of Systematic Bacteriology*, Volume 1, Williams & Wilkins, Baltimore, 1984, page 111.

No.	**Bacterium** *Synonyms* Common names	Characteristics	Habitat Host Transmission	Associated disease
16	**Pseudomonas aeruginosa** (Schroeter) Migula *Bacterium aeruginosum* Blue pus organism	Gram-negative, straight or curved rods, 0.5–0.7 µm wide, 1.5–3.0 µm long. Motile, with 1 polar flagellum. Occur singly, in pairs or in short chains. Optimal growth at 37 °C, still possible at 42 °C. Aerobic. Oxidase-positive. A blue (pyocyanin) and a yellowish-green (fluorescein) dye are produced in cultures (which have a sweetish smell). β-Hemolysis on blood agar. Some strains produce large amounts of extracellular polysaccharides. These mucous strains are isolated in patients with cystic fibrosis, but rarely in children with otitis media. Phage-, pyocyanin- and serotyping possible; 17 serovars and 105 pyocyanin types are known. Produces many factors that may contribute to its virulence (e.g. endotoxin, exotoxin A, exoenzyme S[1,2])	Intestinal tract (feces), water, sewage, skin, air, soil. Ubiquitous saprophyte of increasing importance in hospital-acquired infections: eyedrops, contaminated medication, bottles containing soap solutions, fluid for cleaning of tracheal cannulas, ready-prepared disinfectant solutions, etc.; may remain viable for a considerable time in corked bottles of distilled water, in respirators and humidifiers. Can be introduced to hospitals via fruit and vegetables. Transmission from patient to patient possible	One of the most common and problematic among opportunistic pathogens. Infections occur mainly in critical care settings, immunocompromised patients and patients with cystic fibrosis[3,4]. Nosocomial infections predominate (see Table 4 on page 27). Endocarditis, respiratory tract infections, septicemia (high mortality[5,6]); infections of the central nervous system, urinary tract, gastrointestinal tract (infants), bone and joints; otitis (children, swimmers, divers); dangerous complication of eye injuries *Remarks*. Resistance to antimicrobial drugs may be a problem[7]. The use of an appropriate combination therapy is important[8]. Several types of vaccines are being tested[9]
17	**Pseudomonas fluorescens** (Trevisan) Migula *Bacillus fluorescens*	Morphologically similar to *P. aeruginosa*. No formation of pyocyanin; formation of fluorescein only. Aerobic. Oxidase-positive. Optimal growth at 25 to 30 °C; no growth at 42 °C, but possible at 4 °C	Similar to *P. aeruginosa*. Contaminated blood supplies[10]	Opportunistic pathogen. Infections of respiratory and urogenital tract, septicemia, abscesses[10,11]. Nosocomial infections predominate
18	**Pseudomonas mallei** (Zopf) Redfearn et al. *Bacillus mallei* Glanders bacillus	Gram-negative, slightly curved or straight rods, 0.5 µm wide, 1.4–4.0 µm long, with rounded ends. Occur singly, in end-to-end pairs, in parallel bundles or in agglomerations like Chinese characters. Sometimes filamentous in culture. Nonmotile. Irregular staining, often bipolar. Aerobic; practically no anaerobic growth. Oxidase-positive; optimal temperature 37 °C, growth at 41 °C, not at 4 °C	Parasite in equines (horses, donkeys), less commonly in goats, cats and dogs. Infection in man mainly via skin lesions or nasal mucosa. Laboratory infections are of great concern: cultures of *P. mallei* and *P. pseudomallei* must be handled with extreme care; probably the most dangerous organisms studied in laboratories	Glanders[11]. Incubation period: 1 to 5 days. Fever 40 °C, rigor, nodule formation in muscles, metastases in inner organs, pneumonia. Death after 2–3 weeks. Chronic course lasts for years. Now practically eradicated in western, central and northern Europe as a result of systematic extermination of all infected (mallein-positive) domestic animals
19	**Pseudomonas pseudomallei** (Whitmore) Haynes Whitmore bacillus	Gram-negative, short rods. Motile, with 1–4 flagella at one or both poles. Bipolar staining in fresh cultures is common. Aerobic. Oxidase-positive. Growth at ~37 °C in brain–heart infusion broth, subcultured onto horse blood agar[12]	Natural parasite of rodents. Isolated from blood or lesions in man, also from water. Normal soil organism. Rats likely to be the most frequent source of infection for man. Foodstuffs contaminated by rat droppings. Laboratory infections are a particular concern[13]	Glanders-like infections (melioidosis) in man and animals, almost exclusively in Southeast Asia[11,12,14–16]. Short incubation period. Acute, subacute or chronic septic infection involving also the pleura and lungs, marked by multiple abscesses. Mortality is high in the acute fulminating septicemic form *Remarks*. Resistance to antimicrobial drugs may be a problem; susceptibility tests should be performed[7,17]. The drug of choice may become ceftazidime[12,18]

1 Wick et al., *Ann. Rev. Microbiol.*, **44**, 335 (1990).
2 Iglewski, B.H., in Baron, S. (Ed.), *Medical Microbiology*, 2nd ed., Addison-Wesley, Menlo Park, CA, 1986, page 507.
3 Gould and Wise, *Lancet*, **2**, 1224 (1985).
4 Pollack, M., in Mandell et al. (Eds), *Principles and Practice of Infectious Diseases*, 3rd ed., Churchill Livingstone, New York, 1990, page 1673.
5 Bisbe et al., *Rev. infect. Dis.*, **10**, 629 (1988); Mallolas et al., *Rev. infect. Dis.*, **12**, 718 (1990).
6 Gallagher and Watanakunakorn, *Rev. infect. Dis.*, **11**, 846 (1989).
7 *Med. Lett. Drug. Ther.*, **32**, No. 817 (1990).
8 Hilf et al., *Amer. J. Med.*, **87**, 540 (1989).
9 Pennington, J. E., *Europ. J. clin. Microbiol. infect. Dis.*, **9**, 377 (1990).
10 Khabbaz et al., *Amer. J. Med.*, **76**, 62 (1984).
11 Sanford, J.P., in Mandell et al. (Eds.), *Principles and Practice of Infectious Diseases*, 3rd ed., Churchill Livingstone, New York, 1990, page 1692.
12 White et al., *Lancet*, **2**, 697 (1989).
13 Schlech et al., *New Engl. J. Med.*, **305**, 1133 (1981).
14 Yap et al., *Lancet*, **336**, 376 (1990).
15 Morrison et al., *Amer. J. Med.*, **84**, 965 (1988).
16 Thurnheer et al., *Schweiz. med. Wschr.*, **118**, 558 (1988).
17 Koponen et al., *Arch. intern. Med.*, **151**, 605 (1991).
18 Lam et al., *Lancet*, **2**, 1040 (1989).

No.	**Bacterium** *Synonyms* Common names	Characteristics	Habitat Host Transmission	Associated disease
20	**Pseudomonas cepacia** (ex BURKHOLDER) PALLERONI and HOLMES	GRAM-positive rods, 0.8–1.0 µm wide, 1.6–3.2 µm long. Motile, with 1 or more flagella. Aerobic. Oxidase-positive. Optimal growth at ~30–33 °C. Growth on MACCONKEY's agar or on *Salmonella–Shigella* agar	Mainly found in plants (onions), also in sewage and water supplies, as well as in contaminated hospital solutions and disinfectants[1,2]	Opportunistic pathogen. Infections of respiratory tract (patients with cystic fibrosis), septicemia, endocarditis, wound infections[3,4]. Nosocomial infections predominate
21	Other *Pseudomonas* species of clinical importance: **Pseudomonas stutzeri** **Pseudomonas paucimobilis**			 Nosocomial infections[5] Nosocomial infections[6]
22	**Xanthomonas maltophilia** (HUGH and RYSCHENKOW) HUGH *Pseudomonas maltophilia*	GRAM-negative, straight or curved rods, 0.5 µm wide, 1.5 µm long. Occur singly or in pairs. Motile, with polar multitrichous flagella. Aerobic. Optimal growth at 35 °C	Intestinal tract (feces), water, soil, sewage, milk and frozen foods	Opportunistic pathogen. Infections of respiratory tract (patients with cystic fibrosis), septicemia, endocarditis, wound infections[3,7,8]. Nosocomial infections predominate
23	**Agrobacterium radiobacter** (BEIJERINCK and VAN DELDEN) CONN *Bacillus radiobacter*	GRAM-negative rods, 0.6–1.0 µm wide, 1.5–3.0 µm long. Occur singly or in pairs. Motile, with 1–6 peritrichous flagella. Aerobic	Soil and plant rhizosphere	Sporadic cases of endocarditis, urinary tract infections, septicemia, peritonitis[9]
24	**Legionella pneumophila** BRENNER et al.	GRAM-negative rods, 0.3–0.9 µm wide and 2–20 µm long or longer. Motile. Not acid-fast. Noncapsulated. Aerobic. Gelatine can be dissolved. Urease-negative. Cultured in buffered charcoal–yeast extract agar. Optimal temperature: 36 °C. Optimal pH: 6.8–7.0. 14 serogroups (mainly groups 1, 4 and 6 implicated in human infection)[10]. Diagnosis by culture, by the direct fluorescence antibody (DFA) test[11], by detection of the urinary antigen[12,13] or by use of a DNA probe[14]	Stagnant water, hot water systems[15,16], showers, cooling towers of air conditioning[17]. Droplet infection. Contact infection from person to person very rare[18]. *Legionella* multiplies in amebas, and amebas in water could act as a reservoir of virulent bacteria[19,20]	Usually community- or hospital-acquired infections[10,21,22]: – Legionnaire's disease with pneumonia (poor prognosis in immunocompromised patients, often complication of organ transplantations[23]); incubation period 2–10 days – Nonpneumonic legionellosis (Pontiac fever), an acute febrile condition *Remark*. For treatment, erythromycin without or with rifampin is recommended[21,24]
25	Other *Legionella* species of clinical importance[25,26]: **Legionella bozemanii** **Legionella micdadei** (Pittsburgh pneumonia agent) **Legionella dumoffii** **Legionella gormanii** **Legionella longbeachae** **Legionella feeleii** **Legionella anisa**			 Pneumonia[27] Pneumonia[28], Pontiac-fever-like illness[29] Pneumonia Pneumonia Pneumonia Pontiac fever[30] Pontiac fever[31]

[1] SOBEL et al., *Amer. J. Med.*, **73**, 183 (1982); PALLENT et al., *J. Hosp. Infect.*, **4**, 9 (1983).
[2] HENDERSON et al., *Amer. J. Med.*, **84**, 75 (1984).
[3] SANFORD, J.P., in MANDELL et al. (Eds.), *Principles and Practice of Infectious Diseases*, 3rd ed., Churchill Livingstone, New York, 1990, page 1692.
[4] ISLES et al., *J. Pediat.*, **104**, 206 (1984); TABLAN et al., *J. Pediat.*, **107**, 382 (1985).
[5] GOETZ et al., *Arch. intern. Med.*, **143**, 1909 (1983); ROSENBERG et al., *J. roy. Soc. Med.*, **80**, 457 (1987).
[6] CRANE et al., *J. Amer. med. Ass.*, **246**, 985 (1981); PHILLIPS et al., *Europ. J. clin. Microbiol. infect. Dis.*, **9**, 630 (1990).
[7] KHARDORI et al., *Rev. infect. Dis.*, **12**, 997 (1990).
[8] ELTING and BODEY, *Medicine (Baltimore)*, **69**, 296 (1990).
[9] MCGOWAN and DEL RIO, in MANDELL et al. (Eds.), *Principles and Practice of Infectious Diseases*, 3rd ed., Churchill Livingstone, New York, 1990, page 1782.
[10] YU, V.L., in MANDELL et al. (Eds.), *Principles and Practice of Infectious Diseases*, 3rd ed., Churchill Livingstone, New York, 1990, page 1764.
[11] ZURAVLEFF et al., *J. Amer. med. Ass.*, **250**, 1981 (1983).
[12] SATHAPATAYAVONGS et al., *Amer. J. Med.*, **72**, 576 (1982).
[13] FEHRENBACH et al., *Israel J. med. Sci.*, **22**, 706 (1986).
[14] Editorial, *Lancet*, **2**, 897 (1989).
[15] FISHER-HOCH et al., *Lancet*, **1**, 1073 (1982).
[16] WADOWSKY et al., *Appl. environ. Microbiol.*, **43**, 1104 (1982).
[17] KURTZ et al., *J. Hyg. (Camb.)*, **88**, 369 (1982); GARBE et al., *J. Amer. med. Ass.*, **254**, 521 (1985).
[18] ZIMMERMAN, L., *New Engl. J. Med.*, **301**, 1004 (1979).
[19] VANDENESCH et al., *Zbl. Bakt.*, **272**, 265 (1990).
[20] BREIMAN et al., *J. Amer. med. Ass.*, **263**, 2924 (1990).
[21] FINEGOLD, S. M., *New Engl. J. Med.*, **318**, 571 (1988).
[22] WINN, W. C., *Clin. Microbiol. Rev.*, **1**, 60 (1988).
[23] HORBACH and FEHRENBACH, *Infection*, **18**, 361 (1990).
[24] *Med. Lett. Drug. Ther.*, **32**, No. 817 (1990).
[25] FANG and YU, in MANDELL et al. (Eds.), *Principles and Practice of Infectious Diseases*, 3rd ed., Churchill Livingstone, New York, 1990, page 1774.
[26] FANG et al., *Medicine (Baltimore)*, **68**, 116 (1989).
[27] SOBEL et al., *J. Amer. med. Ass.*, **250**, 383 (1983); PARRY et al., *Ann. intern. Med.*, **103**, 205 (1985); SWIMBURN et al., *Lancet*, **1**, 472 (1988); JAEGER et al., *Mayo Cli. Proc.*, **63**, 72 (1988).
[28] KNUDSEN et al., *Lancet*, **1**, 708 (1983); MUDER et al., *Medicine (Baltimore)*, **62**, 120 (1983); SCHWEBKE et al., *Rev. infect. Dis.*, **12**, 824 (1990).
[29] WING et al., *Amer. J. Med.*, **71**, 836 (1981); GOBBO et al., *Lancet*, **2**, 969 (1986); GOLDBERG et al., *Lancet*, **1**, 316 (1989).
[30] HERWALDT et al., *Ann. intern. Med.*, **100**, 333 (1984).
[31] FENSTERSHEIB et al., *Lancet*, **336**, 35 (1990).

No.	Bacterium *Synonyms* Common names	Characteristics	Habitat Host Transmission	Associated disease
26	**Neisseria gonorrhoeae** (ZOPF) TREVISAN *Merismopedia gonorrhoeae* Gonococcus	GRAM-negative cocci, 0.6–1.0 µm in diameter, occurring singly, but more often in pairs with adjacent sides flattened. Intra- and extracellular location; in fresh cases, mainly intracellular and in clumps; in subacute and chronic cases, mainly extracellular. Affinity for methylene blue. Aerobic to microaerophilic. No growth on ordinary media; requires blood or ascites fluid as well as increased CO_2 pressure for culture. Oxidase- and catalase-positive. For differentiation, see table on page 20	Mucosa of urethra and vagina; conjunctiva (neonates). Transmission usually through sexual intercourse, rarely through contact with infected articles. Perinatal transmission	Gonorrhea. Localized infections: urethritis, prostatitis, epididymitis, bartholinitis, adnexitis, cervicitis, salpingitis, endometritis; conjunctivitis. Disseminated infections: septic arthritis, polyarthritis–dermatitis syndrome, endocarditis, meningitis. Pregnancy associated disease: septic abortion, ophthalmia neonatorum, post-partum endometritis. See also text below
27	**Neisseria meningitidis** (ALBRECHT and GHON) MURRAY *Micrococcus meningitidis*	GRAM-negative cocci, 0.6–1.0 µm in diameter, occurring in pairs with adjacent sides flattened, usually intracellular. Often shows pleomorphism (tetrads) and poor staining. Aerobic to microaerophilic. Media enriched with serum, blood or ascites fluid, required for culture. For differentiation, see table on page 20	Nasopharynx of man	Meningoencephalitis: abrupt onset with headache, meningeal signs and fever Meningococcemia with or without meningitis: thrombosis of small vessels with multiorgan involvement is characteristic. Disseminated intravascular coagulation – including destruction of the adrenal glands – with shock possible (WATERHOUSE–FRIDERICHSEN syndrome) Other syndromes are e.g. pneumonia, arthritis, urethritis. See also text on next page
28	Other *Neisseria* species of clinical importance: **Neisseria lactamica** **Neisseria sicca** **Neisseria subflava** **Neisseria flavescens** **Neisseria mucosa**[2] **Neisseria cinerea**	Morphologically similar to *N. meningitidis*	Saprophytes of mucous membranes of pharynx and upper respiratory tract	Occasionally secondary invaders, rarely primary pathogens of meningitis, pneumonia, septicemia[1]

[1] GRÖSCHEL, D. H., in MANDELL et al. (Eds.), *Principles and Practice of Infectious Diseases*, 3rd ed., Churchill Livingstone, New York, 1990, page 1632.

[2] STOTKA et al., *Rev. infect. Dis.*, **13**, 837 (1991).

Gonorrhea

Epidemiological data on the incidence of gonorrhea are available mainly for industrialized countries[1–4]. In the USA and in Sweden, for example, epidemics emerged in the 1970s (Fig. 1) which have been attributed to changing sexual behavior and an increasing high-risk group of sexually active 15–24 year old men and women[6].

The incidence of gonococcal ophthalmia neonatorum in developing countries in Africa is estimated to be 5–50 cases per 1000 live births, in industrialized countries 0.1–0.6 cases per 1000 live births[7].

Fig. 1 *Incidence of reported gonorrhea in the USA and Sweden*[4,5]

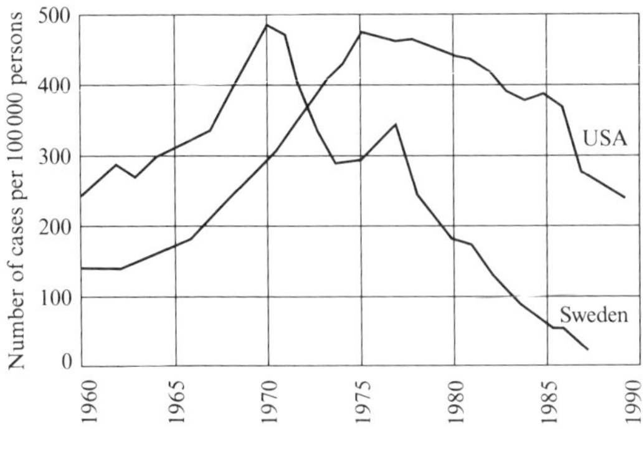

Incubation period. In men who develop urethral discharge, the incubation period is usually 2–5 days, it ranges from 1–10 days or longer[5,6]. It is difficult to determine a meaningful incubation period in women; those who become symptomatic probably do so within 10 days[5].

Diagnosis. Laboratory diagnosis of gonorrhea depends on identification of *Neisseria gonorrhoeae* at an infected site, either by GRAM-stained smear or by culture on gonococcal selective media[5–8]. The diagnostic sensitivity is given in Table 1. Serologic tests and DNA probes for identification of *N. gonorrhoeae* have been developed[8].

Resistance. After the first decade of penicillin treatment for gonorrhea there has been an alarming increase of gonococcal resistance to antimicrobial drugs generated by different mechanisms[6]:

- Plasmid-mediated penicillin resistance due to penicillinase-producing *N. gonorrhoeae* (PPNG). PPNG resulted from the acquisition of a plasmid that carried genes for production of β-lactamase
- Plasmid-mediated, high-level tetracycline resistance. The tetracycline resistant *N. gonorrhoeae* (TRNG) strains arose from the insertion of a streptococcal tetracycline-resistance determinant into the conjugative gonococcal plasmid
- Chromosome-mediated resistance to penicillin, tetracycline, cephalosporin, and other antibiotics. The common molecular mechanism is reduced permeability of the outer cell membrane
- Spectinomycin resistance is caused by a single-step chromosomal mutation that alters the sensitivity of the gonococcal ribosome to spectinomycin, and is highly drug-specific

Penicillinase-producing *N. gonorrhoeae* strains were first documented in 1975–1976 in western Africa, Southeast Asia, the USA

Table 1 *Sensitivity of* GRAM-*stained smear and culture in diagnosing gonorrhea*[6]

Source of specimen	Sensitivity: GRAM-stained smear (%)	Sensitivity: Culture (%)
Local infection		
Urethral discharge, men	98	98
Urethra, asymptomatic men	55–60	80–90
Vagina	Not recommended	50–85
Endocervix	30–60	85–95
Anal canal	Not recommended except for pus	70–85*
Conjunctiva	95	95
Pharynx	Not recommended	50–70*
Disseminated infection		
Blood	Not recommended	25–75
Joints	5–10	25–75
Lesions	5–10	2–5

* Single anorectal or pharyngeal cultures are of undetermined sensitivity, but are probably well below 90%.

Table 2 *Resistance in* N. gonorrhoeae *isolates in the USA (1988–1989)* *[6,9]

	Mean (% of total isolates)	Range (% of total isolates)
Plasmid-mediated		
Penicillinase-producing *N. gonorrhoeae* (PPNG)	7.4	1.2–31.7
Tetracycline-resistant *N. gonorrhoeae* (TRNG)	4.9	0–19.8
PPNG–TRNG	0.9	0–9.7
Chromosome-mediated		
Penicillin resistance	1	–
Tetracycline resistance	8.5	–
Penicillin + tetracycline resistance	2.6	–
Spectinomycin resistance	< 1	–

* Gonococcal Isolate Surveillance Project monitoring antimicrobial susceptibilities at 21 sexually transmitted disease clinics in 21 cities (9309 isolates from primarily black, heterosexual men, median age 25 years).

and western Europe; by 1980 PPNG accounted for up to 50% of gonococcal isolates in some developing countries[5]. Plasmid-mediated tetracycline-resistant strains, first documented in the USA in 1985, apparently have a worldwide distribution[5]. For the prevalence of gonococcal resistance in the USA, see Table 2.

Remarks. Resistance and anatomic site of infection has an impact on efficacy of treatment. A single intramuscular dose of ceftriaxone has been recommended for uncomplicated *N. gonorrhoeae* infections at all anatomic sites[7,10,11], cefixime is an effective oral single-dose alternative[11]. Ciprofloxacin, ofloxacin, spectinomycin, kanamycin, triamphenicol, trimethoprim-sulfamethoxazole may be effective alternatives depending on the prevalence of resistance[7,11]. For treatment of ophthalmia neonatorum, ceftriaxone or cefotaxime plus saline irrigation has been recommended[11].

References

1 ARAL and HOLMES, in HOLMES et al. (Eds.), *Sexually Transmitted Diseases*, 2nd ed., McGraw-Hill, New York, 1990, page 19.
2 WHO Expert Committee on Veneral Diseases and Treponematoses, *Wld Hlth. Org. techn. Rep. Ser.*, No. 736, 1986.
3 DE SCHRYVER and MEHEUS, *Bull. Wld Hlth Org.*, **68**, 639 (1990).
4 *Morb. Mort. wkly Rep.*, **39**, 53 (1990).
5 HANDSFIELD, H. H., in MANDELL et al. (Eds.), *Principles and Practice of Infectious Diseases*, 3rd ed., Churchill Livingstone, New York, 1990, page 1613.
6 JUDSON, F. N., *Med. Clin. N. Amer.*, **74**, 1353 (1990).
7 WHO Study Group on Management of Patients with Sexually Transmitted Diseases, *Wld Hlth Org. techn. Rep. Ser.*, No. 810 (1991).
8 KNAPP, J. S., *Clin. Microbiol. Rev.*, **1**, 415 (1988).
9 *Morb. Mort. wkly Rep.*, **39**, 284 (1990).
10 MORAN and ZENILMAN, *Rev. infect. Dis.*, **12**, Suppl. 6, S633 (1990).
11 *Med. Lett. Drug. Ther.*, **33**, No. 860 (1991).

Meningococcal disease

Neisseria meningitidis can be divided into at least 13 serovars: A, B, C, D, X, Y, Z, E, W-135, H, I, K, L[1]; the serovars A, B, C, Y and W-135 are those most commonly associated with meningococcal disease[2].

The disease is endemic worldwide. Epidemics occur in certain areas, most commonly caused by serovar A, less commonly by serovar C, and rarely by serovar B[3].

Areas with epidemic activity:

- Sahelian area of sub-Saharan Africa, in the so-called meningitis belt, from Mauritania in the West to Ethiopia in the East
- In 1988, epidemic disease spread from Sudan into Egypt and parts of the Middle East
- Saudi Arabia had a recent epidemic during the Haj in 1987 and this spread into some neighboring countries and possibly into sub-Saharan Africa
- Nepal and India
- In late 1989, epidemics in Kenya, Tanzania, Uganda, Malawi, and Mozambique
- Serogroup B epidemics recently in Brazil

The number of meningococcal infections appears to be on the decline in the USA (2727 cases reported in 1989 to the Centers for Disease Control, Atlanta[4]). In New York City, the incidence of meningococcal infections with pathogens of serovar W-135 has increased significantly. A distinct subclone of serovar B-15 has been associated with increased incidence of meningococcal disease in Southwest England[5].

It is most likely that the meningococci are transported via the blood from the nasopharynx to the meninges. Meningococcal meningitis occurs most frequently during the first 6 months of the year. Two-thirds of all cases occur in the first 5 years of life, and of these more than half in children under 1 year of age. In the 4- to 14-year age group, serovar C dominates. Most of the meningococcal carriers are over 21 years of age[6]. The lethality of meningococcal meningitis is lowest in young adults and higher in adults over 40 and in young children[7].

In 1990, commercial vaccines include a quatrivalent product containing polysaccharides of serovars A, C, Y and W-135; there is no vaccine available for prevention of serovar B disease[1].

Remark. For treatment, benzylpenicillin is still the drug of first choice, but a variety of other antibiotic drugs should be considered[1,8].

References

1 APICELLA, M. A., in MANDELL et al. (Eds.), *Principles and Practice of Infectious Diseases*, 3rd ed., Churchill Livingstone, New York, 1990, page 1600.
2 POOLMAN et al., *Lancet*, **2**, 555 (1986).
3 WOLFE, M. S., *Pediat. Clin. N. Amer.*, **37**, 757 (1990).
4 *Morb. Mort. wkly Rep.*, **38**, No. 54, 1 (1989).
5 MCGUINNES et al., *Lancet*, **337**, 514 (1991).
6 MORSE, S. A., in BRAUDE et al. (Eds.), *Infectious Diseases and Medical Microbiology*, 2nd ed., Saunders, Philadelphia, 1986, page 287.
7 TÄUBER and SANDE, *J. Amer. med. Ass.*, **251**, 1877 (1984).
8 *Med. Lett. Drug. Ther.*, **32**, No. 817 (1990).

No.	**Bacterium** *Synonyms* Common names	Characteristics	Habitat Host Transmission	Associated disease
29	**Moraxella (Moraxella) lacunata** (EYRE) BØVRE *Bacillus lacunatus* *Moraxella lacunata* *Moraxella liquefaciens* MORAX–AXENFELD bacillus	GRAM-negative, plump rods, mainly in pairs or short chains. Nonmotile. Growth usually only on media containing blood or serum. Aerobic. Oxidase- and catalase-positive. Biochemically inactive	Conjunctiva; sputum. In pharyngeal and nasal swabs. At present rarely isolated	Eye infections[1,2] (angular blepharoconjunctivitis)
30	Other *Moraxella (Moraxella)* of clinical importance: **Moraxella (Moraxella) nonliquefaciens** **Moraxella (Moraxella) atlantae** **Moraxella (Moraxella) osloensis**	See *Moraxella (Moraxella) lacunata*	Isolated from ear, nose, throat, eye	Rarely pathogenic. Eye infections[1,2]
31	**Moraxella (Branhamella) catarrhalis** (FROSCH and KOLLE) BØVRE *Micrococcus catarrhalis* *Moraxella catarrhalis* *Branhamella catarrhalis*	GRAM-negative cocci, 0.6–1.0 μm in diameter, occurring singly or in pairs. Nonmotile. Aerobic. In contrast to *N. meningitidis*, growth on ordinary media even at room temperature. For differentiation, see table below	Bronchial secretion and pharyngeal mucus	Long considered nonpathogenic. Since 1972, increasingly regarded as a true pathogen especially of pneumonia and other infections of the respiratory tract[3–8]. Laryngitis[3,4], sinusitis and otitis media in children[6,9], neonatal conjunctivitis[9]. Rarely septicemia[9,10] and meningitis[9] *Remarks*. Changes in drug resistance have been reported[10]. Many strains produce β-lactamase. Treatment with amoxicillin plus clavulanic acid has been suggested[11]
32	**Acinetobacter calcoaceticus** (BEIJERINCK) BAUMANN et al. *Acinetobacter anitratus* *Micrococcus calco-aceticus* *Acinetobacter lwoffi*	GRAM-negative, short rods, 0.9 to 1.6 μm wide, 1.5–2.5 μm long. Nonmotile. Bipolar staining. Often coccoid forms, in pairs or in chains of various length. Aerobic. Oxidase- and nitrate-negative; catalase-positive. For differentiation, see table below	Skin and feces of man, in dust and on utensils, also in water, soil and sewage	Usually nonpathogenic, but hospital- or community-acquired infections are reported[12–14]. Pneumonia, sepsis, endocarditis, brain and lung abscesses, meningitis, urinary tract infections

1 GRÖSCHEL, D. H., in MANDELL et al. (Eds.), *Principles and Practice of Infectious Diseases*, 3rd ed., Churchill Livingstone, New York, 1990, page 1632.
2 GRAHAM et al., *Rev. infect. Dis.*, **12**, 423 (1990).
3 Editorial, *Lancet*, **1**, 1056 (1982).
4 MCLEOD et al., *Brit. med. J.*, **287**, 1446, (1983).
5 LE FAOU and RIO, *Presse méd.*, **12**, 2035 (1983).
6 SIMON, C., *Tägl. Prax.*, **30**, 53 (1989).
7 WRIGHT et al., *Amer. J. Med.*, **88**, 5A, 2S (1990).
8 SARUBBI et al., *Amer. J. Med.*, **88**, 5A, 9S (1990).
9 MARCHANT, C. D., *Amer. J. Med.*, **88**, 5A, 15S (1990).
10 WALLACE and OLDFIELD, *Arch. intern. Med.*, **150**, 1332 (1990).
11 *Med. Lett. Drug. Ther.*, **32**, No. 817 (1990).
12 SMEGO, R. A., *Arch. intern. Med.*, **145**, 2174 (1985).
13 HARTSTEIN et al., *Amer. J. Med.*, **85**, 624 (1988).
14 ALLEN and HARTMAN, in MANDELL et al. (Eds.), *Principles and Practice of Infectious Diseases*, 3rd ed., Churchill Livingstone, New York, 1990, page 1696.

Differential characteristics of Neisseria, Moraxella, Acinetobacter *and* Veillonella *species*

	Neisseria gonorrhoeae	*Neisseria meningitidis*	*Neisseria flavescens*	*Moraxella (Branhamella) catarrhalis*	*Acetinobacter calcoaceticus*	*Veillonella* spp.
Anaerobic culture	–	–	–	–	–	+
Catalase activity	+	+	+	+	+	D
Oxidase activity	+	+	+	+	–	
Pigment formation	–	–	+	–	–	–
Growth at 22 °C	–	–	+	v	+	v
Growth on plain agar	–	–	+	+	+	+
Growth with serum or blood supplement	+	+	–	–	–	–
Acids production						
– from glucose	+	+	–	–	+	–
– from lactose	–	–	–	–	+	
– from maltose	–	+	–	–	d	
– from sucrose	–	–	–	–	–	–

\+ 85–100 % of strains are positive. – 85–100 % of strains are negative.
d 16–84 % of strains are positive. D Variable reactions.
v Different reactions in the various strains.

Reference

COWAN, S. T. (Ed.), *Cowan and Steel's Manual for Identification of Medical Bacteria*, 2nd ed., Cambridge University Press, London, 1974.

No.	**Bacterium** *Synonyms* Common names	Characteristics	Habitat Host Transmission	Associated disease
33	**Kingella kingae** HENRIKSEN and BØVRE *Moraxella kingii* *Moraxella kingae*	GRAM-negative rods, ~ 1.0 µm wide and 2.0–3.0 µm long, occurring in pairs or short chains. Nonmotile. Aerobic and facultatively anaerobic. Oxidase-positive, catalase-negative. Acid from glucose. Penicillin-sensitive. β-Hemolysis	Normally in the upper respiratory tract of man	Rare pathogen of bone and joint infections[1,2], septicemia[1,3], epiglottitis[4], endocarditis[1]
34	**Flavobacterium meningosepticum** KING	GRAM-negative rods. Nonmotile. Found in spinal fluid both within and outside the cells (similar to *Haemophilus influenzae*); in cultures mainly filiform and producing a beige or light-yellow pigment. Growth at 25–27 °C. Oxidase-positive. Aerobic, facultatively anaerobic	Widespread in nature: water, soil, humid areas. In hospitals, the organism can be found in water outlets, water baths, air-conditioning plants, ice-making machines, humidifiers[5]	Pathogen mainly causing neonatal meningitis and septicemia (poor prognosis). In adults, sporadic cases of septicemia, subacute endocarditis, pneumonia or meningitis[6,7]
35	**Alcaligenes faecalis** CASTELLANI and CHALMERS *Achromobacter arsenoxydans-tres* *Alcaligenes odorans* *Alcaligenes odorans* var. *viridans*	GRAM-negative, plump rods. Motile, with weakly developed peritrichous flagella. Aerobic. No acid or gas production on usual sugar media. Oxidase- and catalase-positive	Isolated from nematodes and insects in earth and water samples. Contaminant of hospital equipment and fluids[7,8]	Rare pathogen of urogenital tract infections, wounds, abscesses, pleuritis[7]
36	**Brucella melitensis** (HUGHES) MEYER and SHAW *Streptococcus melitensis*	GRAM-negative, short rods, 0.5 to 0.7 µm wide and 1.5 µm long, occurring singly, or in pairs, short chains or small groups. Nonmotile. Aerobic. Do not require increased CO_2 pressure for growth. Catalase-positive. Serum–dextrose agar, trypticase soy agar, tryptose agar, brucella agar are media recommended for primary isolation	Sheep, goats. High pathogenicity in man (cases can assume epidemic proportions). For transmission, see text below	Brucellosis (undulant fever) in man. Known as Malta or Mediterranean fever. See text below
37	**Brucella abortus** (SCHMIDT) MEYER and SHAW *Bacterium abortus* BANG's abortus bacillus	As for *B. melitensis*. Some biovars require CO_2 for growth	Cattle and other bovidae, dogs. Moderate pathogenicity in man. For transmission, see text below	Brucellosis (undulant fever) in man. Known as BANG's disease. See text below
38	**Brucella suis** HUDDLESON	As for *B. melitensis*	Pigs (biovar 1–3), reindeer (biovar 4), rodents (biovar 5). High pathogenicity in man. For transmission, see text below	Brucellosis (undulant fever) in man. See text below
38a	**Brucella canis** CARMICHAEL and BRUNNER	As for *B. melitensis*	Dogs. Low pathogenicity in man (clinical cases are rare)	Brucellosis (undulant fever) in man. See text below

1 GRAHAM et al., *Rev. infect. Dis.*, **12**, 423 (1990).
2 LEWIS and SETTAS, *Postgrad. med. J.*, **59**, 523 (1983).
3 SHANSON and GAZZARD, *Brit. med. J.*, **289**, 730 (1984).
4 KENNEDY and ROSEN, *Amer. J. Med.*, **85**, 701 (1988).
5 WEINSTEIN and YOUNG, in BENNETT and BRACHMAN (Eds.), *Hospital Infections*, Little, Brown, Boston, 1979, page 492.
6 UCHIHARA et al., *Amer. J. Med.*, **85**, 738 (1988); FUJITA et al., *Lancet*, **335**, 544 (1990).
7 MCGOWAN and DEL RIO, in MANDELL et al. (Eds.), *Principles and Practice of Infectious Diseases*, 3rd ed., Churchill Livingstone, New York, 1990, page 1782.
8 BARON and FINEGOLD (Eds.), *Bailey & Scott's Diagnostic Microbiology*, 8th ed., Mosby, St. Louis, 1990, page 402.

Brucellosis

Brucella organisms are strict parasites of animals in all parts of the world. Four species are responsible for infection in man[1–3]. Differential characteristics of these species and their biovars are given in the table on next page.

About 500 000 new cases are reported each year worldwide[3], but in most developed countries the incidence has decreased considerably because of eradication programs against the disease in animals (including milk pasteurization). The disease remains hyperendemic in Kuwait, Saudi Arabia, Iraq, Iran, Algeria, Tunisia, Morocco, Malta, Egypt, Greece, Spain, France, Italy, Mexico, and Peru and in parts of the CIS, China, and India[4]. In the USA, only 89 cases were reported 1991[5].

Man is infected through ingestion of fresh milk, cheese, and cream; through direct contact with infected animals (e.g. shepherds, farmers, and veterinarians); and through inhalation of infectious aerosols (e.g. workers in abattoirs and microbiology laboratories). Transmission via blood and sexual transmission of *B. melitensis* have been reported[6].

B. melitensis and *B. suis* often give rise to a more severe form of infection than does *B. abortus*; however, *B. abortus* infection can also be severe and life-threatening, especially when resistance is low owing to pre-existing disease or malnutrition[1]. The few reported cases of *B. canis* infection, mostly in laboratory workers, dog handlers, and dog owners, have been brief and uncomplicated.

Brucellosis usually presents as a febrile illness with lassitude and muscular pain. In the acute form, the incubation period may be as short as 1–3 weeks, although after long-standing exposure, as in occupational brucellosis, it usually cannot be determined[1]. The illness may be mild and self-limiting or severe and prolonged with

Differential characteristics of some species of the genus Brucella *and their biovars*[1]

	Biovar	Growth enhanced by CO_2	H_2S production	Growth on media containing: Thionine (20 µg/mL)	Growth on media containing: Basic fuchsine (20 µg/mL)	Agglutination with monospecific antisera: A	Agglutination with monospecific antisera: M	Agglutination with monospecific antisera: R
B. melitensis	1	−	−	+	+	−	+	−
	2	−	−	+	+	+	−	−
	3	−	−	+	+	+	+	−
B. abortus	1	(+)	+	−	+	+	−	−
	2	(+)	+	−	−	+	−	−
	3	(+)	+	+	+	+	−	−
	4	(+)	+	−	(+)	−	+	−
	5	−	−	+	+	−	+	−
	6	−	(+)	+	+	+	−	−
	7	−	(+)	+	+	+	+	−
	9	−	+	+	+	−	+	−
B. suis	1	−	+	+	(−)	+	−	−
	2	−	−	+	−	+	−	−
	3	−	−	+	+	+	−	−
	4	−	−	+	(−)	+	+	−
	5	−	−	+	−	−	+	−
B. canis		−	−	+	−	−	−	+

\+ All strains positive.
(+) Most strains positive.
− All strains negative.
(−) Most strains negative.

A Monospecific *B. abortus* antiserum.
M Monospecific *B. melitensis* antiserum.
R Anti-rough *Brucella* serum.

toxemia. In an illness of average severity, natural recovery usually occurs in 1–3 months, although lassitude may persist for very much longer. In prolonged illness, temperature recordings may show an undulating pattern, hence the epithet 'undulant fever'. The illness is labelled 'chronic' when it persists or recurs over a period of 6 months or more[1].

Localized infections have been reported in almost every organ, including bone, central nervous system, lung, testes, liver, spleen, gallbladder, and heart[7].

Diagnosis. This is established by a positive culture of *Brucella* (from blood, bone marrow, lymph glands, abscesses) or serologically, e.g. by positive agglutination and/or complement-fixation tests with standardized antigens[1]. Tests that specifically detect *Brucella* antibodies include radioimmunoassay and enzyme-linked immunosorbent assay[1,8].

Remarks. Vaccines for exposed persons have been tested in the CIS, China and France[1]. The standard therapy is a combination of a tetracycline with streptomycin[4,9]; an alternative is a combination of doxycycline with rifampin[1,4]. Since brucellosis can cause fetal death at any stage of pregnancy, treatment must not be withheld; the drug of choice is rifampin[1]. Localized brucellosis often requires surgery in addition to chemotherapy.

References

1 Joint FAO/WHO Expert Committee on Brucellosis, *Wld Hlth Org. Techn. Rep. Ser.*, No. 740 (1986).
2 SPINK, W. W., in BRAUDE et al. (Eds.), *Infectious Diseases and Medical Microbiology*, 2nd ed., Saunders, Philadelphia, 1986, page 1217.
3 MIKOLICH and BOYCE, in MANDELL et al. (Eds.), *Principles and Practice of Infectious Diseases*, 3rd ed., Churchill Livingstone, New York, 1990, page 1735.
4 HALL, W. H., *Rev. infect. Dis.*, **12**, 1060 (1990).
5 *Morb. Mort. wkly Rep.*, **40**, No. 52, 898 (1991).
6 VANDERCAM et al., *Europ. J. clin. Microbiol. infect. Dis.*, **9**, 303 (1990); RUBEN et al., *Lancet*, **337**, 14 (1991).
7 JACOBS et al., *Rev. infect. Dis.*, **12**, 740 (1990).
8 LULU et al., *Quart. J. Med.*, NS **66**, 39 (1988).
9 *Med. Lett. Drug. Ther.*, **32**, No. 817 (1990).

Bordetella

The genus Bordetella comprises 4 species: *B. pertussis*, *B. parapertussis*, *B. bronchoseptica* and *B. avium*. *B. pertussis* and *B. parapertussis* are pathogens of man; *B. bronchoseptica* is predominantly a pathogen of animals that rarely affects man[1]. *B. avium*, a pathogen of poultry, is not known to infect man.

Differential characteristics of *Bordetella* species pathogenic in man are given in Table 1. In the last decades research has focused on components of *B. pertussis* (the causative agent of pertussis) that induce protective immunity without adverse reactions (Table 2).

Pertussis

Pertussis is still a major respiratory disease in young children in developing countries[4]. In 1986, the World Health Organization estimated the total number of pertussis cases to be 60 million annually and that 0.5–1 million deaths due to pertussis occur every year[5].

In the USA, about 50% of pertussis cases occur in infants less than 1 year old[6]. However, pertussis can occur at any age; it has been reported that about 26% of adults with persistent cough were infected with *B. pertussis*[7]. The disease in adults is usually milder than that seen in children[15].

Pertussis is one of the most highly communicable diseases of man. It is transmitted by respiratory droplets from infected persons; attack rates in unimmunized young children may be higher than 90% in susceptible household contacts[1,3,6]. Attack rates, morbidity and mortality are higher in females than in males[1,5].

The average *incubation period* is 7–10 days (range 5–20 days)[1,8]. Clinical disease develops in 3 stages[1,6,8]:

- Catarrhal phase (1–2 weeks)
- Acute paroxysmal or spasmodic cough phase (1–4 weeks or longer)
- Convalescent stage (1–3 weeks)

No.	Bacterium *Synonyms* Common names	Characteristics	Habitat Host Transmission	Associated disease
39	**Bordetella pertussis** (BERGEY et al.) MORENO-LÓPEZ *Haemophilus pertussis* BORDET–GENGOU bacillus	GRAM-negative, very small coccoid rods, 0.2–0.5 µm wide and 0.5–1.0 µm long. Nonmotile. No growth on usual media at first isolation; needs a complex enriched medium. No growth on tyrosine agar. Aerobic. Produces toxins: the main toxin, the islet-activating protein, is similar to the cholera toxin[1]. For differentiation of *Bordetella* spp., see table below	Respiratory tract of infected persons. Transmission by respiratory droplets	Pertussis (whooping cough). See text on pages 22–24
40	**Bordetella parapertussis** (ELDERING and KENDRICK) MORENO-LÓPEZ *Haemophilus parapertussis* *Bacillus parapertussis*	Similar to *B. pertussis*. Growth more rapid and luxuriant. Urease-positive. Growth on tyrosine agar and ordinary agar. Aerobic. Viable at temperatures of 0 to 10 °C. For differentiation of *Bordetella* spp., see table below	Respiratory tract of infected persons. Transmission by respiratory droplets	Upper respiratory tract infections; occasionally whooping cough[2]
41	**Bordetella bronchiseptica** (FERRY) MORENO-LÓPEZ *Bacillus bronchisepticus* *Bacillus bronchicanis*	Similar to *B. pertussis*. Motile. Good growth on ordinary agar. Urease-positive. Aerobic. For differentiation of *Bordetella* spp., see table below	Respiratory tract of rabbits, guineapigs, dogs and cats. Transmission by contact with animals (e.g. dog saliva)	Respiratory tract infections in animals, but also rarely in man[3]
42	**Francisella tularensis** (McCOY and CHAPIN) DOROFE'EV *Bacterium tularense* *Pasteurella tularensis*	GRAM-negative, small rods, 0.2 µm wide and 0.2–0.7 µm long, some with bipolar staining. Extremely pleomorphic. Nonmotile. Obligately aerobic, but growth enhanced by increased CO_2 pressure. Oxidase-negative. No growth on ordinary media; needs media containing protein with addition of cystine	Mammals, particularly rodents, such as hares, rabbits, muskrats. Transmission by direct contact, less frequently via ticks and deerflies, contaminated water and dust	Tularemia. See text on next page

[1] LENTNER, C. (Ed.), *Geigy Scientific Tables*, 8th ed., Vol. 4, Ciba-Geigy Ltd., Basel, 1986, page 202.
[2] CONNOR, J. D., in BRAUDE et al. (Eds.), *Infectious Diseases and Medical Microbiology*, 2nd ed., Saunders, Philadelphia, 1986, page 787.
[3] REINA et al., *Infection*, **19**, 46 (1991).

Table 1 *Differential characteristics of* Bordetella *species*[2]

	B. pertussis	*B. parapertussis*	*B. bronchiseptica*
Motility	–	–	+
Growth on BORDET-GENGOU medium:			
1–2 days	–	+	+
3–6 days	+		
Growth on MACCONKEY agar	–	+	+
Citrate utilization	–	+	+
Nitrate reduction	–	–	+
Urease activity	–	+	+
Oxidase activity	+	–	+

+ Typically positive. – Typically negative.

B. pertussis is not invasive and does not infect submucosal cells or other sites of the body[1,6]. Persons who recover from pertussis develop a high degree of immunity to the disease that usually lasts for many years.

Diagnosis[9]. The diagnosis is confirmed by identification of the organism in respiratory tract secretions on fresh BORDET–GENGOU medium or other special media. Direct fluorescent-antibody test provides more rapid results, but has limited sensitivity due to the number of organisms necessary for microscopic visualization. Several enzyme-linked immunosorbent assays (ELISA) for detection of *B. pertussis* antibodies or antigens have been developed. DNA probes have been used in clinical studies.

Prophylaxis. Due to widespread use of whole-cell pertussis vaccine since the 1950s, incidence and mortality of pertussis have steadily declined. In recent years immunization has become a topic of public concern because of local and systemic adverse effects of whole-cell vaccine[3,5,6,10], but most developed countries continue to recommend routine pertussis immunization of all infants[5,11]. Of the countries immunizing against pertussis, all but Japan, still rely on whole-cell vaccine[11]. In Denmark monovalent pertussis vaccine is used, in the other countries it is part of diphtheria–tetanus–pertussis (DTP) vaccine[11]. Acellular vaccines have been in general use in Japan since 1981[12], and their introduction in other countries is under discussion[13,14].

Remark. In order to be effective against *B. pertussis*, an antibiotic must penetrate into the respiratory tract, such as erythromycin, trimethoprim–sulfamethoxazole, chloramphenicol[1].

(Continued on next page)

Table 2 *Components of* Bordetella pertussis[3]

Component	Biologic activity	Role of antibody to the component
Pertussis toxin (lymphocytosis-promoting factor, islet-activating protein)	A secreted exotoxin. Histamine sensitization, causes lymphocytosis, pancreatic islet-cell activation, immune enhancement	Protects against respiratory and intracerebral challenge in mice; important for clinical protection in man
Filamentous hemagglutinin	Involved in the attachment to ciliated respiratory epithelium	Protects against respiratory but not intracerebral challenge in mice
Agglutinogens	Surface antigens associated with fimbria involved in attachment	Agglutinates organisms; may contribute to protection against infection
Outer membrane 69-kd protein	Nonfimbrial agglutinogen associated with adenylate cyclase	Induces protection against respiratory challenge in mice
Adenylate cyclase	Extracytoplasmic protein that inhibits phagocytic function	Unknown
Endotoxin	Contributes to fever and local reactions in animals	Unknown
Tracheal cytotoxin	Causes ciliary stasis and cytopathic effects on tracheal mucosa	Unknown
Heat labile toxin	Causes dermal necrosis in animals	Unknown

References

1 HEWLETT, E. L., in MANDELL et al. (Eds.), *Principles and Practice of Infectious Diseases*, 3rd ed., Churchill Livingstone, New York, 1990, page 1756.
2 PITTMAN, M., in KRIEG and HOLT (Eds.), *Bergey's Manual of Systematic Bacteriology*, Vol. 1, Williams & Wilkins, Baltimore, 1984, page 388.
3 EDWARDS and KARZON, *Pediat. Clin. N. Amer.*, **37**, 549 (1990).
4 WRIGHT, P. F., *Rev. infect. Dis.*, **13**, Suppl. 6, S528 (1991).
5 MULLER et al., *Bull. Wld Hlth Org.*, **64**, 321 (1986).
6 CHERRY et al., Report of the Task Force on Pertussis and Pertussis Immunization – 1988, *Pediatrics*, **81**, Suppl., 939 (1988).
7 ROBERTSON et al., *Med. J. Aust.*, **147**, 522 (1987).
8 MARGILETH, A. M., in STICKLAND, G. T. (Ed.), *Hunter's Tropical Medicine*, 7th ed., Saunders, Philadelphia, 1991, page 418.
9 FRIEDMAN, R. L., *Clin. Microbiol. Rev.*, **1**, 365 (1988).
10 *Morb. Mort. wkly Rep.*, **40**, RR–10 (1991).
11 HINMAN and ORENSTEIN, *Lancet*, **335**, 707 (1990).
12 KIMURA and KUNO-SAKAI, *Acta paediat. jap.*, **30**, 143 (1988).
13 BLACKWELDER et al., *Amer. J. Dis. Child.*, **146**, 1285 (1991).
14 American Academy of Pediatrics, Committee on Infectious Diseases, *Pediatrics*, **88**, 401 (1991).
15 Editorial, *Lancet*, **339**, 526 (1992).

Tularemia

Francisella tularensis is widely distributed in nature and is found on all continents except Australia and Antarctica. The two main regions in which numerous infections of humans have occurred over a relatively large area are the USA and southern regions of the CIS. Two biovars are recognized and differ in virulence (Table 1). One appears only in North America, where it is predominant and highly virulent for numerous hosts. The other is found in Europe and Asia, as well as in North America, but causes a milder disease in humans and domestic rabbits[1,2].

F. tularensis is a very virulent pathogen capable of initiating infection with as few as 10 cells inoculated subcutaneously or 10–50 cells by inhalation[3,4].

The clinical picture and severity of tularemia vary appreciably according to the route of infection and the virulence of the organism (Table 2)[2,3,5].

The *incubation period* of tularemia is usually 3–5 days (range ~ 1–14 days)[1,2].

No specific laboratory tests characterize tularemia, and cultures of the pathogen are often difficult to obtain because of the special growth requirements of *F. tularensis* and the inability of many clinical laboratories to handle the dangerous pathogen. A four-fold rise in hemagglutination titers or a single titer ≥ 1:160 in the presence of compatible clinical illness are still the best diagnostic indicators[4].

Remarks. For treatment, streptomycin or gentamicin have been suggested as drugs of first choice[6,7]. A live vaccine strain of *F. tularensis* has been developed and may be of use for laboratory workers exposed to the organism[4].

Table 1 *Differentiation between* Francisella tularensis, *biovar tularensis and biovar palaearctica*[2]

Characteristic	Biovar tularensis (Jellison A; nearctica)	Biovar palaearctica (Jellison B)
Geographic distribution	North America	Europe, Asia, the Americas
Acid formation from glycerol	+	–
Citrulline ureidase	+	–
Source of infection	Ticks, rabbits	Contaminated water or rodents
Human disease	Severe	Mild

Table 2 *Manifestations of tularemia**[2]

Type of disease	Infections (%)	Characteristics
Ulceroglandular	75–85	Ulcers at the site of exposure and adenopathy of the draining lymph nodes
Glandular	5–10	Adenopathy, but no ulcers
Typhoidal	5–15	Systemic signs, but no adenopathy or ulcers
Oculoglandular	1–2	Eye involvement
Oropharyngeal	< 1	Oropharyngeal involvement (primarily in children)

* Pleuropulmonary complications are seen in 30–80% of the typhoidal cases and in 10–18% of the ulceroglandular cases[3].

References

1 EIGELSBACH and MCGANN, in KRIEG and HOLT (Eds.), *Bergey's Manual of Systematic Bacteriology*, Volume 1, Williams & Wilkins, Baltimore, 1984, page 394.
2 MURRAY et al., *Medical Microbiology*, Wolfe, London, 1990, page 149.
3 BOYCE, J. M., in MANDELL et al. (Eds.), *Principles and Practice of Infectious Diseases*, 3rd ed., Churchill Livingstone, New York, 1990, page 1742.
4 EVANS et al., *Medicine (Baltimore)*, **64**, 251 (1985).
5 BATES, J. H., in BRAUDE et al. (Eds.), *Infectious Diseases and Medical Microbiology*, 2nd ed., Saunders, Philadelphia, 1986, page 1503.
6 PARKHURST and SAN JOAQUIN, *Amer. J. Dis. Child.*, **144**, 1070 (1990).
7 *Med. Lett. Drug. Ther.*, **32**, No. 817 (1990).

No.	Bacterium *Synonyms* Common names	Characteristics	Habitat Host Transmission	Associated disease
43	**Escherichia coli** (MIGULA) CASTELLANI and CHALMERS *Bacillus coli* Colon bacillus Coli bacillus	GRAM-negative rods, 1.1–1.5 µm wide and 2.0–6 µm long, with rounded ends, and shape varying from coccoid to long. Some motile (peritrichous flagella), some nonmotile. Most strains have fimbriae (pili) extending from the surface (width 5–9 nm), some of them function as adhesive organs. Some strains show β-hemolysis on blood agar. Aerobic, facultatively anaerobic. Oxidase- and urease-negative. Citrate cannot be used as sole carbon source. Lactose is fermented by most strains	Intestinal tract of man and animals. Sewage, contaminated food, drinking water	Most frequent cause of some common bacterial infections: diarrhea, dysentery, urinary tract infections, septicemia; also a leading cause of neonatal meningitis and a cause of other clinical infections including pneumonia. See text below

Escherichia coli infections

Escherichia coli serovars can be differentiated on the basis of 3 major types of antigens: the heat-stable somatic (O) antigen, the heat-labile capsular (K) antigen, and the flagellar (H) antigen for motile organisms. 171 O antigens and 53 H antigens have been recognized[1], as well as more than 80 K antigens[2]. In pathogenic strains, virulence results from the cumulative impact of special properties of the cell (Fig. 1).

Enteric infections. Since the 1920s, pathogenic strains of *E. coli* are known as an etiologic agent of infant diarrhea; more recently, they have been recognized as a major cause of gastrointestinal disease in tourists (Table 1). Enteric infections caused by *E. coli* may be due to at least 4 different categories of the organism operating through different mechanisms (Table 2)[5–8]. Transmission occurs mainly via contaminated foodstuffs or drinking water, rarely directly from man to man[7]. Incubation period for 'travellers' diarrhea' in adults in a Mexican study was 1–2 days[9]; the duration is usually 1–5 days, occasionally longer[4]. Adequate fluid and electrolyte replacement is essential when fluid loss is prominent.

Urinary tract infection. E. coli is the most frequently isolated organism in urinary tract infection[2, 10–12]. In outpatients 50–85% of cases are due to *E. coli*[12], in hospitalized patients the relative fre-

Fig. 1 *Schematic representation of an* E. coli *cell interacting with host tissue*[3]

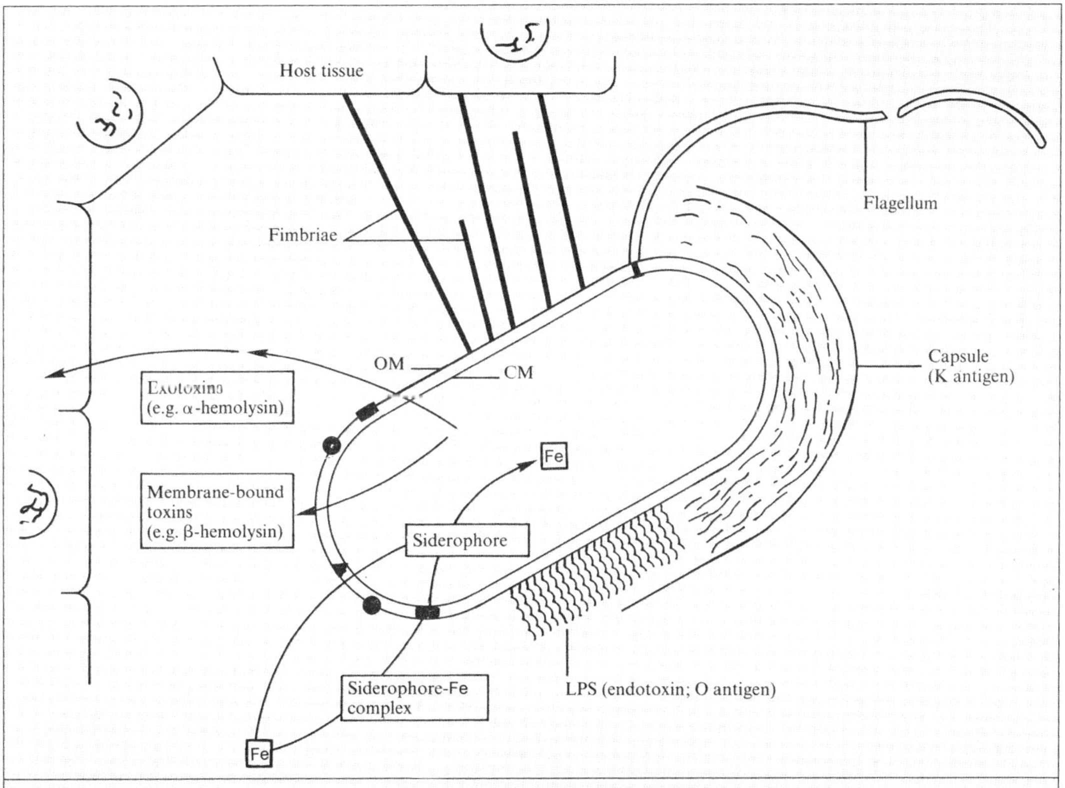

OM Outer membrane.
CM Cytoplasmic membrane.
LPS Lipopolysaccharide.

Membrane proteins involved in transport, serum resistance, etc., are indicated by solid, black circles, triangles and rectangles. Siderophores: high-affinity iron-chelating compounds (e.g. aerobactin system) promoting bacterial growth in the limiting iron concentration during infection.

Table 1 *Pathogens causing travellers' diarrhea*[4]

Organism	Latin America (8 studies) Median	Latin America (8 studies) Range	Africa (3 studies) Median	Africa (3 studies) Range	Asia (8 studies) Range
	%				
Enterotoxic					
Escherichia coli	46	28–72	36	31–75	20–34
Shigella spp.	0	0–30	0	0–15	4–7
Salmonella spp.	0	0–16	0	0–0	11–15
Campylobacter jejuni	–	–	–	–	2–15
Vibrio parahaemolyticus	–	–	–	–	1–13

Table 2 *Pathogens isolated in urine of patients with urinary tract infections (Swiss study)*[13]

Organism	Hospital patients Number	Hospital patients %	Outpatients Number	Outpatients %
Escherichia coli	2935	56.1	1967	67.1
Staphylococci (coagulase-positive and coagulase-negative)	858	16.4	327	11.2
Enterococci	529	10.1	242	8.3
Proteus spp. (mainly *P. mirabilis*)	383	7.3	230	7.9
Klebsiella spp.	297	5.7	113	3.9
Pseudomonas aeruginosa	229	4.4	54	1.8

Table 3 *Enteric infections caused by* Escherichia coli[8]

Organism	Site of action	Disease	Pathogenesis	Predominant serovars
Enterotoxigenic *E. coli* (ETEC)	Small intestine	Travellers' diarrhea; infant diarrhea in developing countries; watery diarrhea, cramps, nausea, low-grade fever	Heat-stable (ST) and/or heat-labile (LT) enterotoxins; stimulates guanylate- or adenylate cyclase activity with fluid and electrolyte loss	Heat-labile: O6:K15; O8:K40 Heat-labile + heat-stable: O11:H27; O15; O20:K79; O25:K7; O27; O63; O80; O85; O139 Heat-stable: O12; O78; O115; O148; O149; O153; O159; O166; O167
Enteroinvasive *E. coli* (EIEC)	Large intestine	Fever, cramps, watery diarrhea followed by development of dysentery with scant, bloody stools	Plasmid-mediated invasion and destruction of epithelial cells lining colon	O11; O28c; O29; O112; O115; O124; O136; O144; O147; O152; O164
Enterohemorrhagic *E. coli* (EHEC)	Large intestine	Hemorrhagic colitis with severe abdominal cramps, watery diarrhea initially followed by grossly bloody diarrhea, little or no fever	Mediated by cytotoxic 've-rotoxin' (inhibits protein synthesis)	O157:H7; O26:H11/H⁻; O128; O139; O111:K58:H8/H⁻; O113:K75:H7/H21; O121:H⁻; O145:H⁻, rough
Enteropathogenic *E. coli* (EPEC)	Small intestine	Infant diarrhea with fever, nausea, vomiting, non-bloody stools	Plasmid-mediated adherence and destruction of epithelial cells	Class I: O55:K59(B5):H⁻/H6/H7; O111ab:K58(B4):H⁻/H5/H12; O119:K69(B14); O125ac:K70(B15):H21; O126:K71(B16):H⁻/H27; O127a:K63(B8):H6; O128ab:K67(B12):H12; O142; O158 Class II: O44:K74; O86a:K61(B7); O114:H2

quency of pathogens isolated in urine differs from that in outpatients (Table 3)[10,13]. A major proportion of *E. coli* infections is caused by the O antigen types O1, O2, O4, O6, O7, O8, O16, O18, O25, O50, and O75[2,10].

In patients with symptoms of urinary tract infection, a bacterial number concentration in urine of $\geq 10^5$/mL indicates a 95% probability of true bacteruria, in those with recurrent infections a lower number concentration is already of diagnostic importance[10].

Septicemia. E. coli is the most frequently GRAM-negative organism isolated in septicemia[14]. Most strains of *E. coli* are not invasive and septicemia rarely occurs from underlying enteric infection[6]. Septicemia is much more commonly associated with urinary tract infection, particularly when there is obstruction to urinary flow[6,15]. In children in St. Thomas Hospital, London, the most common underlying conditions were found to be immunodeficiencies, urinary tract infection, and lesions of the gastrointestinal tract (the O antigen types identified most frequently were O1, O2, O4, O6, O15, and O75)[16].

Meningitis. E. coli is the most frequently isolated organism in neonatal meningitis, followed by type B streptococci and rarely *Listeria monocytogenes*. Neonatal meningitis remains a serious problem with high mortality (30–60%)[17,18]. In contrast to adult meningitis due to *E. coli*, in neonates there is a strong association between the presence of K1 antigen strains in meningitis, and, to a lesser extent, with septicemia; increased colonization with K1 strains occurs during pregnancy and these strains are the ones involved in the subsequent neonatal meningitis[6].

Nosocomial infections. E. coli is a leading cause of nosocomial infections (see Table 4 on next page).

Remarks. Resistance is often a problem and susceptibility tests should be performed. In treatment of *E. coli* infections, a cephalosporin is the drug of choice – in severe illness combined with gentamicin, tobramycin or amikacin[20]. A wide variety of other antimicrobial drugs have been listed as alternatives[20]. In meningitis, as well as in septicemia, prompt treatment is essential and antimicrobial drugs should not be withheld until laboratory tests are performed[20]. For treatment of neonatal meningitis and septicemia directed against *E. coli*, group B streptococci and *Listeria monocytogenes*, ampicillin plus gentamicin or tobramycin is used; ampicillin plus cefotaxine is an alternative[20]. For acute, uncomplicated urinary tract infection, before the infecting organism is known, an oral sulfonamide is the drug of choice, otherwise ampicillin or amoxicillin may be effective[20].

References

1 CLEARLY, T. G., *Pediat. Clin. N. Amer.*, **35**, 485 (1988).
2 JOHNSON, J. R., *Clin. Microbiol. Rev.*, **4**, 80 (1991).
3 EISENSTEIN and JONES, *Advanc. intern. Med.*, **33**, 231 (1988).
4 GUERRANT, R. L., in MANDELL et al. (Eds.), *Principles and Practice of Infectious Diseases*, 3rd ed., Churchill Livingstone, New York, 1990, page 851.

Table 4 *Pathogen distribution for major sites of nosocomial infection (US National Surveillance System, 1986–1989)*[19]

Organism	Total		Urinary tract infection		Surgical wound infection		Pneumonia		Septicemia	
	Number	%	Number	%	Number	%	Number	%	Number	%
Escherichia coli	14765	16	11135	26	1951	10	946	6	733	6
Enterococci	10744	12	6720	16	2645	13	342	2	1037	8
Pseudomonas aeruginosa	9936	11	5127	12	1668	8	2598	17	543	4
Staphylococcus aureus	8647	10	823	2	3439	17	2401	16	1984	16
Coagulase-negative staphylococci	7783	9	1634	4	2472	12	293	2	3384	27
Enterobacter spp.	6103	7	2339	6	1529	8	1625	11	610	5
Klebsiella pneumoniae	4872	5	2664	6	618	3	1042	7	548	4
Candida albicans	4691	5	2978	7	481	2	615	4	617	5
Proteus mirabilis	3632	4	2312	5	712	4	503	3	105	1
Streptococcus spp.	1442	2	207	0	539	3	231	1	465	4
Citrobacter spp.	1441	2	812	2	321	2	226	1	82	1
Candida spp.	1373	2	853	2	81	0	109	1	330	3
Serratia marcescens	1369	2	367	1	271	1	579	4	152	1

[5] LEVINE, M. M., *J. infect. Dis.*, **155**, 377 (1987).
[6] EISENSTEIN, B. I., in MANDELL et al. (Eds.), *Principles and Practice of Infectious Diseases*, 3rd ed., Churchill Livingstone, New York, 1990, page 1658.
[7] DOYLE, M. P., *Lancet*, **336**, 1111 (1990).
[8] GUERRANT, R. L., in MANDELL et al. (Eds.), *Principles and Practice of Infectious Diseases*, 3rd ed., Churchill Livingstone, New York, 1990, page 837.
[9] GORBACH et al., *New Engl. J. Med.*, **292**, 933 (1975).
[10] SOBEL and KAYE, in MANDELL et al. (Eds.), *Principles and Practice of Infectious Diseases*, 3rd ed., Churchill Livingstone, New York, 1990, page 582.
[11] STAMM et al., *Rev. infect. Dis.*, **13**, 77 (1991).
[12] GLAUSER, M. P., in BRAUDE et al. (Eds.), *Infectious Diseases and Medical Microbiology*, 2nd ed., Saunders, Philadelphia, 1986, page 1009.
[13] BRODHAGE, H., unpublished data.
[14] KREGER et al., *Amer. J. Med.*, **68**, 332 (1980).
[15] GRANSDEN et al., *Rev. infect. Dis.*, **12**, 1008 (1990).
[16] BONADIO et al., *Amer. J. Dis. Child.*, **145**, 671 (1991).
[17] MULDER and ZANEN, *J. Infect.*, **9**, 177 (1984).
[18] BELL et al., *Arch. Dis. Childh.*, **64**, 873 (1989).
[19] SCHABERG et al., *Amer. J. Med.*, **91**, Suppl. 3B, 3B–72S (1991).
[20] *Med. Lett. Drug. Ther.*, **32**, No. 817 (1990).

Shigella infections

The genus *Shigella* consists of 4 species: *S. dysenteriae* with 10 serovars, *S. flexneri* with 8 serovars, *S. boydii* with 15 serovars, and *S. sonnei* with 1 serovar (see following table).

Shigellosis is found in all parts of the world, although man is practically the only source of infection. As few as 10 cells can produce infection[2], which means that man-to-man transmission can easily occur, particularly via contaminated foodstuffs, objects, or water (even by swimming in polluted water[3]).

From 1986 to 1988 the reported infection rate of *Shigella* in the USA increased from 5.4 to 10.1 cases per 100000 persons[4].

Although individuals of all ages are susceptible to bacterial dysentery, it occurs mainly in children aged 6 months to 10 years[5].

In the early 1960s, *S. flexneri* was by far the most commonly isolated *Shigella* organism in the USA; this position is now occupied by *S. sonnei*[4] (66% of cases in 1981[6]). *S. sonnei* is the most frequently isolated *Shigella* organism in other areas, such as northwestern Europe and Japan. Of the *Shigella* organisms isolated over the past years in central Switzerland, 53.2% were *S. sonnei*, 42.3% *S. flexneri* and 4.5% *S. boydii*; most of the carriers were tourists from North America and tropical countries[7]. In 1985, a water-born epidemic of 1000 cases of *S. sonnei* infections occurred in the Haifa Bay (Israel)[8].

Dysentery from *S. dysenteriae* did not play any significant role in Western countries; it was mainly found in regions of the Middle and Far East and in some tropical countries. *S. dysenteriae* did not recur in Central America until 1968, giving rise to severe infections of pandemic extent in five countries[9].

The *incubation period* is 2–7 days, rarely 8–12 hours. Frequent watery stools with mucus, blood or pus, or an ordinary watery diarrhea are typical features of the disease. The latter lasts a few days, and the bacterial excretion a few days to a few weeks. Bacterial excretion (*S. flexneri* and *S. sonnei*) lasting over one year has also been observed[10]. One member of a family with the disease usually causes the infection to spread to other members of the same family.

Shigella bacteremia is rare, occurring in children, but also in adult patients[11].

Remarks. Vaccines, mainly for *S. sonnei* and *S. flexneri*, are in development but were still at the stage of clinical trials in 1990[12]. Multiple resistance to antibacterial drugs may be a problem[13–15], but trimethoprim–sulfamethoxazole has been suggested as the drug of choice[16]. Oral or intravenous rehydration is advocated when fluid loss is prominent[5, 15].

Differential characteristics of species of the genus Shigella[1]

	S. dysenteriae		*S. flexneri*		*S. boydii*	*S. sonnei*
	Serovars					
	1	2–10	1–5	6	1–15	
Catalase activity	−	+	+	+	+	+
Urease activity	−	−	−	−	−	−
Indole production	−	d	d	−	d	−
H_2S production	−	−	−	−	−	−
Gas production from glucose	−	−	−	d	−	−
Acid production from glucose	+	+	+	+	+	+
– from mannitol	−	−	+	+	+	+
– from lactose	−	−	−	−	−	(+)

\+ 85–100% of strains are positive.
− 85–100% of strains are negative.
d 16–84% of strains are positive.
(+) Positive after prolonged incubation (aerobic cultivation).

References

[1] COWAN and STEEL, *Manual for the Identification of Medical Bacteria*, 2nd ed., Cambridge University Press, London, 1974.
[2] DUPONT et al., *J. infect. Dis.*, **159**, 1126 (1989).
[3] ROSENBERG et al., *J. Amer. med. Ass.*, **236**, 1849 (1976).
[4] *Morb. Mort. wkly Rep.*, **39**, 509 (1990).
[5] DUPONT, H. L., in MANDELL et al. (Eds.), *Principles and Practice of Infectious Diseases*, 3rd ed., Churchill Livingstone, New York, 1990, page 1716.
[6] World Health Organization, *Wkly epidem. Rec.*, **58**, 87 (1983).
[7] BRODHAGE, H., unpublished.
[8] EGOZ et al., *J. Infect.*, **22**, 87 (1991).
[9] KANTOR, H. S., in BRAUDE et al. (Eds.), *Infectious Diseases and Medical Microbiology*, 2nd ed., Saunders, Philadelphia, 1986, page 897.
[10] BREDE, H. D., *Münch. med. Wschr.*, **128**, 61 (1986).
[11] MORDUCHOWICZ et al., *Arch. intern. Med.*, **147**, 2034 (1987).
[12] LEVINE, M. M., *Lancet*, **335**, 958 (1990).
[13] PARSONNET et al., *Lancet*, **2**, 543 (1989).
[14] KATOULI et al., *Scand. J. infect. Dis.*, **21**, 415 (1989).
[15] OLDFIELD et al., *Rev. infect. Dis.*, **13**, Suppl. 3, S 199 (1991).
[16] *Med. Lett. Drug. Ther.*, **32**, No. 817 (1990).

No.	**Bacterium** *Synonyms* Common names	Characteristics	Habitat Host Transmission	Associated disease
44	**Shigella dysenteriae** (SHIGA) CASTELLANI and CHALMERS *Bacillus dysenteriae*	GRAM-negative, straight rods, similar in morphology to other *Enterobacteriaceae*. Nonmotile. Aerobic		
	Serovar 1: *Shigella shigae*	For biochemical properties, see table on page 27. Produces an exotoxin in high concentration	In feces of infected persons. Contaminated milk and ice cream. Flies. Transmission via contact or contaminated foods	Severe epidemic dysentery. Often marked toxemia. Convalescence takes months. Occurs in the tropics, also in the temperate zone of East Asia. Epidemic in Central America since the end of 1968[1]. See text on page 27
	Serovars 2–10: *Shigella schmitzii* *Shigella ambigua* *Shigella largei* *Shigella arabinotarda*	For biochemical properties, see table below. Serovar 2 always indole-positive, other serovars vary in indole production	In feces of infected persons	Rare cause of dysentery. Occurs in eastern Europe and Asia, occasionally imported into other European countries. See text on page 27
45	**Shigella flexneri** CASTELLANI and CHALMERS FLEXNER's bacillus Pseudodysentery bacillus STRONG's bacillus	Similar to *S. dysenteriae*. For biochemical properties, see table on page 27. No formation of exotoxin	In feces of infected persons	Worldwide distribution. Epidemic in times of war and catastrophe. The second most common cause of dysentery in the USA and Europe in 1981, accounting for 29% of cases[2]. See text on page 27
46	**Shigella boydii** EWING	Similar to *S. dysenteriae*. For biochemical properties, see table on page 27. No formation of exotoxin	In feces of infected persons	Rare cause of dysentery, mainly in tropical countries. See text on page 27
47	**Shigella sonnei** (LEVINE) WELDIN *Bacterium sonnei* SONNE's bacillus DUVAL's bacillus	Similar to *S. dysenteriae*. For biochemical properties, see table on page 27. No formation of exotoxin	In feces of infected persons. Occasionally in contaminated foods and milk and in drinking water	Worldwide distribution; in the USA and Europe commonest cause of a comparatively mild form of dysentery, especially in children, known and feared in Japan as 'ekiri'
48	**Salmonella anatum** (RETTGER and SCOVILLE) BERGEY et al.	GRAM-negative, straight rods, 0.7–1.5 µm wide and 2.0–2.5 µm long. Motile, with peritrichous flagella. Acid and gas production from glucose and mannitol. Formation of H_2S. Growth on citrate agar. Aerobic, facultatively anaerobic. Indole- and urease-negative. For antigenic formula, see Table 1 on page 30	Mainly in ducks and dried-egg products from various sources. Mesenteric lymph nodes of healthy pigs; silver foxes	Food poisoning, febrile gastroenteritis
49	**Salmonella bareilly** BRIDGES and SCOTT	As for *S. anatum*	Chickens, turkeys, dried-egg products, fish meal; rarely dogs and cats	Food poisoning, gastroenteritis; clinical picture occasionally resembles typhoid. See text on pages 30 and 31
50	**Salmonella bovismorbificans** (BASENAU)	As for *S. anatum*	Dried-egg products, cats; less often cattle	Food poisoning, gastroenteritis. See text on pages 30 and 31
51	**Salmonella choleraesuis** (SMITH) WELDIN *Bacillus cholerae suis*	As for *S. anatum*. H_2S formation variable. Arabinose and trehalose are not fermented. Ferments dulcitol slowly and irregularly. For antigenic formula, see Table 1 on page 30	Commonest *Salmonella* organism in pigs. Secondary pathogen in viral cholera of pigs	Enteritis; clinical picture often resembles typhoid. Complications: pneumonia, arthritis, meningitis, endocarditis, abscesses. See text on pages 30 and 31
52	**Salmonella dublin** WARREN and SCOTT	As for *S. anatum*	Calves, more rarely older cattle; silver foxes	Food poisoning, gastroenteritis; clinical picture sometimes resembles typhoid. Meningitis, cholecystitis. See text on pages 30 and 31
53	**Salmonella enteritidis** (GÄRTNER) CASTELLANI and CHALMERS *Bacillus enteritidis* GÄRTNER's bacillus	As for *S. anatum*. For antigenic formula, see Table 1 on page 30	Common in animals, especially cattle, pigs, ducks, chickens	One of the commonest causes of food poisoning. Febrile gastroenteritis; very rarely septicemia or a typhoid-like clinical picture. See text on pages 30 and 31

[1] KANTOR, H. S., in BRAUDE et al. (Eds.), *Infectious Diseases and Medical Microbiology*, 2nd ed., Saunders, Philadelphia, 1986, page 897.

[2] World Health Organization, *Wkly epidem. Rec.*, **58**, 87 (1983).

No.	Bacterium *Synonyms* Common names	Characteristics	Habitat Host Transmission	Associated disease
54	**Salmonella hirschfeldii** WELDIN *Salmonella paratyphi* C Paratyphoid C bacillus HIRSCHFELD's bacillus	As for *S. anatum*. Ferments dulcitol and trehalose. Arabinose fermentation is variable. For antigenic formula, see Table 1 on next page	In feces and urine of infected persons and carriers	Typhoid-like symptoms, often of septicemic character. Found in eastern Europe and China. See text on pages 30 and 31
55	**Salmonella newport** SCHÜTZE	As for *S. anatum*. For antigenic formula, see Table 1 on next page	Chickens, turkeys, lymph nodes of healthy pigs; dried-egg products, fish meal	Common cause of food poisoning. Gastroenteritis, rarely meningitis. See text on pages 30 and 31
56	**Salmonella panama** KAUFFMANN	As for *S. anatum*. For antigenic formula, see Table 1 on next page	Natural host unknown. In various animals	Food poisoning, gastroenteritis, also meningitis, especially in children. See text on pages 30 and 31
57	**Salmonella paratyphi** A (BRION and KAYSER) CASTELLANI and CHALMERS *Bacterium paratyphi* *Bacterium paratyphi* typus A Paratyphoid A bacillus	Similar to *S. anatum*. Most strains do not produce H_2S. No growth on citrate agar. For antigenic formula, see Table 1 on next page	In feces of infected persons and carriers. Contaminated foods and water	Obligatory pathogen in man. Acute gastroenteritis, typhoid-like clinical picture. Found in Asia, Middle East, Africa, also in southern Europe. See text on pages 30 and 31
58	**Salmonella schottmuelleri** (WINSLOW et al.) BERGEY et al. *Salmonella paratyphi* B *Bacterium paratyphi* B Paratyphoid B bacillus	Similar to *S. anatum*. For antigenic formula, see Table 1 on next page	As for *S. paratyphi*	Obligatory pathogen in man. Typhoid-like symptoms, rarely acute gastroenteritis (food poisoning). See text on pages 30 and 31
59	**Salmonella thompson** SCOTT	As for *S. anatum*. For antigenic formula, see Table 1 on next page	Dried-egg products. Often causes epidemic disease in hens	Food poisoning, gastroenteritis. See text on pages 30 and 31
60	**Salmonella typhi** (SCHRÖTER) WARREN and SCOTT *Bacillus typhi* Typhoid bacillus	As for *S. anatum*. No gas production from glucose or other sugars. No growth on citrate agar. For antigenic formula, see Table 1 on next page	In feces, urine and bile of infected persons and carriers. Contaminated foods and water	Typhoid fever in man. See text on pages 30 and 31
61	**Salmonella typhimurium** (LOEFFLER) CASTELLANI and CHALMERS *Bacillus typhimurium*	As for *S. anatum*. For antigenic formula, see Table 1 on next page	In feces of infected persons and animals. Ducks, duck eggs, pigs, cattle, mice, rats, chickens, hen's eggs, dried-egg products, fish meal	Pathogenic to man and animals. Commonest cause of food poisoning. Gastroenteritis. In rare cases typhoid-like symptoms. See text on pages 30 and 31
62	Other *Salmonella* serovars (subgenus I): **Salmonella bredeney** **Salmonella cerro** **Salmonella derby** **Salmonella give** **Salmonella havana** **Salmonella heidelberg** **Salmonella minnesota** **Salmonella mississippi** **Salmonella muenchen** **Salmonella newington** **Salmonella reading** **Salmonella saint-paul** **Salmonella schwarzengrund** **Salmonella sendai** **Salmonella sundsvall** **Salmonella waycross**	As for *S. anatum*. For antigenic formulae, see Table 1 on next page		See text on pages 30 and 31
63	**Salmonella arizonae** (BORMAN) KAUFFMANN *Paracolobactrum arizonae*	GRAM-negative, straight rods, 0.7–1.5 µm wide and 2.0–2.5 µm long. Motile. Acid and gas production from glucose, acid from lactose. Aerobic. Liquefies gelatin at 36°C. On the basis of 34 O and 43 H antigens, about 400 serovars have been identified[2]	Often isolated from reptiles, less frequently from warm-blooded animals	Food poisoning, gastroenteritis, occasionally septicemia[1]

[1] RILEY et al., *Arch. intern. Med.*, **148**, 1207 (1988).

[2] LE MINOR, L., in KRIEG and HOLT (Eds.), *Bergey's Manual of Systematic Bacteriology*, Vol. 1, Williams & Wilkins, Baltimore, 1984, page 427.

Salmonella infections

All *Salmonella* are so closely related in genetic or evolutionary terms that there is no species differentiation[1,2]. Nevertheless, *Salmonella* strains demonstrate sufficient differences in biochemical reactions, antigenic structure, host adaptation and geographic distribution to be grouped by DNA hybridization into 7 distinct subgroups with numerous serovars[2]. *Nos. 48–62* of the tabulation on pages 28 and 29 are members of subgroup 1, and *S. arizona* (*No. 63*) represents subgroups 3a and 3b.

So far, approximately 2200 different serovars have been described[2], which can be differentiated by their somatic (O) and flagellar (H) antigens (selected serovars are given in Table 1). There are no natural saprophytes among the salmonellae. All are pathogenic

Table 1 *Selected* Salmonella *serovars according to the Kauffmann–White scheme*[3]

Serovar	Clinical features	O group	O antigens	H antigens	
				Phase 1	Phase 2
S. paratyphi A	S	A	1, 2, 12	a	–
S. schottmuelleri	S, E	B	1, 4, [5], 12	b	1, 2
S. schwarzengrund	E, (S)	B	1, 4, 12, 27	d	1, 7
S. saint-paul	E, (S), M	B	1, 4, [5], 12	e, h	1, 2
S. reading	E	B	4, [5], 12	e, h	1, 5
S. typhimurium	E, M, (S)	B	1, 4, [5], 12	i	1, 2
S. heidelberg	E	B	1, 4, [5], 12	r	1, 2
S. indiana	E	B	1, 4, 12	z	1, 7
S. hirschfeldii	S, M	C_1	6, 7, [Vi]	c	1, 5
S. choleraesuis	E, S, M	C_1	6, 7	c	1, 5
S. montevideo	E, (S)	C_1	6, 7	g, m, s	–
S. oranienburg	E, (S)	C_1	6, 7	m, t	–
S. thompson	E, (S)	C_1	6, 7	k	1, 5
S. virchow	E, (S)	C_1	6, 7	r	1, 2
S. infantis	E	C_1	6, 7	r	1, 5
S. muenchen	E, M	C_2	6, 8	d	1, 2
S. newport	E, M, (S)	C_2	6, 8	e, h	1, 2
S. sendai	S	D_1	1, 9, 12	a	1, 5
S. typhi	S, M	D_1	9, 12, [Vi]	d	–
S. enteritidis	E, (S), M	D_1	1, 9, 12	g, m	–
S. panama	E, M, (S)	D_1	1, 9, 12	l, v	1, 5
S. napoli	E	D_1	1, 9, 12	l, z_{13}	e, n, x
S. anatum	E, (S)	E_1	3, 10	e, h	1, 6
S. give	E	E_1	3, 10	l, v	1, 7
S. newington	E, (M)	E_2	3, 15	e, h	1, 6
S. mississippi	E	G_2	1, 13, 23	b	1, 5
S. havana	E, M	G_2	1, 13, 23	f, g	–
S. sundsvall	E	H	1, 6, 14, 25	z	e, n, x
S. cerro	E	K	6, 14, 18	z_4, z_{23}	[1,5]
S. minnesota	E	L	21	b	e, n, x
S. ealing	E	O	35	g, m, s	–
S. waycross	E, (S)	S	41	z_4, z_{23}	–

E Predominantly enteritic.
M Meningeal localization possible.
S Predominantly septicemic.
(S) Septicemic infection possible.
[ ] Antigen may be absent.

for one (e.g. *S. typhi* in man, *S. abortus-equi* in the horse) or several hosts.

In man, *Salmonella* infections usually occur by the oral route; the bacteria either colonize the intestine directly and cause gastroenteritis (enteritic salmonellae), or they reach the mesenteric lymph nodes via the submucosa of the lymphatics in the small intestine, where they multiply and produce a general infection via the bloodstream. Localization may occur in almost any organ or tissue (according to several studies with a predominance of *S. typhimurium* or *S. choleraesuis*[4]).

The *incubation period* of enteritic salmonellae is between 6 and 48 hours[5]. Transmission is caused by contaminated foodstuffs: meat products, duck eggs, dried-egg products, milk (also pasteurized milk), poultry, etc., as well as animal feed[1], garden manure[6], reptiles[7], rectal thermometers in neonates[8]. Sometimes the vector is indicated by the type of *Salmonella* isolated, e.g. *S. hadar* originating from imported turkeys, and *S. dublin* with raw cow's milk[9]. Direct contact infections are rarer; however, they can occur in adults and particularly in children[10,11].

A large number of *Salmonella* must be swallowed in most instances to produce disease in healthy human beings; in general, 10^6–10^9 organisms must be ingested to produce symptomatic infection[1]. However, in the event of infection with unusually virulent organisms or in patients with reduced resistance, symptomatic infection may result from extremely small inocula, e.g. 50 organisms in 1 g chocolate for *S. napoli* and less than 10 organisms in 1 g cheddar cheese for *S. typhimurium*[2].

In recent decades the number of enteritic *Salmonella* infections officially notified has increased markedly, although the true figures may well be considerably higher[2]. In the USA, 47812 cases (excluding typhoid fever) were reported in 1989[12] compared with approximately 30000 cases in 1980[13].

Some recent outbreaks of food-borne salmonellosis are given in Table 2. A nation-wide outbreak of infection by *S. enteritidis* type 4 has been taking place in Britain with hen's eggs and contaminated poultry meat as a vehicle of infection[14,15].

Table 2 *Food-borne salmonellosis, 1981–1985*[2]

Year	Country	Food	Serovar	Cases*
1981	Netherlands	Cold buffet	*S. indiana*	700
	Scotland	Raw milk	*S. typhimurium*	654
	England	Chicken	*S. montevideo*	500
1982	England	Chocolate	*S. napoli*	245
	Norway	Black pepper	*S. oranienburg*	126
1984	Global◊	Aspic glaze	*S. enteritidis*	766
	England	Cooked meats	*S. virchow*	274
	Canada	Cheddar cheese	*S. typhimurium*	2000
	England	Cold roast beef	*S. typhimurium*	450
1985	England	Cooked meats	*S. infantis*	150
	USA	Pasteurized milk	*S. typhimurium*	20000
	England	Infant dried milk	*S. ealing*	60

* Approximate numbers.
◊ Airline meals prepared in London.

Enteric fever. Enteric fever produced by *S. typhi* is called 'typhoid fever' and that produced by *Salmonella* serovars other than *S. typhi* is termed 'paratyphoid fever'. Besides *S. typhi*, the pathogens that most often produce a clinical picture of enteric fever are *paratyphi* A, *S. schottmuelleri* and *S. hirschfeldii*, as well as *S. choleraesuis*. In a few cases, however, other enteritic salmonellae can be responsible for septic infections (see table on selected serovars).

The *incubation period* of typhoid fever is usually 10–14 days, but may vary from 7 to 21 days[1]. The incubation period is influenced by the number of organisms ingested.

Typhoid fever is a severe prolonged disease with a high rate of complications. The clinical features of typhoid and paratyphoid fevers are essentially the same, although paratyphoid tends to be a milder illness than typhoid[1]. In clinically untreated typhoid, the fever worsens by stages, usually associated with relative bradycardia and possibly constipation. Because this is a systemic infection, the pathogens can be demonstrated in the blood, and initial diagnosis can be made from blood cultures. From the second week, stool examination is mostly negative in treated patients, and after the third week WIDAL's test is positive.

No.	**Bacterium** *Synonyms* Common names	Characteristics	Habitat Host Transmission	Associated disease
64	**Citrobacter freundii** (BRAAK) WERKMAN and GILLEN *Bacterium freundii*	Similar to *Escherichia coli*. GRAM-negative, straight rods, ~ 1.0 µm wide and 2.0–6.0 µm long. Motile, with peritrichous flagella. Forms H_2S, utilizes citrate. Indole- and oxidase-negative	Soil, water; intestinal tract in man and animals	Urinary tract and wound infections, septicemia[1]. Nosocomial infections[2] (see Table 4 on page 27)
65	**Citrobacter diversus** (BURKEY) WERKMAN and GILLEN *Aerobacter diversum* *Citrobacter koseri*	Similar to *Escherichia coli*. GRAM-negative, straight rods, ~ 1.0 µm wide and 2.0–6.0 µm long. Motile, with peritrichous flagella. No H_2S production. Indole-positive, oxidase-negative	Water, sewage, foodstuffs; intestinal tract in man and animals	Urinary tract and wound infections, septicemia[1]; meningitis in neonates[3,4]. Nosocomial infections[2] (see Table 4 on page 27)
66	**Klebsiella pneumoniae** (SCHROETER) TREVISAN *Bacillus pneumoniae* *Bacterium pneumoniae crouposae* FRIEDLÄNDER's bacillus NEUMANN's bacillus Pneumobacillus	GRAM-negative, straight rods, 0.3 to 1.0 µm wide and 0.6–6.0 µm long, occurring singly, in pairs and in short chains. Capsulated. Nonmotile. Facultatively anaerobic. Urease-positive. Oxidase-negative, no H_2S formation *Remark*. Most strains of *Klebsiella* spp. produce a capsular layer surrounding the bacterial cell. Of the 82 capsular (K) antigens known, 77 are used for serological typing. The O-antigens are less heterogeneous and 12 serogroups have been described[5]	Upper respiratory and intestinal tract in man. Transmission from man to man via contaminated hands and foodstuffs[6]	FRIEDLÄNDER's pneumonia, especially hospital- and community-acquired[7,8] (see Table 4 on page 27); urinary tract infections, septicemia (high lethality in neonates and old patients[9]), meningitis *Remark*. For treatment, a cephalosporin may be tried[10], but multiple antibiotic resistance could be a problem[11]
67	**Klebsiella pneumoniae** subsp. **ozaenae** subsp. nov. (ABEL) BERGEY et al. *Klebsiella ozaenae* *Bacillus mucosus ozaenae* *Bacillus ozaenae* ABEL's bacillus	Similar to *K. pneumoniae*. Often no gas formation in glucose degradation	As for *K. pneumoniae*	Isolated with other organisms in ozena (atrophic rhinitis)
68	**Klebsiella pneumoniae** subsp. **rhinoscleromatis** subsp. nov. TREVISAN *Klebsiella rhinoscleromatis* *Bacterium rhinoscleromatis*	Similar to *K. pneumoniae*	As for *K. pneumoniae*. Very low pathogenicity	Isolated in rhinoscleroma, occurring in eastern Europe, also in Asia, Indonesia and Central America

1 DRELICHMAN and BAND, *Arch. intern. Med.*, **145**, 1808 (1985).
2 GUENTZEL, M.N., in BARON, S. (Ed.), *Medical Microbiology*, 2nd ed., Addison-Wesley, Menlo Park, CA, 1986, page 495.
3 PARRY et al., *Pediatrics*, **65**, 1105 (1980).
4 KLINE, M.W., *J. Pediat.*, **113**, 430 (1988).
5 AYLING-SMITH and PITT, *J. Hosp. Infect.*, **16**, 287 (1990).
6 COOKE et al., *J. Hyg. (Camb.)*, **84**, 97 (1980).
7 EISENSTEIN, B.I., in MANDELL et al. (Eds.), *Principles and Practice of Infectious Diseases*, 3rd ed., Churchill Livingstone, New York, 1990, page 1658.
8 CARPENTER, J.L., *Rev. infect. Dis.*, **12**, 672 (1990).
9 MONTGOMERIE and OTA, *Arch. intern. Med.*, **140**, 525 (1980).
10 *Med. Lett. Drug. Ther.*, **32**, No. 817 (1990).
11 ARLET et al., *Europ. J. clin. Microbiol. infect. Dis.*, **9**, 797 (1990).

Transmission is the result of direct contact or contaminated water and food. Man always starts the chain of infection (either as a typhoid sufferer or as a chronic carrier)[16–18].

Approximately 3% of typhoid patients (in contrast to about 0.1% of patients with enteritic *Salmonella* infection) become chronic carriers[19]; very few of them are children.

Remarks. For immunization against typhoid fever, 2 vaccines are generally available: a parenteral heat–phenol-inactivated vaccine and an oral live-attenuated vaccine, derived from the Ty21a strain of *S. typhi*[20,21].

The use of antibacterial drugs is extensively discussed[1]; chloramphenicol is still of value. For *S. typhi* infections, ceftriaxone seems to be the drug of choice; ampicillin or amoxicillin may be effective in milder cases. For other *Salmonella* infections (especially meningitis), cefotaxime or ceftriaxone has been recommended, but most cases of *Salmonella* gastroenteritis subside spontaneously without antimicrobial therapy[22].

References

1 HOOK, E.W., in MANDELL et al. (Eds.), *Principles and Practice of Infectious Diseases*, 3rd ed., Churchill Livingstone, New York, 1990, page 1700.
2 WHO Expert Committee on Salmonellosis Control, *Wld Hlth Org. techn. Rep. Ser.*, No. 774 (1988).
3 KAUFFMANN, F., *The Bacteriology of Enterobacteriaceae*, Munksgaard, Copenhagen, 1966.
4 COHEN et al., *Medicine (Baltimore)*, **66**, 349 (1987).
5 KANTOR, H.S., in BRAUDE et al. (Eds.), *Infectious Diseases and Medical Microbiology*, 2nd ed., Saunders, Philadelphia, 1986, page 897.
6 SMITH et al., *J. Hyg. (Camb.)*, **89**, 125 (1982).
7 Editorial, *Lancet*, **2**, 130 (1981).
8 MCALLISTER et al., *Lancet*, **1**, 1262 (1986).
9 ST. LOUIS et al., *J. Amer. med. Ass.*, **259**, 2103 (1988).
10 PALMER et al., *Lancet*, **1**, 881 (1981).
11 WILSON et al., *Pediatrics*, **69**, 436 (1982).
12 *Morb. Mort. wkly Rep.*, **38**, No. 54 (1990).
13 *Morb. Mort. wkly Rep.*, **31**, 613 (1981).
14 COYLE et al., *Lancet*, **2**, 1295 (1988).
15 RAMPLING et al., *Lancet*, **2**, 436 (1989).
16 KLOTZ et al., *Arch. intern. Med.*, **144**, 533 (1984).
17 BREDE, H.D., *Münch. med. Wschr.*, **128**, 64 (1986).
18 *Morb. Mort. wkly Rep.*, **39**, 749 (1990).
19 GIANELLA, R.A, in BARON, S. (Ed.), *Medical Microbiology*, 2nd ed., Addison-Wesley, Menlo Park, CA, 1986, page 452.
20 *Morb. Mort. wkly Rep.*, **39**, No. RR-10 (1990).
21 WOODRUFF et al., *J. Amer. med. Ass.*, **265**, 756 (1991).
22 *Med. Lett. Drug. Ther.*, **32**, No. 817 (1990).

No.	Bacterium *Synonyms* Common names	Characteristics	Habitat Host Transmission	Associated disease
69	**Klebsiella oxytoca** (FLÜGGE) LAUTROP *Bacillus oxytocus perniciosus*	Similar to *K. pneumoniae*. Urease- and indole-positive. Growth at 10 °C	Intestinal tract in man and animals	Clinical importance uncertain
70	Other *Klebsiella* species of clinical importance: **Klebsiella terrigena** **Klebsiella planticola** **Klebsiella trevisanii**	Similar to *K. pneumoniae*. Growth at 10 °C	Soil, water, plants	Rarely implicated in human infections
71	**Enterobacter cloacae** (JORDAN) HORMAECHE and EDWARDS *Bacillus cloacae*	GRAM-negative, straight rods, 0.6 to 1.0 µm wide and 1.2–3.0 µm long. Capsulated. Motile, with peritrichous flagella. Facultatively anaerobic. Liquefies gelatine slowly. Urease- and indole-negative	Soil, sewage, water, meat products. Intestinal tract in man and animals	Opportunistic pathogen. Can be isolated in respiratory tract, urinary tract, surgical wounds[1]. Nosocomial infections, e.g. septicemia[2-5] (see Table 4 on page 27) *Remark*. Resistance to antimicrobial drugs may be a problem; susceptibility tests should be performed[6]
72	**Enterobacter aerogenes** (KRUSE) HORMAECHE and EDWARDS *Aerobacter aerogenes* *Bacillus aerogenes*	Similar to *E. cloacae*	Soil, sewage, water, dairy products. Intestinal tract in man and animals	Opportunistic pathogen. Can be isolated in respiratory tract, urinary tract. Nosocomial infections, e.g. septicemia[3] (see Table 4 on page 27)
73	Other *Enterobacter* species of clinical importance: **Enterobacter sakazakii** **Enterobacter agglomerans**	Similar to *E. cloacae*	Soil, water, plants, foodstuffs	Opportunistic pathogens. Nosocomial infections, e.g. septicemia, meningitis[7,8]
74	**Serratia marcescens** BIZIO *Chromobacterium prodigiosum*	GRAM-negative, straight rods, 0.5 to 0.8 µm wide and 0.9–2.0 µm long. Motile. Aerobic, facultatively anaerobic. Colonies white, pink or red. Certain strains form various pigments: (1) prodigiosin (water-insoluble, red), (2) pyrimine (water-soluble, white or pink). Strains isolated from hospital infections form very little pigment	Soil, water, foodstuffs (especially milk and salads); insects, contaminated detergents and disinfectant solutions	Alone or combined with other pyogenic organisms in wound infections, urinary tract infections, pulmonary infections, septicemia, meningitis. Particularly important as pathogen in nosocomial infections[9-13] (associated with intravenous, intraperitoneal, urinary catheters, etc.); septic arthritis associated with intra-articular intervention[14]. See Table 4 on page 27 *Remark*. Resistance to antimicrobial drugs may be a problem; susceptibility tests should be performed
75	**Serratia liquefaciens** (GRIMES and HENNERTY) BASCOMB et al. *Aerobacter liquefaciens*	Similar to *S. marcescens*. No prodigiosin formation	The most wide-spread *Serratia* species found in the natural environment (plants, intestinal tract of rodents)	Nosocomial infections[15]
76	**Edwardsiella tarda** EWING and MCWHORTER Asakusa group Bartholomew group	GRAM-negative, small straight rods, 1 µm wide and 2–3 µm long. Motile, with peritrichous flagella. Facultatively anaerobic. Catalase-, indole- and citrate-positive. Oxidase-negative. H_2S is produced	Soil, sewage, water; intestinal tract of animals, rarely found in man	Opportunistic pathogen in man; may cause wound infections, diarrhea, septicemia[16,17]

[1] ANDERSEN et al., *Scand. J. infect. Dis.*, **21**, 181 (1989).
[2] JOHN et al., *Rev. infect. Dis.*, **4**, 13 (1982).
[3] BOUZA et al., *Arch. intern. Med.*, **145**, 1024 (1985).
[4] GALLAGHER, P. G., *Rev. infect. Dis.*, **12**, 808 (1990).
[5] WATANAKUNAKORN and WEBER, *Scand. J. infect. Dis.*, **21**, 1 (1989).
[6] *Med. Lett. Drug. Ther.*, **32**, No. 817 (1990).
[7] CLARK et al., *Diagn. Microbiol. infect. Dis.*, **13**, 467 (1990).
[8] MAKI and MARTIN, *J. infect. Dis.*, **131**, 267 (1975).
[9] YU, V. L., *New Engl. J. Med.*, **300**, 887 (1979).
[10] BROOKS et al., *J. Hyg. (Camb.)*, **82**, 31 (1979).
[11] WATANAKUNAKORN, C., *Scand. J. infect. Dis.*, **21**, 477 (1989).
[12] SAITO et al., *Rev. infect. Dis.*, **11**, 912 (1989).
[13] ARRIBAS et al., *Rev. infect. Dis.*, **12**, 563 (1990).
[14] NAKASHIMA et al., *J. clin. Microbiol.*, **25**, 1014 (1987).
[15] COOKSON et al., *Lancet*, **2**, 1276 (1982).
[16] FARMER and MCWHORTER, in KRIEG and HOLT (Eds.), *Bergey's Manual of Systematic Bacteriology*, Volume 1, Williams & Wilkins, Baltimore, 1984, page 486.
[17] WILSON et al., *Arch. intern. Med.*, **149**, 208 (1989).

No.	Bacterium *Synonyms* Common names	Characteristics	Habitat Host Transmission	Associated disease
77	**Proteus vulgaris** HAUSER	GRAM-negative, straight rods, 0.4–0.8 μm wide and 1–3 μm long. Motile, with peritrichous flagella. Culture on ordinary media; luxuriant growth on solid media. Aerobic, facultatively anaerobic. Some strains show hemolysis on blood agar. See also table below	Soil, sewage, water; intestinal tract in man and animals	Urinary tract infections, wound infections (e.g. burns); septicemia, meningitis. Nosocomial infections predominate[1] *Remarks.* *P. vulgaris* is not as commonly isolated in clinical material as *P. mirabilis*. Treatment with antimicrobial drugs is difficult; susceptibility tests should be performed[2,3]
78	**Proteus mirabilis** HAUSER	Similar to *P. vulgaris*. Indole-negative. See also table below	As for *P. vulgaris*	Urinary tract infections. See also *P. vulgaris* and Table 4 on page 27. May cause diarrhea[4] *Remarks.* For treatment ampicillin has been recommended[3]. Resistance to antimicrobial drugs may be a problem; susceptibility tests should be performed
79	**Providencia stuartii** (BUTTIAUX et al.) EWING *Proteus stuartii* *Proteus inconstans*	GRAM-negative, straight rods, 0.6–0.8 μm wide and 1.5–2.5 μm long. Motile, with peritrichous flagella. No swarming capacity. Aerobic, facultatively anaerobic. See also table below	Soil, sewage, water	Urinary tract infections (especially catheterized patients[5]), wound infections (e.g. burns); septicemia. Nosocomial infections predominate *Remark.* Treatment with antimicrobial drugs is difficult; susceptibility tests should be performed[3]
80	**Providencia rettgeri** (HADLEY et al.) BRENNER et al. *Bacterium rettgeri* *Proteus rettgeri*	Similar to *Providencia stuartii*. See also table below	Soil, sewage, water	As for *Providencia stuartii*
81	**Morganella morganii** (WINSLOW et al.) BRENNER et al. *Bacillus morgani* *Proteus morganii*	GRAM-negative, straight rods, 0.6–0.7 μm wide and 1.0–1.7 μm long. Motile, with peritrichous flagella; above 30 °C, certain strains do not grow flagella. Aerobic, facultatively anaerobic. See also table below	Soil, sewage, water; intestinal tract in man and animals	As for *Providencia stuartii*

[1] PENNER, J. L., in KRIEG and HOLT (Eds.), *Bergey's Manual of Systematic Bacteriology*, Volume 1, Williams & Wilkins, Baltimore, 1984, page 491.
[2] EISENSTEIN, B. I., in MANDELL et al. (Eds.), *Principles and Practice of Infectious Diseases*, 3rd ed., Churchill Livingstone, New York, 1990, page 1658.
[3] *Med. Lett. Drug. Ther.*, **32**, No. 817 (1990).
[4] MÜLLER, H. E., *Zbl. Bakt.*, **272**, 30 (1989).
[5] WARREN, J. W., *Rev. infect. Dis.*, **8**, 61 (1986).

Differential characteristics of Proteus, Providencia *and* Morganella

	Proteus vulgaris	*Proteus mirabilis*	*Providencia stuartii*	*Providencia rettgeri*	*Morganella morganii*
Swarming on moist media	+	+	–	–	[illegible]
H_2S production	+	+	–	–	–
Gelatine liquefaction	+	+	–	–	–
Indole production	+	–	+	+	+
Urease activity	+	+	d	+	+
Lipase activity (corn oil)	d	+	–	–	–
Ornithine decarboxylase activity	d	d	–	–	+
Gas production from glucose	+	+	+	–	d
Acid production from mannitol	–	–	d	+	–
– from maltose	+	–	–	–	–

\+ 90% or more of strains are positive.
– 90% or more of strains are negative.
d 11–89% of strains are positive.

Reference

PENNER, J. L., in KRIEG and HOLT (Eds.), *Bergey's Manual of Systematic Bacteriology*, Volume 1, Williams & Wilkins, Baltimore, 1984, page 491.

No.	**Bacterium** *Synonyms* Common names	Characteristics	Habitat Host Transmission	Associated disease
82	**Yersinia pestis** (LEHMANN and NEUMANN) VAN LOGHEM *Pasteurella pestis* *Bacterium pestis* *Yersinia pseudotuberculosis* (subsp. *pestis*)	GRAM-negative, pleomorphous rods with rounded ends. Nonmotile. Characteristic bipolar staining with methylene blue, carbolfuchsine or carbolthionine solution. Aerobic. Optimal growth at 25–30 °C, retarded at 37 °C. Uncapsulated in animal tissue and serum-agar cultures, envelope formation at 37 °C. See also table below	Rodents, particularly rats. Man. Transmission by fleas	Pathogenic to all rodents and man. For the various plague syndromes in man, see text below
83	**Yersinia pseudotuberculosis** (PFEIFFER) SMITH and THAL *Bacillus pseudotuberculosis* *Yersinia pseudotuberculosis* subsp. *pseudotuberculosis*	GRAM-negative, pleomorphous rods, 0.5–0.8 μm wide and 1–3 μm long. Nonmotile at 37 °C, but motile with peritrichous flagella when grown below 30 °C. Bipolar staining is not a constant feature. Aerobic, facultatively anaerobic. Optimal growth at 25–30 °C. See also table below	Rodents, especially guinea pigs. Enteral route of infection probable	In man[1-4]: fever, mesenteric lymphadenitis, gastroenteritis, invasive ileitis, septicemia, hemolytic uremic syndrome[5], exanthema[6]. Incubation period in an outbreak was 4–9 days
84	**Yersinia enterocolitica** (SCHLEIFSTEIN and COLEMAN) FREDERIKSEN *Bacterium enterocoliticum*	GRAM-negative, pleomorphous rods, 0.5–0.8 μm wide and 1–3 μm long. Nonmotile at 37 °C, but motile with peritrichous flagella when grown below 30 °C. Bipolar staining is not a constant feature. Aerobic, facultatively anaerobic. Optimal growth at 25–30 °C. Detection by polymerase chain reaction[7]. Characterization by biotyping (biogroups)[8] or serotyping (according to O and H antigens)[9]. See also table below	Pigs, cattle, sheep, goats, horses, monkeys, also birds, fishes, frogs. Transmission to man by ingestion of contaminated foods[10] (e.g. outbreaks via raw pork[11], tofu[12]), contaminated water and various milk products	In man[1,10]: fever, mesenteric lymphadenitis, abdominal pain mimicking appendicitis, severe gastroenteritis, invasive ileitis, septicemia, reactive arthritis, erythema, pharyngitis, abscess formation[13]. Incubation period ranges from 1–11 days[10]. Worldwide distribution, especially northern Europe, USA, Japan, Australia

[1] BUTLER, T., in MANDELL et al. (Eds.), *Principles and Practice of Infectious Diseases*, 3rd ed., Churchill Livingstone, New York, 1990, page 1748.
[2] KNAPP, W., *Münch. med. Wschr.*, **121**, 239 (1979).
[3] ATTWOOD et al., *Lancet*, **1**, 529 (1987).
[4] TOBIN et al., *J. roy. Soc. Med.*, **81**, 423 (1988).
[5] DAVENPORT and FINN, *Lancet*, **1**, 358 (1988).
[6] NAKANO et al., *Scand. J. infect. Dis.*, **21**, 175 (1989).
[7] THORPE et al., *Lancet*, **337**, 496 (1991).
[8] WAUTERS et al., *Contr. Microbiol. Immunol.*, **9**, 14 (1987).
[9] WAUTERS, G., in BOTTONE, E. J. (Ed.), *Yersinia enterocolitica*, CRC Press, Boca Raton, FL, 1981, page 41.
[10] COVER and ABER, *New Engl. J. Med.*, **321**, 16 (1989).
[11] LEE et al., *J. infect. Dis.*, **163**, 660 (1991).
[12] *Morb. Mort. wkly Rep.*, **31**, 562 (1982).
[13] ALBRECHT et al., *Dtsch. med. Wschr.*, **116**, 331 (1991).

Differential characteristics of several species of the genus Yersinia *and* Pasteurella multocida

	Yersinia pestis	*Yersinia enterocolitica*	*Yersinia pseudotuberculosis*	*Pasteurella multocida*
Motility	–	+ (at 22 °C)	+ (at 22 °C)	–
Growth on MCCONKEY agar	+	+	+	–
Growth at 5 °C	–	+	–	–
Urease activity	–	+	+	–
Ornithin decarboxylase activity	–	+	–	+
Indole production	–	variable	–	+
Acid production from sucrose	–	+	–	+
Esculin hydrolysis	+	–	+	–

Reference

CHEN, T. H., in BRAUDE et al. (Eds.), *Infectious Diseases and Medical Microbiology*, 2nd ed., Saunders, Philadelphia, 1986, page 333.

Plague

The regions where wild plague is endemic among rodents and where, as a result, the disease is often seen to recur in man (either in isolated individuals or in groups) are at present the southern and western part of the USA, South Africa, southeastern Russia, Central Asia and South America[1,2]. In 1989, 770 cases were reported from 11 countries (see table below)[3]. In 1991, 10 cases were reported from the USA[11].

The transmission of plague among rodents, and from the domestic rat (*Rattus rattus*) and the sewer rat (*Rattus norvegicus*) to man occurs almost exclusively via fleas, children under 16 years of age being particularly affected[4,5]. Man-to-man direct transmission of uncomplicated bubonic plague does not occur. The disease can also be transmitted via catscratch lesions[6]. Pneumonic plague is highly contagious.

The *incubation period* is 2–8 days for bubonic plague, 1–2 days for primary pneumonic plague. Onset is sudden and characterized by fever, rigor, severe headaches and acute pain in the limbs. One of the manifestations of bubonic plague is swelling of the lymph nodes (distribution: groin ca. 70%, axilla 20% and, in children especially,

No.	**Bacterium** *Synonyms* Common names	Characteristics	Habitat Host Transmission	Associated disease
85	**Kluyvera ascorbata** FARMER et al.	GRAM-negative, small rods, 0.5 to 0.7 µm wide and 2–3 µm long. Motile, with scant peritrichous flagella. Aerobic, facultatively anaerobic. Acid production from glucose and L-ascorbate. Catalase- and indole-positive, oxidase-negative	Water, sewage, soil, foodstuffs	Infrequent opportunistic pathogen in man. Peritonitis[1] and urinary tract infections[2] in children
86	**Ewingella americana** Enteric group 40	GRAM-negative rods. Acid production from lactose. Lipase-negative	No environmental source known; isolated from respiratory tract or blood[3]	Nosocomial infections[4]

[1] YOGEV and KOZLOWSKI, *Rev. infect. Dis.*, **12**, 399 (1990).
[2] DOLLBERG et al., *Europ. J. clin. Microbiol. infect. Dis.*, **9**, 281 (1990).
[3] FARMER et al., *J. clin. Microbiol.*, **21**, 46 (1985).
[4] PIEN and BRUCE, *Arch. intern. Med.*, **146**, 111 (1986).

Number of plague cases reported between 1975 and 1989[3]

Year	Africa		USA and South America		Asia		Europe		World total	
	Cases	Deaths	Cases	Deaths	Cases	Deaths	Cases	Deaths	Cases	Deaths
1975	147	41	521	9	811	52	–	–	1479	102
1976	93	35	146	9	1266	60	–	–	1505	104
1977	172	41	48	11	1258	26	–	–	1478	78
1978	203	15	97	5	485	14	–	–	785	34
1979	251	15	23	2	387	16	–	–	661	33
1980	86	22	142	7	283	29	–	–	551	58
1981	59	19	128	12	13	0	–	–	200	31
1982	290	43	182	4	281	1	–	–	753	48
1983	594	59	225	12	248	21	–	–	1067	92
1984	650	59	500	42	196	6	–	–	1346	107
1985	215	41	128	9	143	8	–	–	486	58
1986	729	90	162	19	112	6	–	–	1003	115
1987	853	198	88	9	114	8	–	–	1055	215
1988	1109	138	52	5	202	10	–	–	1363	153
1989	315	55	30	0	423	48	2*	1*	770	104

* Kazakhstan.

submaxilla 10%[4]); oval swellings vary from 1–10 cm in length[1]. Heart rate increases to 110–140 min^{-1} and blood pressure is characteristically low (~100/60 mmHg) due to extreme vasodilatation[1]. The early features of primary pneumonic plague are dyspnea, cyanosis, heavy cough with occasional expectoration of hemorrhagic sputum and circulatory collapse.

Remarks. Vaccination with a commercially available vaccine is recommended for persons exposed to possible plague infection[7].

Rapid diagnosis of suspected plague infection may be difficult. Confirmation by culture of *Y. pestis* from appropriate clinical specimens usually requires 36–72 hours[8]. Rapid presumptive diagnosis of plague can be obtained by staining smears of appropriate material[2,8]. The value of an enzyme-linked immunosorbent assay has been discussed[9].

Because of the high mortality and risk of pneumonic transmission when treatment of plague is delayed, presumptive antimicrobial therapy should be instituted urgently on clinical and epidemiologic grounds without awaiting bacteriologic confirmation[2]. Streptomycin is the drug of choice, with a tetracycline as the first alternative[1,10].

References

[1] BUTLER, T., in MANDELL et al. (Eds.), *Principles and Practice of Infectious Diseases*, 3rd ed., Churchill Livingstone, New York, 1990, page 1748.
[2] KISCH, A. L., in BRAUDE et al. (Eds.), *Infectious Diseases and Medical Microbiology*, 2nd ed., Saunders, Philadelphia, 1986, page 1506.
[3] *Wkly epidem. Rec.*, **65**, 321 (1990).
[4] MANSON-BAHR and BELL (Eds.), *Manson's Tropical Diseases*, 19th ed., Saunders, Philadelphia, 1988.
[5] MANN et al., *Pediatrics*, **69**, 762 (1982).
[6] WENIGER et al., *J. Amer. med. Ass.*, **251**, 927 (1984).
[7] *Morb. Mort. wkly Rep.*, **37**, 653 (1988).
[8] MANN et al., *J. Amer. med. Ass.*, **251**, 953 (1984).
[9] WILLIAMS et al., *Bull. Wld Hlth Org.*, **66**, 77 (1988).
[10] *Med. Lett. Drug. Ther.*, **32**, No. 817 (1990).
[11] *Morb. Mort. wkly Rep.*, **40**, No. 52, 898 (1991).

No.	**Bacterium** *Synonyms* Common names	Characteristics	Habitat Host Transmission	Associated disease
87	**Vibrio cholerae** SPACINI Cholera vibrio Comma bacillus	GRAM-negative, slightly curved rods, 0.5–0.8 µm wide and 1.4 to 2.6 µm long. Very motile, with a single polar flagella. Primary smear: fish-shoal-like arrangement of cells. Grows well in alkaline peptone water. Growth at 40 °C. No absolute requirement for NaCl. Oxidase-positive. Utilization of sucrose and 2-oxoglutarate. Aerobic, facultatively anaerobic. For differentiation of the biovars, see Table 1 on next page. Produces a potent enterotoxin (choleragen)[1]	Marine environment (surface waters, estuaries). Intestinal tract of infected persons. For transmission, see text on next page	Cholera (serovar O1). See text on next page. Gastroenteritis, occasionally extra-intestinal infections (serovar non-O1)[2]
88	**Vibrio parahaemolyticus** (FUJINO et al.) SAKAZAKI et al. *Pasteurella parahaemolytica* *Beneckea parahaemolytica*	GRAM-negative, straight rods, 0.5–0.8 µm wide and 1.4–2.6 µm long. Motile, with lateral flagella on solid medium. Growth at 40 °C. Culture still possible in an 8% NaCl solution. Oxidase-positive. Utilization of ethanol, but not of sucrose. Aerobic, facultatively anaerobic. Usually KANAGAWA positive (hemolytic for human erythrocytes). Produces enterotoxin	Marine environment (surface waters, estuaries). Transmission by ingestion of raw or undercooked seafood	Food-borne gastroenteritis. Particularly common in Japan. Rarely reported from the USA and other countries[2]. Incubation period may be as short as 2.5 hours (mean: 15 hours)[3]. Rarely wound infections[4]
89	**Vibrio vulnificus** (REICHELT et al.) FARMER *Beneckea vulnifica*	GRAM-negative, slightly curved rods, 0.5–0.8 µm wide and 1.4 to 2.6 µm long. Growth at 40 °C. Culture still possible in a 6% NaCl solution. Oxidase- and lactose-positive. Produces enterotoxin	Marine environment (surface waters, estuaries). Transmission by ingestion of raw or undercooked seafood	Primary septicemia, commonly associated with liver disease[2,5]; wound infections[2,4]. Mean incubation period for septicemia after ingestion of raw oysters 83 hours[2]. Rarely gastroenteritis[6], sporadic cases of meningitis[7], osteomyelitis[8] *Remark*. Treatment with a tetracycline or benzylpenicillin[9]
90	Other *Vibrio* species of clinical importance: see table below	Morphologically similar to other *Vibrio* species	Marine environment (surface waters, estuaries). Transmission by ingestion of raw or undercooked seafood	

[1] LENTNER, C. (Ed.), *Geigy Scientific Tables*, 8th ed., Vol. 4, Ciba-Geigy Ltd., Basel, 1986, page 201.
[2] JANDA et al., *Clin. Microbiol. Rev.*, **1**, 245 (1988).
[3] FINKELSTEIN, R. A., in BARON, S. (Ed.), *Medical Microbiology*, 2nd ed., Addison-Wesley, Menlo Park, CA, 1986, page 473.
[4] PLOTKIN et al., *J. infect. Dis.*, **161**, 364 (1990).
[5] HOFFMANN et al., *Arch. intern. Med.*, **148**, 1825 (1988).
[6] JOHNSTON et al., *Amer. J. Med.*, **80**, 336 (1986).
[7] KATZ, B. Z., *Pediatrics*, **82**, 784 (1988).
[8] VARTIAN and SEPTIMUS, *J. infect. Dis.*, **161**, 363 (1990).
[9] *Med. Lett. Drug. Ther.*, **32**, No. 817 (1990).

Anatomical distribution of Vibrio *species recovered from man**

	Sites of recovery (frequency)
V. cholerae O1	Gastrointestinal tract (97%)
V. cholerae non-O1	Gastrointestinal tract (49%), blood (22%), ear (13%)
V. mimicus	Gastrointestinal tract (81%), ear (15%)
V. hollisae	Gastrointestinal tract (94%)
V. damsela	Wounds (100%)
V. fluvialis	Gastrointestinal tract (100%)
V. furnissii	Gastrointestinal tract (94%)
V. alginolyticus	Wounds (42%), ear (34%), respiratory tract (11%)
V. parahaemolyticus	Gastrointestinal tract (90%)
V. vulnificus	Blood (66%), wounds (24%)
V. metschnikovii	Blood◊
V. cincinnatiensis	Blood◊

* Based on isolates submitted to the Centers for Disease Control, Atlanta, GA, USA.
◊ Only one clinical isolate of each species recovered.

Reference

JANDA et al., *Clin. Microbiol. Rev.*, **1**, 245 (1988).

Cholera

Vibrio cholera possesses heat labile flagellar (H) and heat stable somatic (O) antigens. On the basis of its O antigens, *V. cholerae* can be subdivided into 72 serovars or more[1]. The serovar O1 – all strains responsible for pandemic and epidemic cholera fall into this serovar – can be divided into 2 biovars (for characteristics, see Table 1) or into 3 serologic subtypes (Ogawa, Inaba, Hikojima)[1,2]:

Biovar	El Tor			Classical		
Serologic subtype	Ogawa	Inaba	(Hikojima)	Ogawa	Inaba	(Hikojima)
O antigens	A,B	A,C	(A,B,C)	A,B	A,C	(A,B,C)

Table 1 *Characteristics of the biovars of* Vibrio cholerae[1]

	Classical biovar	El Tor biovar
Hemolysis	–	±*
(Sheep erythrocytes, brain-heart-thioglycolate-cystine agar)		
Hemagglutination	–	+
(Chicken erythrocytes, slide test)		
Sensitivity to		
– polymyxin B (50 IU)	+	–
– classical phage IV..................	+	–
– El Tor phage V.....................	–	+

* Original El Tor strains were very hemolytic, those isolated in recent years have been poorly hemolytic or even nonhemolytic.

Over the last 25 years, the El Tor biovar has replaced the classical biotype as the main pathogen of cholera; the classical biovar was earlier endemic in the Ganges and Brahmaputra deltas as well as in certain areas of Indonesia and Burma. The biotype El Tor spread from Sulawesi in 1961 to South-East Asia (1963), India (1964), to the Middle East (1965–1966), eastern Europe/southern Russia (1970), West Africa (1971), North Africa (1972), and even to East Africa and southern Europe (Italy, Portugal)[3,4]. Since 1982, the classical cholera pathogen has again been found in rapidly increasing numbers in Bangladesh; during the epidemic in 1982, 90% of isolates were of the classical biovar of *V. cholerae*[5]. An epidemic starting in Peru in 1991 has been due to the biovar El Tor, serologic subtype Inaba[6].

Unreliability in the reporting of cholera cases makes it difficult to give accurate incidence data, but an annual incidence in the world can be assumed to be more than a million[7].

Transmission occurs by the fecal–oral route; usually by ingestion of water contaminated with human feces. Less commonly by contaminated food – increasingly reported after ingestion of raw oysters and other seafood[8]. Man-to-man transmission is unusual because of the high inoculum required (e.g. 10^8 to 10^{10} organisms)[9].

The *incubation period* is usually 1–2 days[7]. The extent and duration of water and electrolyte losses (Table 2) – mainly due to the production of the enterotoxin choleragen – as well as the severity of circulatory shock determine the fate of the patient (Table 3). A healthy person may become hypotensive within an hour of the onset of symptoms and may die within 2–3 hours if no treatment is provided[10].

Remarks. Replacement of water and electrolyte losses is of vital importance. Solutions can be administered orally[10,11] or intravenously[10,12]. Antibiotics will shorten the duration of diarrhea and thereby shorten the fluid loss. A tetracycline is the drug of choice in most instances; alternative drugs are trimethoprim–sulfamethoxazole, ciprofloxacin, etc.[10,13]. Prophylactic immunization by a parenteral vaccine has been available for nearly 100 years; its use is not encouraged because of short-lasting immunity (3–6 months) and significant side effects[7]. Therefore, in 1988 WHO eliminated the requirement of cholera vaccine for travellers[14]. A live attenuated cholera vaccine (deleted by the virulent A-subunit of the enterotoxin) is in trial[15].

Table 2 *Composition of cholera stool**[10]

	Na^+	K^+	Cl^-	HCO_3^-
	mmol/L			
Adults	135	15	100	45
Children	105	25	90	30

* Daily purging rate related to body mass 50 mL/kg or more.

References

1 BAUMANN et al., in KRIEG and HOLT (Eds.), *Bergey's Manual of Systematic Bacteriology*, Vol. 1, Williams & Wilkins, Baltimore, 1984, page 518.
2 FINKELSTEIN, R. A., in BARON, S. (Ed.), *Medical Microbiology*, 2nd ed., Addison-Wesley, Menlo Park, CA, 1986, page 473.
3 Editorial, *Lancet*, **2**, 601 (1973).
4 MANSON-BAHR and BELL (Eds.), *Manson's Tropical Diseases*, 19th ed., Saunders, London, 1987.
5 SAMADI et al., *Lancet*, **1**, 805 (1983).
6 *Morb. Mort. wkly Rep.*, **40**, 108 (1991).
7 BUTLER and SACK, in WARREN and MAHMOUD (Eds.), *Tropical and Geographical Medicine*, 2nd ed., McGraw-Hill, New York, 1990, page 745.
8 LOWRY et al., *Arch. intern. Med.*, **149**, 2079 (1989); *Morb. Mort. wkly Rep.*, **40**, 225 (1991); *Morb. Mort. wkly Rep.*, **40**, 287 (1991).
9 MURRAY et al., *Medical Microbiology*, Wolfe, London, 1990, page 127.
10 GREENOUGH, W. B., in MANDELL et al. (Eds.), *Principles and Practice of Infectious Diseases*, 3rd ed., Churchill Livingstone, New York, 1990, page 1636.
11 CASTEEL and FIEDOREK, *Pediat. Clin. N. Amer.*, **37**, 295 (1990).
12 KALLEN, R. J., *Pediat. Clin. N. Amer.*, **37**, 265 (1990).
13 *Med. Lett. Drug. Ther.*, **32**, No. 817 (1990).
14 WOLFE, M. S., *Pediat. Clin. N. Amer.*, **37**, 757 (1990).
15 BART and LIN, *Pediat. Clin. N. Amer.*, **37**, 735 (1990).

Table 3 *Symptoms and signs of cholera correlated with severity of dehydration*[7]

	Mild form	Moderate form	Severe form
Symptoms...	Thirst	Thirst, weakness, lethargy, shortness of breath	Prostration, obtundation, labored breathing
Signs of dehydration	None	Dry mucous membranes, loss of skin turgor	Marked dryness of mucous membranes, loss of skin turgor
Heart rate..	Normal	Increased	Greatly increased
Blood pressure	Normal	Diminished with orthostatic changes	More diminished or absent
Respiration...	Normal	Hyperpnea	KUSSMAUL's respiration

No.	Bacterium *Synonyms* Common names	Characteristics	Habitat Host Transmission	Associated disease
91	**Aeromonas hydrophila** (CHESTER) STANIER *Bacillus hydrophilus*	GRAM-negative, straight rods, 0.3–1.0 µm wide and 1.0–3.5 µm long, with rounded edges. Motile, with single polar flagellum, peritrichous flagella may be formed on solid media. Facultatively anaerobic. Oxidase- and catalase-positive. Acid and gas production from glucose. Some types of *Aeromonas* produce enterotoxins which are thermolabile and can be neutralized by cholera antitoxins	Water, sewage, seafood	In man[1,2]: (1) wound infection related to exposure to water or soil; (2) gastroenteritis (acute diarrheal syndrome of short duration, travellers' diarrhea[3]); (3) septicemia, mostly in association with hematologic malignancies, solid tumors, hepatic dysfunction, hepatobiliary disorders and traumatic injuries; (4) other infections (osteomyelitis, peritonitis, cholecystitis, obstetric gynecologic infections, meningitis, otitis, ocular infections, endocarditis) *Remark*. Treatment usually with trimethoprim–sulfamethoxazole or gentamicin[2,4,5]
92	Other motile *Aeromonas* species of clinical importance: **Aeromonas caviae**[6] **Aeromonas veronii** biogroup **sobria** (formerly *Aeromonas sobria*)[6,7] **Aeromonas jahdaei**[7,8]	Similar to *A. hydrophilia*	Water, sewage, seafood	Gastroenteritis, wound infection
93	**Plesiomonas shigelloides** (BADER) HABS and SCHUBERT *Pseudomonas shigelloides*	GRAM-negative, straight rods, 0.8–1.0 µm wide and 3.0 µm long. Motile, with polar flagella. Facultatively anaerobic. Oxidase-, catalase- and indole-positive, H_2S- and urease-negative. Acid production from glucose	Fishes, pigs, dogs, cats, goats, sheep and monkeys. Transmission via direct contact or, indirectly, via contaminated water and seafood	In man[1,9,10]: gastroenteritis, very rarely septicemia, meningitis, osteomyelitis
94	**Pasteurella multocida** (LEHMANN and NEUMANN) ROSENBUSCH and MERCHANT *Pasteurella gallicida* *Bacterium multocidum*	GRAM-negative, small, pleomorphous rods, frequently showing bipolar staining. Nonmotile. Good growth on usual media (but not MACCONKEY agar), preferably with addition of blood. Aerobic. Catalase- and oxidase-positive. Optimal growth at 37 °C. See table on page 34, for differentiation from *Yersinia* spp.	Worldwide distribution. Isolated from the nasopharynx or gastrointestinal tract of many domestic and wild animals (e.g. dogs, cats – including lions and tigers, swine, cattle) and birds. Transmission by animal bites in most cases of human infection	In man[11–13]: (1) focal soft tissue infection after animal contact; (2) chronic respiratory infections; (3) septicemia with or without metastatic lesions. Local complication of infected bites includes osteomyelitis, tenosynovitis, arthritis. Rarely brain abscess (children), endocarditis, meningitis[14] *Remark*. For treatment, benzylpenicillin is the drug of choice[5,13]
95	**Haemophilus influenzae** (LEHMANN and NEUMANN) WINSLOW et al. *Bacterium influenzae* Influenza bacillus PFEIFFER's bacillus	GRAM-negative, pleomorphic rods, 0.3–0.5 µm wide and 0.5 to 3.0 µm long. Nonmotile. Aerobic, facultatively anaerobic. No growth on ordinary agar, requires X and V factor for growth. Symbiotic growth with other bacteria, e.g. staphylococci. See also table on next page	Respiratory tract, to a lesser extent conjunctiva and genital surfaces	Meningitis, respiratory tract infections, etc., predominantly during childhood. See text on next page
96	**Haemophilus aegyptius** (TREVISAN) PITTMAN and DAVIS *Bacillus aegyptius* KOCH–WEEKS bacillus	Similar to *H. influenzae*. See table on next page	Conjunctiva	Conjunctivitis in warm countries. Rare in temperate zones. Brazilian purpuric fever, an often fatal childhood illness[15,16]

[1] MCGOWAN and DEL RIO, in MANDELL et al. (Eds.), *Principles and Practice of Infectious Diseases*, 3rd ed., Churchill Livingstone, New York, 1990, page 1782.
[2] SIRE et al., *Europ. J. clin. Microbiol. infect. Dis.*, **9**, 904 (1990).
[3] GRACEY et al., *Brit. med. J.*, **289**, 658 (1984).
[4] ALTWEGG and GEISS, *CRC Crit. Rev. Microbiol.*, **16**, 253 (1989).
[5] *Med. Lett. Drug. Ther.*, **32**, No. 817 (1990).
[6] GEISS et al., *Immun. Infekt.*, **16**, 115 (1988).
[7] JOSEPH et al., *J. clin. Microbiol.*, **29**, 565 (1991).
[8] CARNAHAN et al., *J. clin. Microbiol.*, **29**, 560 (1991).
[9] REINHARDT and GEORGE, *J. Amer. med. Ass.*, **253**, 3294 (1985).
[10] *Morb. Mort. wkly Rep.*, **38**, 617 (1989).
[11] WEBER et al., *Medicine (Baltimore)*, **63**, 133 (1984).
[12] RYAN, J. L., in BRAUDE et al. (Eds.), *Infectious Diseases and Medical Microbiology*, 2nd ed., Saunders, Philadelphia, 1986, page 1499.
[13] BOYCE, J. M., in MANDELL et al. (Eds.), *Principles and Practice of Infectious Diseases*, 3rd ed., Churchill Livingstone, New York, 1990, page 1746.
[14] KUMAR et al., *Rev. infect. Dis.*, **12**, 440 (1990).
[15] Editorial, *Lancet*, **2**, 761 (1987).
[16] MCINTYRE et al., *Lancet*, **2**, 112 (1987).

No.	Bacterium *Synonyms* Common names	Characteristics	Habitat Host Transmission	Associated disease
97	**Haemophilus ducreyi** (Neveu-Lemaire) Bergey et al. *Coccobacillus ducreyi* Ducrey's bacillus	Gram-negative, slender, noncapsulated rods, 0.5 µm wide and 1.5–2.0 µm long. Nonmotile. Located both intra- and extracellularly, often forming parallel chains between cells. Requires X factor and 5% CO_2 for growth. See also table below	External genitalia of infected persons	Chancroid (soft chancre, ulcus molle). See text on next page
98	**Haemophilus parainfluenzae** Rivers	Similar to *H. influenzae*. Requires V factor but not X factor for growth. See table below	Upper respiratory tract, genital surfaces	Usually nonpathogenic, but may cause infections similar to those of *H. influenzae*
98a	Other *Haemophilus* species of clinical importance: **Haemophilus parahaemolyticus** **Haemophilus haemolyticus**	Similar to *H. influenzae*	Upper respiratory tract Upper respiratory tract	Rare cause of infections similar to those of *H. influenzae* Pathogenicity not reported

Differential characteristics of Haemophilus *species*[1,2]

	H. influenzae	*H. aegyptius*	*H. ducreyi*	*H. parainfluenzae*
Requirement				
– of X factor*	+	+	+	–
– of V factor◊	+	+	–	+
Growth enhanced by CO_2	–	–	+	–
Indole production	+	–	–	–
Hemolysis	–	–	+/–	–

\+ 90% or more of strains are positive.
– 90% or more of strains are negative.
+/– Some strains show weak β-hemolysis.
* Hemin or protoporphyrin IX.
◊ NAD, NADP or the nucleosides.

References
1 Mannheim et al., *Zbl. Bakt.*, **272**, 87 (1989).
2 Kilian and Biberstein, in Krieg and Holt (Eds.), *Bergey's Manual of Systematic Bacteriology*, Volume 1, Williams & Wilkins, Baltimore, 1984, page 558.

Haemophilus influenzae infections

The majority of *H. influenzae* strains can be assigned to 6 biovars on the basis of biochemical characteristics[1]. The organisms may be noncapsulated (nontypable) or capsulated; according to capsular polysaccharide structures 6 serovars (a–f) have been identified. The relationship between biovars and capsular serovars is given in Table 1.

Haemophilus species most commonly colonize the upper respiratory tract and are indigenous to man. Virtually all individuals aged 1 year or more are carriers of one or more *Haemophilus* species (Table 2), and up to 80% of healthy persons are carriers of *H. influenzae*[3,4]. In the USA, children under 6 months of age are rarely colonized, whereas early, heavy colonization of infants may be common in developing countries[3,5]. Colonization with noncapsulated strains predominate and only 3–5% of healthy persons in the USA and the United Kingdom are colonized with *H. influenzae* serovar b; the frequency of colonization with serovar b in developing countries seems to be higher[6,7] (Table 3).

H. influenzae is transmitted by respiratory droplets or occasionally by direct contagion with secretions.

Capsulated strains of *H. influenzae*, notably 9 clones of serovar b[8], are a major cause of meningitis and other systemic infections in young children in many parts of the world (Table 4), the incidence being highest in children less than 5 years of age[9,10]. In developing countries, the mortality from meningitis may be as high as 40%[7]. In noninvasive disease, mainly caused by noncapsulated strains, the organisms extend from their normal site of colonization; these infections are generally not associated with bacteremia[3,4,7].

Confirmation of provisional clinical diagnosis of meningitis, epiglottitis, septic arthritis, etc. requires isolation of the pathogen by culture of blood, CSF or other body fluids. Detection of capsular polysaccharide in serum, CSF or concentrated urine by immunoelectrophoresis, latex agglutination or enzyme-linked immunosorbent assay may be diagnostic and can be found in 90% of culture-proven cases of meningitis[4].

Immunity and prophylaxis. Human immunity to *H. influenzae* serovar b (Hib) is mediated by humoral antibodies against the capsular polysaccharide polyribosylribitol phosphate (PRP) and all the vaccines against Hib are designed to induce antibodies against PRP[11]. Vaccines derived from PRP alone (polysaccharide vaccines) have not been effective in children less than 18 months old[11,12]. The

(Continued on next page)

Table 1 *Relationship between biovar and capsular serovar of 423 clinical isolates of* Haemophilus influenzae[1]

Biovar	Non-capsulated strains	Capsulated strains Total	a	b	c	d	e	f
I	32	195	3	182	0	0	0	10
II	75	12	0	8	3	0	0	1
III	59	0	0	0	0	0	0	0
IV	12	22	0	4	0	8	10	0
V	16	0	0	0	0	0	0	0

Table 2 *Nasopharyngeal carriage of* Haemophilus *species in children**[2]

	% of total *Haemophilus* isolates
H. influenzae	49
H. parainfluenzae	25
H. haemolyticus	12
H. parahaemolyticus	11
V factor-independent species	3

* 130 hospitalized Danish children aged 1–7 years (colonization close to 100%).

Table 3 *Nasopharyngeal carriage of* Haemophilus influenzae *in children in various populations*[7]

	Non-capsulated strains	Capsulated strains		
		Serovar		
		a	b	Other
	%			
Alaska (Eskimos)				
< 3 years	–	–	5	–
Papua New Guinea				
2 weeks to 5 years	51	11	10	28
6 months to 5 years	74	7	5	14
Gambia				
< 5 years	65	3	0–33	11
USA				
< 1 year	13	0.7	0.6	2
1 year	24	0.6	2	4
2 years	23	0.3	6	6
3 years	15	0.8	6	7
4 years	19	0	1	2
< 5 years	19	2	9	9

Table 4 *Pathogenicity of* Haemophilus influenzae[3,4,7]

Clinical manifestation of pathogenicity	*H. influenzae* strains
Systemic infections (commonly in young children) Meningitis Epiglottitis Cellulitis Empyema Pericarditis Septic arthritis Osteomyelitis Tissue abscess Occult bacteremia	Serovar b strains
Noninvasive infections (commonly in adults) Acute or chronic respiratory tract infections Otitis media Sinusitis Urinary tract infection	Mainly noncapsulated, rarely non-serovar b strains
Pneumonia	Serovar b, noncapsulated or non-serovar b strains

Table 5 *Characteristics of* Haemophilus influenzae *serovar b conjugate vaccines*[11–14]

Vaccine	Polysaccharide	Carrier protein	Linkage
PRP-D	Heat-sized (M_r 200–2000)	Diphtheria toxoid	6-carbon spacer
HbOC	20-unit oligosaccharide	CRM 197 mutant *Corynebacterium diphtheriae* protein	No spacer
PRP-OMP	Native polysaccharide	*Neisseria meningitidis* outer membrane protein complex	Complex thioether
PRP-T	Native polysaccharide	Tetanus toxoid	6-carbon spacer

immunogenicity of the vaccines has been improved by covalent linkage (conjugation) of PRP with T-cell dependent protein antigens. Conjugate vaccines differ by polysaccharide size, carrier protein and method of chemical conjugation (Table 5). In 1990, the US Food and Drug Administration stated that a specific (HbOC) conjugate vaccine was safe and effective for administration to infants beginning at 2 months of age[13]. Recommendations for immunization of infants and children have been published in 1991 by the Immunization Practices Advisory Committee[12] and by the American Academy of Pediatrics[13].

Remarks. Resistance to ampicillin (especially β-lactamase mediated) or/and chloramphenicol is often a problem[15] and susceptibility tests should be performed. For treatment of systemic diseases, cefotaxime or ceftriaxone have been recommended[16]. Chloramphenicol plus ampicillin can be used initially for treatment of meningitis in children more than 1 month old until the organism is identified and susceptibility is determined[4,16]. For treatment of upper respiratory tract infections and bronchitis, ampicillin or amoxicillin are the drugs of choice, but a variety of other antimicrobial drugs have been listed as alternatives[16].

References

1 KILIAN and BIBERSTEIN, in KRIEG and HOLT (Eds.), *Bergey's Manual of Systematic Bacteriology*, Vol. 1, Williams & Wilkins, Baltimore, 1984, page 558.
2 KILIAN et al., *Acta path. microbiol. scand.*, Section B, **80**, 571 (1972).
3 MOXON and WILSON, *Rev. infect. Dis.*, **13**, Suppl. 6, S518 (1991).
4 MOXON, E. R., in MANDELL et al. (Eds.), *Principles and Practice of Infectious Diseases*, 3rd ed., Churchill Livingstone, New York, 1990, page 1722.
5 SHANN et al., *Lancet*, **2**, 537 (1984).
6 BIJLMER et al., *Trans. roy. Soc. trop. Med. Hyg.*, **83**, 831 (1989).
7 FUNKHOUSER et al., *Rev. infect. Dis.*, **13**, Suppl. 6, S542 (1991).
8 MUSSER et al., *Rev. infect. Dis.*, **12**, 75 (1990).
9 COCHI et al., *J. Amer. med. Ass.*, **253**, 521 (1985).
10 PELTOLA et al., *Rev. infect. Dis.*, **12**, 708 (1990).
11 SHAPIRO, E. D., *Pediat. Clin. N. Amer.*, **37**, 567 (1990).
12 *Mort. Morb. wkly Rep.*, **40**, RR-1 (1991).
13 PETER et al., Committee on Infectious Diseases, *Pediatrics*, **88**, 169 (1991).
14 KÄYHTY et al., *Amer. J. Dis. Child.*, **145**, 223 (1991).
15 NEEDHAM, C. A., *Clin. Microbiol. Rev.*, **1**, 218 (1988).
16 *Med. Lett. Drug. Ther.*, **32**, No. 817 (1990).

Chancroid

Taxonomic position of *Haemophilus ducreyi* has not been settled[1], e.g. there is lack of significant DNA hybridization with other *Haemophilus* species and higher requirement of X factor. Essentially *H. ducreyi* does not utilize sugars, but extensively produces aminopeptidases. See table for differential characteristics of *Haemophilus* spp.

Chancroid can be found worldwide, the number of cases exceed that of syphilis[2]. Until the 1970s it was thought that the occurrence of chancroid was limited to tropical countries and that only a few cases were introduced into temperate countries[3]. An increasing number of cases, sometimes of epidemic proportions, have been reported in temperate regions, such as northwestern Europe (i.e. Britain[2,4], Netherlands, France, Germany) and North America[5,6].

Chancroid is transmitted almost exclusively by sexual intercourse. The *incubation period* in men ranges from 2 to 35 days, with a mean of 7 days[1]; in women it is probably similar to men. The portal entry of *H. ducreyi* is a break in the integrity of the epithelium. Within 2 or 3 days a pustula forms that soon ruptures, resulting in a sharply circumscribed ulcer. Tender, regional lymphadenopathy is characteristic and occurs in about half of the patients a few days after the primary lesion[7]. The isolation of the pathogen is essential for diagnosis, this can be done with special culture media and appropriate incubation. A satisfactory serological method is not yet available[1,5].

Remarks. Resistance to penicillins and ampicillin because of β-lactamase production is common. Erythromycin or ceftriaxone are the drugs of choice[8,9]. Sexual partners must be treated as well[7].

References

1 JESSAMINE and RONALD, *Med. Clin. N. Amer.*, **74**, 1417 (1990).
2 Editorial, *Lancet*, **2**, 747 (1982).
3 NEUBERT, U., *Münch. med. Wschr.*, **124**, 15 (1982).
4 MCENTEGAST et al., *J. Hyg. (Camb.)*, **89**, 467 (1982).
5 MORSE, S. A., *Clin. Microbiol. Rev.*, **2**, 137 (1989).
6 SCHMID et al., *J. Amer. med. Ass.*, **258**, 3265 (1987).
7 HAND, W. L., in MANDELL et al. (Eds.), *Principles and Practice of Infections Diseases*, 3rd ed., Churchill Livingstone, New York, 1990, page 1729.
8 *Med. Lett. Drug. Ther.*, **33**, No. 860 (1991).
9 SCHMID, G. P., *Rev. infect. Dis.*, **12**, Suppl. 6, S580 (1990).

No.	**Bacterium** *Synonyms* Common names	Characteristics	Habitat Host Transmission	Associated disease
99	**Actinobacillus lignieresii** BRUMPT	GRAM-negative. In young cultures small and rod-like, in older cultures a more coccoid form. Streptobacillary forms in serum broth. Nonmotile. Often bipolar staining. Aerobic, facultatively anaerobic. Grows at 20–39 °C. Optimal growth at 37 °C. No growth at 44 °C	Cattle and sheep	Actinobacillosis of cattle and sheep. Very rarely responsible for infections in man
100	**Actinobacillus actinomycetemcomitans** (KLINGER) TOPLEY and WILSON *Bacterium actinomycetem comitans*	GRAM-negative, spherical or rod-shaped cells in dense masses. Nonmotile. Growth promoted by addition of blood or serum. Aerobic, facultatively anaerobic	Part of the normal flora of the mouth. Isolated from lesions in actinomycosis, of which it is the commonest associate	Pathogen of periodontitis. Rare cause of acute endocarditis, wound infections, meningitis, osteomyelitis, urinary tract infections[1]
101	**Chromobacterium violaceum** BERGONZINI	GRAM-negative rods, 0.6–0.9 µm wide and 1.5–3.0 µm long. Bipolar staining. Motile. Aerobic, facultatively anaerobic. Oxidase- and catalase-positive. Growth at 10–37 °C, optimal growth at 25 °C. Formation of a violet pigment not soluble in water and chloroform, but soluble in ethanol. No growth at 4 °C	Water and soil, mainly in tropical areas	Septicemia, urinary tract infection, abscess formation reported[2]
102	**Cardiobacterium hominis** SLOTNICK and DOUGHERTY	GRAM-negative rods, 0.5–0.75 µm wide and 1.0–3.0 µm long, with rounded ends. Nonmotile. Oxidase-positive, catalase-negative. No growth on MACCONKEY agar. Facultatively anaerobic. CO_2 required for culture	Part of the normal flora of the nose and pharynx	Endocarditis, meningitis reported[2–4]
103	**Calymmatobacterium granulomatis** ARAGÃO and VIANNA	GRAM-negative, mostly encapsulated rods, 0.5–1.5 µm wide and 1.0–2.0 µm long. Tendency to pleomorphism. Nonmotile. Growth in yolk sac of chicken embryo, or yolk-containing special culture media	In lesions, mostly of genitals but also of mouth, nose and throat. The role of sexual transmission is controversial[5]	Donovanosis (granuloma inguinale, granuloma venereum). Widespread in the tropics. Extremely rare in Europe and the USA[6]. Both sexes affected. Incubation period probably 8–80 days[5] *Remark*. Treatment with a tetracycline is usually effective[5,7]
104	**Gardnerella vaginalis** (GARDNER and DUKES) GREENWOOD and PICKETT *Haemophilus vaginalis*	GRAM-negative to GRAM-variable, pleomorphic rods, ~ 0.5 µm wide and 1.5–2.5 µm long. No capsule, no endospores. Nonmotile. Facultatively anaerobic. Catalase- and oxidase-negative. β-Hemolysis occurs on human and rabbit blood media, but not on sheep blood media	Natural habitat is the vagina (infrequently also isolated from the urinary tract[8]). The possibility of sexual transmission is discussed[9,10]	Pathogen of nonspecific bacterial vaginosis[8,9,11]. Septicemia and upper genitourinary infections in obstetric and gynecologic patients[8] *Remarks*. Treatment with metronidazole is effective in bacterial vaginosis; ampicillin is advocated for septic infections[7,8]

[1] MCGOWAN and DEL RIO, in MANDELL et al. (Eds.), *Principles and Practice of Infectious Diseases*, 3rd ed., Churchill Livingstone, New York, 1990, page 1782.
[2] WORMSER and BUTTONE, *Rev. infec. Dis.*, **5**, 680 (1983).
[3] CHRISTEN, R. D., *Infection*, **18**, 291 (1990); PRITCHARD et al., *Amer. J. Med.*, **90**, 516 (1991).
[4] FRANCIOLI et al., *Arch. intern. Med.*, **143**, 1483 (1983).
[5] HART, G., in MANDELL et al. (Eds.), *Principles and Practice of Infectious Diseases*, 3rd ed., Churchill Livingstone, New York, 1990, page 1872.
[6] DE SCHRYVER and MEHEUS, *Bull. Wld Hlth Org.*, **68**, 639 (1990).
[7] *Med. Lett. Drug. Ther.*, **32**, No. 817 (1990).
[8] SPIEGEL, C. A., in MANDELL et al. (Eds.), *Principles and Practice of Infectious Diseases*, 3rd ed., Churchill Livingstone, New York, 1990, page 1733.
[9] BUMP and BUESCHING, *Amer. J. Obstet. Gynec.*, **158**, 935 (1988).
[10] WEST et al., *Brit. med. J.*, **296**, 1163 (1988).
[11] SOBEL, J. D., *Ann. intern. Med.*, **111**, 551 (1989).

No.	**Bacterium** *Synonyms* Common names	Characteristics	Habitat Host Transmission	Associated disease
105	**Eikenella corrodens** (EIKEN) JACKSON and GOODMAN *Bacteroides corrodens*	GRAM-negative, straight rods, 0.3–0.4 µm wide and 1.5–4.0 µm long, with rounded ends. Nonmotile. Oxidase-positive; catalase-, urease- and indole-negative. Facultatively anaerobic. See also table below	Part of normal oropharyngeal flora in man	Increasingly isolated in lung infections, sinusitis, osteomyelitis, wound infections, peritonitis, meningitis, endocarditis, gynecological infections[1–4] *Remark*. Treatment with ampicillin is usually effective[1,5]
106	**Streptobacillus moniliformis** LEVADITI et al. *Haverhillia multiformis*	GRAM-negative rods, 0.1–0.7 µm wide and 1–5 µm long. Extremely pleomorphic, in long filaments; sometimes also coccoid forms. Nonmotile. No growth on ordinary media, but requires addition of serum, ascites fluid or blood. Requirement of 10% CO_2 for primary isolation. Anaerobic or aerobic	Part of normal nasopharyngeal flora in rats. Transmission by rat bite, also via contaminated foods, especially milk and water	One type of rat-bite fever, sometimes described as erythema arthriticum. Incubation period usually less than 10 days[6]. Manifestations: high fever, morbilliform rash, polyarthritis. For classical rat-bite fever (sodoku), see *Spirillum minus* (*No. 12*). The consumption of contaminated milk or water leads to a clinical syndrome referred to as Haverhill fever[7,8] (according to an outbreak in Haverhill, MA) *Remark*. For treatment, benzylpenicillin is the drug of choice[5,6]
107	**Bacteroides fragilis** (VEILLON and ZUBER) CASTELLANI and CHALMERS *Bacillus fragilis* *Ristella fragilis* *Fusiformis fragilis*	GRAM-negative, capsulated rods, 0.8–1.3 µm wide and 1.6–8.0 µm long, occurring singly or in pairs. Nonmotile, or motile with peritrichous flagella. Obligately anaerobic. Good growth on blood agar plates. β-Hemolysis on sheep blood agar by very few strains (less than 1%)	Mouth, pharynx, intestinal tract	Isolated in intra-abdominal infections, brain abscesses, oral and pleuropulmonary infections, septicemia, urinary tract, skin and bone infections[9,10] *Remarks*. Treatment of infections by oropharyngeal strains with benzylpenicillin (increasing frequency of resistance to penicillin reported; clindamycin may be an alternative)[5]. Treatment of infections by gastrointestinal strains with metronidazole. When infection is in the central nervous system, either intravenous metronidazole or chloramphenicol is recommended[5]
108	**Bacteroides vulgatus** EGGERTH and GAGNON *Pasteurella vulgata*	As for *B. fragilis*. Some strains are capsulated. No hemolysis on sheep blood agar	Intestinal tract	As for *B. fragilis*

1 MCGOWAN and DEL RIO, in MANDELL et al. (Eds.), *Principles and Practice of Infectious Diseases*, 3rd ed., Churchill Livingstone, New York, 1990, page 1782.
2 SUWANAGOOL et al., *Arch. intern. Med.*, **143**, 2265 (1983).
3 POLIN and SHULMAN, *Pediatrics*, **70**, 462 (1982).
4 RICHE et al., *Lancet*, **2**, 1089 (1987); DROUET et al., *Lancet*, **2**, 1089 (1987).
5 *Med. Lett. Drug. Ther.*, **32**, No. 817 (1990).
6 WASHBURN, R. G., in MANDELL et al. (Eds.), *Principles and Practice of Infectious Diseases*, 3rd ed., Churchill Livingstone, New York, 1990, page 1762.
7 MCEVOY et al., *Lancet*, **2**, 1361 (1987).
8 SHANSON et al., *Lancet*, **2**, 92 (1983).
9 ZALEZNIK and KASPER, in MANDELL et al. (Eds.), *Principles and Practice of Infectious Diseases*, 3rd ed., Churchill Livingstone, New York, 1990, page 1860.
10 HOFSTAD, T., in BRAUDE et al. (Eds.), *Infectious Diseases and Medical Microbiology*, 2nd ed., Saunders, Philadelphia, 1986, page 417.

Differentiation of the genus Eikenella *from superficially similar Gram-negative bacteria*

	Eikenella	*Actinobacillus*	*Bordetella*	*Brucella*	*Cardiobacterium*	*Haemophilus*	*Moraxella*	*Kingella*	*Pasteurella*	*Yersinia*
Oxidase activity (dimethyl-*p*-phenylenediamine)	+	−					+	+	+	
Catalase activity	−	+	+*	+			+	−	+	+
Indole production	−				+					
Acid production from glucose	−	+			+	+		+	+	+
Urease activity	−			+						
Strictly anaerobic	−									
Motility	−									+◊

\+ 90% or more of strains are positive.
− 90% or more of strains are negative.
* *Bordetella bronchiseptica* excluded.
◊ *Yersinia pestis* excluded.

Reference

JACKSON and GOODMAN, in KRIEG and HOLT (Eds.), *Bergey's Manual of Systematic Bacteriology*, Volume 1, Williams & Wilkins, Baltimore, 1984, page 591.

No.	**Bacterium** *Synonyms* Common names	Characteristics	Habitat Host Transmission	Associated disease
109	**Bacteroides thetaiotaomicron** (DISTASO) CASTELLANI and CHALMERS *Bacillus thetaiotaomicron* *Sphaerocillus thetaiotaomicron*	As for *B. fragilis*. No hemolysis on sheep blood agar	Intestinal tract	As for *B. fragilis*
110	**Bacteroides melaninogenicus** (OLIVER and WHERRY) ROY and KELLY *Bacterium melaninogenicum*	As for *B. fragilis*. β-Hemolysis occasionally possible	Mouth, nose, pharynx, intestinal and respiratory tracts, ear	Isolated from purulent lesions in the mouth and nasopharynx, also in mixed flora in lung gangrene and lung abscesses, appendicitis, subphrenic abscesses. Often accompanies actinomycosis *Remark*. Increasing frequency of resistance to penicillin reported[1]
111	**Bacteroides pneumosintes** (OLITSKY and GATES) HOLDEMAN and MOORE *Bacterium pneumosintes* *Dialister pneumosintes*	GRAM-negative, extremely short rods, 0.2–0.4 µm wide and 0.3 to 0.6 µm long, occurring singly, in pairs and in short chains. Obligately anaerobic. Filtrable through BERKEFELD V and N filters	Nose, pharynx and respiratory tract	As for *B. fragilis*
112	**Bacteroides putredinis** (WEINBERG et al.) KELLY *Bacillus putredinis* *Ristella putredinis*	As for *B. fragilis*	Intestinal tract (appendix)	In mixed flora in appendicitis, rectal abscesses
113	Other *Bacteroides* species of clinical importance[2, 3]: **Bacteroides oris** **Bacteroides distasonis** **Bacteroides ovatus** **Bacteroides gingivalis** **Bacteroides bivius** **Bacteroides disiens** **Bacteroides ureolyticus**			May play a role in nongonococcal urethritis[4]
114	**Fusobacterium nucleatum** KNORR *Bacillus fusiformis* *Fusobacterium polymorphum*	GRAM-negative, slender, fusiform rods, 0.4–0.7 µm wide and 3–10 µm long, with pointed ends and plumper middle part, often slightly curved. Nonmotile. Obligately anaerobic. No β-hemolysis. Exotoxin formation	Mucosa of oropharynx, urogenital tract, intestinal tract in man	Upper airway and pleuropulmonary infections[5, 6]. Found in polymicrobial infections[6, 7]
115	**Fusobacterium necrophorum** (FLÜGGE) MOORE and HOLDEMAN *Bacillus necrophorus* *Fusiformis necrophorus* *Sphaerophorus necrophorus* BANG's necrosis bacillus SCHMORL's bacillus	Primary cultures (pus smears): GRAM-negative, short rods, either straight or slightly curved; also coccoid forms in pairs or chains. Very pleomorphous in cultures, with rods up to 100 µm long. Nonmotile. Obligately anaerobic. Produces gas in media containing peptones (fetid odor). β-Hemolysis. Endotoxin formation	Mucosa of oropharynx, urogenital tract, intestinal tract in man	Upper airway and pleuropulmonary infections[5, 6]. Septicemia following oropharyngeal infection, with local thrombophlebitis (LEMIERRE syndrome), lung and liver abscesses, septic arthritis, osteomyelitis[8–10]. Found in polymicrobial infections[6, 7]
116	Other *Fusobacterium* species of clinical importance: **Fusobacterium gonidiaformans** **Fusobacterium naviforme**	GRAM-negative, pleomorphous rods	As for *F. necrophorum*	Pleuropulmonary infections[5]

[1] GUDIOL et al., *Arch. intern. Med.*, **150**, 2525 (1990).
[2] ZALEZNIK and KASPAR, in MANDELL et al. (Eds.), *Principles and Practice of Infectious Diseases*, 3rd ed., Churchill Livingstone, New York, 1990, page 1860.
[3] HOLDEMAN et al., in SNEATH et al. (Eds.), *Bergey's Manual of Systematic Bacteriology*, Vol. 2, Williams & Wilkins, Baltimore, 1986, page 604.
[4] BENNETT et al., *Europ. J. clin. Microbiol. infect. Dis.*, **9**, 825 (1990).
[5] FINEGOLD, S. M., in MANDELL et al. (Eds.), *Principles and Practice of Infectious Diseases*, 3rd ed., Churchill Livingstone, New York, 1990, page 560.
[6] LANCASTER and ATTEBERY, in BRAUDE et al. (Eds.), *Infectious Diseases and Medical Microbiology*, 2nd ed., Saunders, Philadelphia, 1986, page 421.
[7] HENRY et al., *Amer. J. Med.*, **75**, 225 (1983).
[8] SEIDENFELD et al., *J. Amer. med. Ass.*, **248**, 1348 (1982).
[9] GUBLER et al., *Schweiz. med. Wschr.*, **120**, 440 (1990).
[10] SINAVE et al., *Medicine (Baltimore)*, **68**, 85 (1989).

No.	**Bacterium** *Synonyms* Common names	Characteristics	Habitat Host Transmission	Associated disease
117	**Leptotrichia buccalis** (ROBIN) TREVISAN *Leptothrix buccalis*	GRAM-negative, straight or slightly curved rods, 0.8–1.5 µm wide and 5–15 µm long, often arranged in pairs, chains or septate filaments. Nonmotile. Anaerobic culture in blood agar or tryptone and yeast extract agar (KASAI). Optimal growth at 35 to 37 °C. Colorless colonies, 2 to 3 mm in diameter, after 2–3 days	Oral cavity	Pathogen of VINCENT's angina, together with *Treponema vincentii*[1] *Remark*. Treatment with benzylpenicillin; a tetracycline or clindamycin as an alternative[2]
117a	**Mobiluncus** spp.	GRAM-variable, curved rods, 1.7 to 2.9 µm long. Motile, with subpolar flagella. No spore formation. Anaerobic. Produce succinic acid[3]	Intestinal tract, genital tract (?)	Bacterial vaginosis, vaginal bleeding[4,5]. Breast abscess[6]. The clinical significance of *Mobiluncus* is not yet established
117b	**Helicobacter pylori** MARSHALL and GOODWIN *Campylobacter pyloridis* *Campylobacter pylori*	GRAM-negative, curved or helical rods, 0.5–1.0 µm wide and 2.5 to 5 µm long. Motile, with 4–6 polar flagella[7]. The cells have smooth surfaces and rounded ends. Catalase-, oxidase-, urease-positive. No nitrate reduction. For biochemical characteristics, see also table on page 15. Microaerophilic. Grows on blood agar, chocolate agar, SKIRROW medium and THAYER–MARTIN medium[8]	Upper gastrointestinal tract of man. Worldwide occurrence. Mode of transmission unknown[8,9]	Gastritis, antral gastritis in children, peptic ulcers, nonulcer dyspepsia, epidemic hypochlorhydria[8–10]. Longlasting *H. pylori* infection is strongly associated with an increased risk of gastric carcinoma[17–19] *Remark*. The organism is sensitive *in vitro* to many antibiotics and bismuth components, but eradiction of the organism *in vivo* is difficult[11,12]
118	**Veillonella parvula** (VEILLON and ZUBER) PRÉVOT *Staphylococcus parvulus*	GRAM-negative, small diplococci. Nonmotile. Strictly anaerobic. Some gas formation in peptone media (fetid odor). Oxidase- and catalase-negative. For differentiation, see also table on page 20	Saliva of man; respiratory and intestinal tract; vagina	Usually harmless saprophyte. The role of *Veillonella* in human clinical infections is not well established[13]. Rare cause of gangrenous and fetid suppuration, osteomyelitis[14]
119	**Rickettsia prowazekii** DA ROCHA-LIMA *Rickettsia exanthematotyphi* *Rickettsia kairo* *Rickettsia prowazeki* var. *prowazeki*	GRAM-negative, short rods, 0.3 to 0.5 µm wide and 0.8–2.0 µm long. Pleomorphic. Nonmotile. Aerobic. Staining by GIMÉNEZ method. Intracellular growth exclusively in the cytoplasm of sensitive cells (louse intestine, conjunctival epithelium of infected animals), not in the nucleus. Massive spread of rickettsiae follows rupture of the cells. Grows readily on the yolk sac membrane of chicken embryos *Serological diagnosis*. For WEIL–FELIX test, see table on page 47. Complement fixation; indirect immunofluorescent antibody test[15]	Man. Transmitted by human body louse (*Pediculus humanus*). Extrahuman reservoir: flying squirrel. Mode of infection: louse feces rubbed into the skin by scratching	Epidemic typhus (typhus fever, louse-borne typhus); worldwide epidemic disease of varying severity. Incubation period 7–14 days, shorter after a massive infection, sometimes much longer in latent infections. Rash appears between 3rd and 5th days of fever, which lasts about 3 weeks. Relapses may occur years after the primary infection (BRILL–ZINSSER disease)[16] *Remarks*. Prophylaxis by vermin control. Prophylactic vaccination. Treatment with a tetracycline, or with chloramphenicol as an alternative[2,16]

1 NAUMANN et al., *Medizinische Mikrobiologie und Immunologie für Stomatologen*, Barth, Leipzig, 1983, page 132.
2 *Med. Lett. Drug. Ther.*, **32**, No. 817 (1990).
3 SPIEGEL and ROBERTS, *Int. J. syst. Bacteriol.*, **34**, 177 (1984).
4 LARSSON and BERGMAN, *Amer. J. Obstet. Gynecol.*, **154**, 107 (1986).
5 HOLST, E., *J. clin. Microbiol.*, **28**, 2035 (1990).
6 BENNETT et al., *Lancet*, **1**, 564 (1989).
7 GOODWIN et al., *Int. J. system. Bact.*, **39**, 397 (1989).
8 BUCK, G. E., *Clin. Microbiol. Rev.*, **3**, 1 (1990).
9 BLASER, M. J., *Rev. infect. Dis.*, **12**, Suppl. 1, S99 (1990).
10 DOOLEY and COHEN, *Ann. intern. Med.*, **108**, 70 (1988).
11 CHAMBERLAIN and PEURA, *Arch. intern. Med.*, **150**, 951 (1990).
12 MORRIS et al., *Ann. intern. Med.*, **114**, 662 (1991).
13 LANCASTER and ATTEBERY, in BRAUDE et al. (Eds.), *Infectious Diseases and Medical Microbiology*, 2nd ed., Saunders, Philadelphia, 1986, page 426.
14 BARNHART et al., *Amer. J. Med.*, **74**, 902 (1983).
15 *Bull. Wld Hlth Org.*, **66**, 409 (1988).
16 SAAH, A. J., in MANDELL et al. (Eds.), *Principles and Practice of Infectious Diseases*, 3rd ed., Churchill Livingstone, New York, 1990, page 1476.
17 FORMAN et al., *Brit. med. J.*, **302**, 1303 (1991).
18 PARSONNET et al., *New Engl. J. Med.*, **325**, 1127 (1991).
19 NOMURA et al., *New Engl. J. Med.*, **325**, 1132 (1991).

No.	**Bacterium** *Synonyms* Common names	Characteristics	Habitat Host Transmission	Associated disease
120	**Rickettsia typhi** (WOLBACH and TODD) PHILIP *Dermacentroxenus typhi* *Rickettsia mooseri*	Morphologically similar to *R. prowazekii*. Good growth in yolk sac of chicken embryos *Serological diagnosis*. For WEIL-FELIX test, see table on page 47. Complement fixation; indirect immunofluorescent antibody test[1]	Rats and other rodents. Transmitted by the rat flea (*Xenopsylla cheopis*) and rat louse (*Polyplax spinulosus*), possibly also by the human flea (*Pulex irritans*). Mode of infection: infected feces rubbed into the skin by scratching; inhalation of air-borne rickettsiae	Endemic typhus (murine typhus); worldwide distribution (especially America, the CIS, Mediterranean coast, Far East, northern Australia, West and South Africa); sporadic and limited to endemic foci. Clinically similar to epidemic typhus, but much more benign. Incubation period 6–14 days, duration of fever 9–14 days[2]. In 1989, 41 cases of murine typhus were reported in the USA[3] *Remarks*. Prophylaxis by flea and rodent control. Treatment as for *R. prowazekii*
121	**Rickettsia rickettsii** (WOLBACH) BRUMPT *Dermacentroxenus rickettsii*	GRAM-negative rods, slightly smaller than *R. prowazekii*. Staining by GIMÉNEZ method. Intracellular (in cytoplasm and nucleus). Can be grown on yolk sac of chicken embryos. Rapidly inactivated at 50 °C *Serological diagnosis*. For WEIL-FELIX test, see table on page 47. Complement fixation; indirect immunofluorescent antibody test; indirect hemagglutination test; latex agglutination[4]	Reservoirs: ticks of the genera *Dermacentor*, *Amblyomma*, *Haemaphysalis*, *Rhipicephalus*; various American rodents, dogs, foxes, raccoons, opossums, etc. Transovarian transmission from tick to tick. Transmission to man by tick bite	Rocky Mountain spotted fever[5] (mountain fever, tick fever, São Paulo exanthematic typhus, Tobia fever, Minas Gerais typhus, Brazilian macular fever) in the USA, Canada, Mexico, Brazil, Colombia; sporadic disease of varying severity. Incubation period 2–14 (average 7) days. The rash appears 2–6 (usually 4) days after the onset of fever, which lasts 15–20 days[4]. Gastrointestinal manifestation in early stage[5]. Complications: pneumonia, circulatory failure. In 1989, 623 cases were reported in the USA[3] *Remarks*. Prophylaxis by tick control. Treatment as for *R. prowazekii*
122	**Rickettsia sibirica** ZDRODOVSKII	Morphologically similar to *R. rickettsii* *Serological diagnosis*. For WEIL-FELIX test, see table on page 47. Complement fixation; indirect immunofluorescent antibody test[1]	Reservoirs: ticks of genera *Dermacentor* and *Haemaphysalis*, rodents. Transovarian transmission from tick to tick. Transmission to man by tick bite	North Asian tick typhus or tick fever in Pacific maritime regions of the CIS, from northern and southern Siberia to the Armenian Republic. Sporadic. Benign course. Similar to boutonneuse fever *Remark*. Treatment as for *R. prowazekii*
123	**Rickettsia conorii** BRUMPT	Morphologically similar to *R. rickettsii* *Serological diagnosis*. For WEIL-FELIX test, see table on page 47. Complement fixation; indirect immunofluorescent antibody test[1]	Reservoirs: dog ticks (*Rhipicephalus sanguineus*), also ticks of genera *Amblyomma*, *Dermacentor*, *Ixodes*, *Haemaphysalis*; various rodents, especially rats (*Rattus rattus*), dogs. Transovarian transmission from tick to tick. Transmission to man by tick bite	Boutonneuse fever (Mediterranean spotted fever, Kenya tick typhus, Indian tick typhus or other names that designate the locality of occurrence) in Mediterranean area, Black Sea, Caspian Sea, Central and South Africa, parts of India. Sporadic. Benign course. Incubation period 5–9 days. Maculopapular rash appears 3–5 days after onset of fever, which lasts 8–14 days[6]. From 1977 to 1986, 67 cases of *R. conorii* infections were reported in the USA[6] *Remark*. Treatment as for *R. prowazekii*
124	**Rickettsia australis** PHILIP	Morphologically similar to *R. rickettsii* *Serological diagnosis*. For WEIL-FELIX test, see table on page 47	Reservoirs: probably rodents and small marsupials. Transmission to man by tick bite (*Ixodes holocyclus*)	North Australian or Queensland tick typhus. Sporadic. Benign course. Similar to boutonneuse fever *Remark*. Treatment as for *R. prowazekii*

[1] *Bull. Wld Hlth Org.*, **66**, 409 (1988).
[2] SAAH, A. J., in MANDELL et al. (Eds.), *Principles and Practice of Infectious Diseases*, 3rd ed., Churchill Livingstone, New York, 1990, page 1478.
[3] *Morb. Mort. wkly Rep.*, **38**, No. 54 (1989).
[4] RAOULT and WALKER, in MANDELL et al. (Eds.), *Principles and Practice of Infectious Diseases*, 3rd ed., Churchill Livingstone, New York, 1990, page 1465.
[5] SEXTON, D. J., *Arch. intern. Med.*, **145**, 2173 (1985).
[6] MCDONALD et al., *Amer. J. Med.*, **85**, 799 (1988).

No.	Bacterium *Synonyms* Common names	Characteristics	Habitat Host Transmission	Associated disease
125	**Rickettsia akari** HUEBNER et al.	Morphologically similar to *R. rickettsii*, but can be differentiated immunologically. Only *Rickettsia* species not pathogenic to monkeys *Serological diagnosis.* For WEIL–FELIX test, see table on next page. Complement fixation; indirect immunofluorescent antibody test[1]	Reservoirs: mice, rats. Transmitted by mice and mites (*Allodermanyssus sanguineus*)	Rickettsialpox (vesicular rickettsiosis), sporadically in the USA and some regions of the CIS and Central Africa. Benign course. Incubation period (up to appearance of the initial lesion at the site of a mite bite) 9 to 14 days[1,2]. Sudden onset of fever a few days later, followed by a papulovesicular rash and lasting 2–3 weeks if untreated. Relapses are uncommon *Remark.* Treatment as for *R. prowazekii*
126	**Rickettsia tsutsugamushi** (HAYASHI) OGATA *Theileria tsutsugamushi* *Rickettsia orientalis*	GRAM-negative, short rods, about 1.2 µm long. Staining by GIMÉNEZ method. Pleomorphic. Intracellular (in cytoplasm). Can be grown in yolk sac of chicken embryos *Serological diagnosis.* For WEIL–FELIX test, see table on next page. Complement fixation; indirect immunofluorescent antibody test[3]	Reservoirs: trombiculid mites (*Leptostrombidium deliense*, *L. akamushi*, *L. fletcheri*); rodents (rats, voles, bandicoots), possibly birds. Transovarian transmission from mite to mite. Transmission to man (or rodent) by introduction of *R. tsutsugamushi* into the skin through the bite of an infected larval mite	Scrub typhus (tsutsugamushi disease, mite-borne typhus) in Japan, Southeast Asia, South Pacific, northern Australia; endemic with varying severity and mortality, most severe in Japan. Incubation (6–)10–12(–18) days[4]. The rash appears 5–8 days after onset of fever, which lasts 2–3 weeks if untreated. Complications such as pneumonia, encephalitis and peripheral circulatory collapse are possible[5,6]. Relapses may occur *Remarks.* Prophylaxis by mite control. Treatment as for *R. prowazekii*
127	**Rochalimaea quintana** (SCHMINCKE) KRIEG *Rickettsia quintana*	GRAM-negative, short rods, 0.3 to 0.5 µm wide and 1.0–1.7 µm long. Staining by GIMÉNEZ and GIEMSA methods. Multiplies extracellularly on epithelial cells of louse gut, also on blood agar. Increased CO_2 pressure and an erythrocyte factor are essential for growth *Serological diagnosis.* The WEIL–FELIX test is negative. Complement fixation	Man; the pathogen may be present in the blood for months after infection. Transmitted by human body louse (*Pediculus humanus*). The life of the louse is not shortened by the infection, but the organism is not transmitted to the progeny. Transmission by louse excreta or bites, possibly by inhaled dust	Trench fever (5-day fever, quintan fever, shinbone fever, Volhynian fever, HIS–WERNER disease) occurring epidemically in central Europe, Balkans, the CIS (especially during World Wars I and II). Incubation period 14–30 days, followed by several bouts of fever at intervals of 5 days and sometimes roseola-like rashes[7]. Lethality practically nil. Late relapses possible
128	**Coxiella burnetii** (DERRICK) PHILIP *Rickettsia burneti*	GRAM-negative, short rods, 0.2 to 0.4 µm wide and 0.4–1.0 µm long. Staining by GIMÉNEZ method. Undergoes phase variation, giving phase I and phase II antigens. Intracellular growth preferentially in the vacuoles of the host cell. Grows well in the yolk sac of chicken embryos. Resistant to drying, heat and chemical agents *Serological diagnosis.* The WEIL–FELIX test is negative. Microagglutination; complement fixation; indirect immunofluorescent antibody test; enzyme-linked immunosorbent assay[8]	Reservoirs: ticks (transovarian transmission), rodents, birds, domestic animals. Infection by inhalation of *C. burnetii* with dust or droplets, by ingestion of foods containing the organisms, by exposure to products of feline parturition[9], possibly also through tick bites	Q fever (query fever, Queensland fever, nine-mile fever, quadrilateral fever). Worldwide distribution, with high incidence in cattle-breeding areas. Incubation period 14–39 days[8]. Usually an acute self-limited febrile illness (2–14 days)[8,10]; pneumonia as complication[11] (often a community-acquired infection[9,12]); no rash. Chronic course involving heart[8] (very rare in children[13]), liver, bone, uterus and placenta[14] *Remarks.* Prophylaxis by pasteurization of milk and vaccination of persons at risk[15]. Treatment with a tetracycline is effective[8,9]

[1] SAAH, A. J., in MANDELL et al. (Eds.), *Principles and Practice of Infectious Diseases*, 3rd ed., Churchill Livingstone, New York, 1990, page 1471.
[2] BRETTMANN et al., *Medicine (Baltimore)*, **60**, 363 (1981).
[3] *Bull. Wld Hlth Org.*, **66**, 409 (1988).
[4] SAAH, A. J., in MANDELL et al. (Eds.), *Principles and Practice of Infectious Diseases*, 3rd ed., Churchill Livingstone, New York, 1990, page 1480.
[5] MCDONALD et al., *Amer. J. Med.*, **85**, 799 (1988).
[6] CHAYAKUL et al., *Quart. J. Med.*, N.S. **68**, 595 (1988).
[7] WARREN, J., in HORSFALL and TAMM (Eds.), *Viral and Rickettsial Infections of Man*, 4th ed., Pitman, London, 1965, page 1161.
[8] MARRIE, T. J., in MANDELL et al. (Eds.), *Principles and Practice of Infectious Diseases*, 3rd ed., Churchill Livingstone, New York, 1990, page 1472.
[9] LANGLEY et al., *New Engl. J. Med.*, **319**, 354 (1988).
[10] SAWYER et al., *Rev. infect. Dis.*, **9**, 935 (1987).
[11] CLEMENTS and WOODWARD, in BARON, S. (Ed.), *Medical Microbiology*, 2nd ed., Addison-Wesley, Menlo Park, CA, 1986, page 618.
[12] SPICER, A. J., *J. roy. Soc. Med.*, **71**, 762 (1978).
[13] LAUFER et al., *J. Pediat.*, **108**, 535 (1986).
[14] RIECHMAN et al., *Amer. J. Med.*, **85**, 253 (1988).
[15] MARMION et al., *Lancet*, **2**, 1411 (1984); Editorial, *Lancet*, **2**, 1435 (1984).

No.	**Bacterium** *Synonyms* Common names	Characteristics	Habitat Host Transmission	Associated disease
129	**Ehrlichia canis** (DONATIENS and LESTOQUARD) MOSHKOVSKI *Rickettsia canis*	Small, pleomorphic, coccoid to ellipsoidal organisms occurring intracytoplasmatically in circulating leucocytes. Nonmotile. Not cultivable in cell-free media or chicken embryos. Pathogen not isolated from human material until 1990[1] *Serological diagnosis.* Indirect fluorescent antibody test for *E. canis* has been adapted for human ehrlichiosis[2]	Dogs, ticks. Transmission to man by ticks suggested[3]	Possibly pathogen of human ehrlichiosis. Febrile illness, myalgia, in some cases rash[1,4–6] *Remark.* Treatment with a tetracycline seems to be effective[3,4]
130	**Ehrlichia sennetsu** (MISAO and KOBAYASHI) *Rickettsia sennetsu*	Similar to *E. canis* *Serological diagnosis.* The WEIL–FELIX test is negative. Indirect fluorescent antibody test	Vectors, if known, are ticks	Sennetsu rickettsiosis, glandular fever, Hyuga fever, Kagami fever. The disease is limited to western Japan and Malaysia[6]
131	**Bartonella bacilliformis** (STRONG et al.) STRONG et al.	GRAM-negative, slender, straight or bent rods occurring singly or in pairs, chains or clusters. Motile, with unipolar flagella. Seen in blood films inside the erythrocytes. In progressive infections up to 90% of the erythrocytes contain bacteria in varying numbers. Aerobic. May be cultivated in cell-free media. GIEMSA or ROMANOWSKY staining	Transmitted by certain species of *Phlebotomus* flies. Occurrence: western and central Cordillera ranges of the Andes in Peru, Ecuador and Colombia	Oroya fever (fever with hypochromic anemia), followed in many cases by superficial papular eruptions (verruga peruana)[7,8]. The latter often appear unheralded by fever *Remark.* Prophylaxis by sandfly control. Treatment with chloramphenicol, penicillin or a tetracycline is effective[7,8]

[1] ENG et al., *J. Amer. med. Ass.*, **264**, 2251 (1990).
[2] DAWSON et al., *J. infect. Dis.*, **163**, 564 (1991).
[3] *Morb. Mort. wkly Rep.*, **37**, 270 and 275 (1988).
[4] SAAH, A. J., in MANDELL et al. (Eds.), *Principles and Practice of Infectious Diseases*, 3rd ed., Churchill Livingstone, New York, 1990, page 1482.
[5] DORAN et al., *J. Pediat.*, **114**, 809 (1989).
[6] TACHIBANA, N., in LEIVE, L. (Ed.), *Microbiology–1986*, American Society for Microbiology, Washington DC, 1986, page 182.
[7] CUADRA, M., in BRAUDE et al. (Eds.), *Infectious Diseases and Medical Microbiology*, 2nd ed., Saunders, Philadelphia, 1986, pages 444 and 1219.
[8] ROBERTS, N. J., in MANDELL et al. (Eds.), *Principles and Practice of Infectious Diseases*, 3rd ed., Churchill Livingstone, New York, 1990, page 1870.

Rickettsiaceae *associated with human disease*[1–4]

Pathogen	Vector	Reservoir	Disease	Distribution	Observations	WEIL–FELIX agglutination test		
						OX-19	OX-2	OX-K
R. prowazekii	Human body louse	Man	Epidemic typhus	Worldwide (except Australia)	Late relapse	+++	+	–
R. typhi	Rat flea	Rats	Endemic typhus	Worldwide	–	+++	+	–
R. rickettsii	Ticks	Rodents, ticks	Rocky Mountain spotted fever	Western hemisphere	Late relapse (?)	+++	+	–
R. sibirica	Ticks	Rodents, ticks	North Asian tick typhus	Siberia, Mongolia	–	+	+++	–
R. conorii	Ticks	Rodents, ticks	Boutonneuse fever	Mediterranean countries, Africa, India	–	+	+++	–
R. akari	Mites	Rodents	Rickettsialpox	USA, CIS, Korea, Africa	–	–	–	–
R. australis	Ticks	Rodents, ticks	North Australian tick typhus	Australia	–	+	+++	–
R. tsutsugamushi	Mites	Rodents, birds, mites	Scrub typhus	South Pacific, Asia, Australia	Secondary illness	–	–	+++
Rochalimaea quintana	Human body louse	Man	Trench fever	North America, Europe, Africa	Late relapse	–	–	–
Coxiella burnetii	Ticks	Domestic animals, ticks	Q fever	Worldwide	Possible chronic course	–	–	–
Ehrlichia sennetsu	Ticks	Dogs, raw fish	Glandular fever	Western Japan	–	–	–	–

References
[1] WHO Working Group on Rickettsial Diseases, *Bull. Wld Hlth Org.*, **60**, 157 (1982).
[2] SAAH, A. J., in MANDELL et al. (Eds.), *Principles and Practice of Infectious Diseases*, 3rd ed., Churchill Livingstone, New York, 1990, page 1463.
[3] RAPMUND, G., in BRAUDE et al. (Eds.), *Infectious Diseases and Medical Microbiology*, 2nd ed., Saunders, Philadelphia, 1986, page 432.
[4] CLEMENTS and WOODWARD, in BARON, S. (Ed.), *Medical Microbiology*, 2nd ed., Addison-Wesley, Menlo Park, CA, 1986, page 618.

No.	Bacterium *Synonyms* Common names	Characteristics	Habitat Host Transmission	Associated disease
131a	**Agent of bacillary angiomatosis** *Rochalimaea henselae* sp. nov.	Closely related to *Rochalimaea quintana*		Bacillary angiomatosis (epithelioid angiomatosis); most often in immunocompromised persons[1]
131b	**Agent of cat-scratch disease** *Afipia felis* gen. nov., sp. nov. ENGLISH–WEAR bacillus	GRAM-negative rods, 0.3–1.0 µm wide and 0.6–3.0 µm long. Pleomorphic, not acid-fast. Acid production from D-xylose in a delayed, weak reaction. Nitrate reduction. Catalase-negative. Intracellular growth[2-4, 19]	Cats or dogs. Transmission by bites or scratches, possibly also contact. Direct transmission from man to man improbable	Cat-scratch disease (benign infectious lymphoreticulosis)[5-7]. Worldwide distribution. Infected cats show no symptoms. In man, incubation period of 1–2 weeks[5, 6], followed by lymphadenitis, fever, malaise, headache; occasionally generalized lymphadenopathy with rashes; complications such as encephalopathy[8]
132	**Chlamydia trachomatis** (BUSACCA) RAKE *Rickettsia trachomae*	GRAM-negative, coccoid organisms, 0.2–1.5 µm in diameter. Nonmotile. Elementary bodies are round, 0.2–0.4 µm in diameter (for developmental cycle, see text below). Cannot be cultured on artificial media. Culture possible in white mice (i.p.), in yolk sac of chicken embryo and in some cell cultures	Man is the only source of infection Biovar trachoma: transmission through direct contact from fingers, handtowels, flies, etc. Biovar lymphogranuloma venereum: transmission through sexual intercourse	For the wide range of infections, see text on next page
133	**Chlamydia psittaci** (LILLIE) PAGE *Rickettsia psittaci*	As *C. trachomatis*	Birds, cows, sheep. Transmission through contact with the excreta (dust) of diseased birds and animals, rarely from man to man (e.g. nursing staff)	Psittacosis (parrot disease, parrot fever, ornithosis). Worldwide distribution. In man[9, 10], incubation period 7–14 days. Onset with fever and headache; influenza-like or typhus-like course, often bronchopneumonia, rarely meningeal involvement, septicemia[11], abortion[12]. Family outbreaks have been reported[13] *Remark.* A tetracycline is considered the most effective antimicrobial agent, with chloramphenicol as an alternative[9, 14]
134	**Chlamydia pneumoniae** TWAR (Taiwan acute respiratory agent)	As *C. trachomatis*. Characteristically pear-shaped elementary bodies	No bird or animal reservoir known. Transmission from man to man	Influenza-like illness, bronchopneumonia, pharyngitis[15, 16], induction of GUILLAIN–BARRÉ syndrome[18]. Community-aquired infections reported from Scandinavia, North America and Japan[16, 17] *Remark.* A tetracycline is considered the most effective antimicrobial agent, with erythromycin as an alternative[14]

[1] RELMAN et al., *New Engl. J. Med.*, **323**, 1573 (1990); REGNERY et al., *J. clin. Microbiol.*, **30**, 265 (1992); WELCH et al., *J. clin. Microbiol.*, **30**, 275 (1992).
[2] WEAR et al., *Science*, **221**, 1403 (1983).
[3] KITCHELL et al., *New Engl. J. Med.*, **313**, 1090 (1985).
[4] ENGLISH et al., *J. Amer. med. Ass.*, **259**, 1347 (1988).
[5] CARITHERS, H. A., *Amer. J. Dis. Child.*, **139**, 1124 (1985).
[6] FISHER, G. W., in MANDELL et al. (Eds.), *Principles and Practice of Infectious Diseases*, 3rd ed., Churchill Livingstone, New York, 1990, page 1874.
[7] SCHÄDELIN, J., *Schweiz. med. Wschr.*, **120**, 738 (1990).
[8] CARITHERS and MARGILETH, *Amer. J. Dis. Child.*, **145**, 98 (1991).
[9] SCHAFFNER, W., in MANDELL et al. (Eds.), *Principles and Practice of Infectious Diseases*, 3rd ed., Churchill Livingstone, New York, 1990, page 1440.
[10] FREEDMAN, S. D., in BRAUDE et al. (Eds.), *Infectious Diseases and Medical Microbiology*, 2nd ed., Saunders, Philadelphia, 1986, page 808.
[11] MCKINLEY et al., *Quart. J. Med.*, N.S. **57**, 689 (1985).
[12] JOHNSON et al., *Brit. med. J.*, **290**, 592 (1985).
[13] HUMINER et al., *Lancet*, **2**, 615 (1988).
[14] *Med. Lett. Drug. Ther.*, **32**, No. 817 (1990).
[15] SCHAFFNER, W., in MANDELL et al. (Eds.), *Principles and Practice of Infectious Diseases*, 3rd ed., Churchill Livingstone, New York, 1990, page 1443.
[16] GRAYSTON, J. T., *Chest*, **95**, 664 (1989).
[17] KOBAYASHI et al., *J. infect. Dis.*, **163**, 417 (1991).
[18] HAIDL et al., *New Engl. J. Med.*, **326**, 576 (1992).
[19] BRENNER et al., *J. clin. Microbiol.*, **29**, 2450 (1991).

Chlamydia trachomatis infections

In the current taxonomy, the genus *Chlamydia* comprises 3 species: *C. trachomatis*, *C. psittaci* and *C. pneumoniae*. *C. trachomatis* is further divided into 3 biovars, namely biovar trachoma, biovar lymphogranuloma venereum and biovar mouse, only the first two being pathogenic in man. Microimmunofluorescent techniques permit identification of numerous antigenic types (see table)[1].

The individual species of *Chlamydia* do not differ in morphology and developmental cycle[2]. The latter, lasting 24–28 hours, comprises a change from small cells (elementary bodies, approximately 0.3 µm in diameter) to large cells (reticulate bodies, approximately 0.5–1 µm in diameter). At the beginning of the cycle the highly infectious elementary body invades the host cell by endocytosis; the invading cell retains its morphological integrity and does not undergo eclipse. The small cell enlarges, without losing its individuality, into a reticulate body, and the latter then multiplies by binary fission. The cycle is completed when most reticulate bodies have been transformed into elementary particles ready, in their turn, to infect a host cell.

Individual serovars are associated with specific diseases (see table)[2–4].

Trachoma. This is the most common cause of preventable blindness in the world, particularly in Africa, the Middle East, and Asia. The current (in the late 1980s) prevalence is unknown but is probably lower than that given two decades ago by the WHO (500 million)[6]. The disease is characterized by chronic keratoconjunctivitis with formation of granular follicles, corneal lesions, pannus, corneal clouding, eyelid deformities, and frequent blindness in older adults.

Inclusion conjunctivitis. In the USA, 2–6% of neonates develop neonatal chlamydial ophthalmia; in London the prevalence has been estimated as less than 1%[6]. According to the WHO, 2.5 million cases of neonatal chlamydial infection occur every year. The reported incidence in neonates born to infected women ranges between 18% and 74%[7]. Onset of the disease is usually 1 week after birth (range 1–40 days)[6]. It usually presents as mucopurulent conjunctivitis. Follicles can occur several weeks after onset of infection.

Adult chlamydial ophthalmia follows the transfer of infected discharges from the genital tract to the eye. 1 in 300 of those with genital chlamydial infection may develop ophthalmia[6]. The incubation period is about 1 week (range 2–21 days)[6]. Onset presents as acute papillary conjunctivitis, followed by a chronic follicular conjunctivitis.

Genital infections. In many industrialized countries the prevalence of genital *C. trachomatis* infection in the 1980s exceeds that of gonococcal infection[8,9]. In the USA, it is at present the most common sexually transmitted bacterial disease; the number of infections (1986) was estimated to be higher in women (2.6 million) than among men (1.8 million)[9].

Nongonococcal urethritis is diagnosed when urethritis is present, but gonococci are not detected. With acute presentation of an untreated episode of nongonococcal urethritis, *C. trachomatis* can be isolated from 25% to 40% of men, *Ureaplasma urealyticum* from 40% to 50% (often with *C. trachomatis*), and neither organism from 20% to 30%. When it can be calculated, the incubation period for gonorrhea is often less than 1 week; for nongonococcal urethritis, it peaks at 2 to 3 weeks. The range varies considerably, however, and in many men the incubation period appears to be much longer[10]. The most frequently recognized complications of nongonococcal urethritis are epididymitis and prostatitis (in 1–3% of cases[5]).

The prevalence of chlamydial infections in women varies according to the population and the laboratory techniques used to identify the organism[5]. In a recent study in Glasgow, a prevalence of 12% has been reported[11]. The infection is frequently asymptomatic and many infected women harbor the organism for a long period of time with few or no symptoms. Clinical signs of the infection are given in the table. The major long-term complications are obstructive infertility and ectopic pregnancy[12].

Lymphogranuloma venereum. Worldwide distribution, especially in the tropics and seaports. Incubation period 3–20 days[4]. First stage: primary lesion with small papule; second stage (after 2 weeks): swelling of lymph glands, occasionally with formation of fistulae, pyrexia, sometimes arthritis, conjunctivitis (no follicle formation), and meningoencephalitis.

Detection. Cell culture isolation of *C. trachomatis* is still the most sensitive and specific method for identifying the organism. Immunochemical detection is possible by direct immunofluorescent antibody test and enzyme-linked immunoassay[13,14].

Remarks. A tetracycline is the drug of choice, erythromycin or ofloxacin are alternatives[15,16].

References

1 WANG and GRAYSTON, *J. infect. Dis.*, **163**, 403 (1991).
2 MOULDER, J. W., in KRIEG and HOLT (Eds.), *Bergey's Manual of Systematic Bacteriology*, Vol. 1, Williams & Wilkins, Baltimore, 1984, page 729.
3 BECKER, Y., in BARON, S. (Ed.), *Medical Microbiology*, 2nd ed., Addison-Wesley, Menlo Park, CA, 1986, page 633.
4 BOWIE and HOLMES, in MANDELL et al. (Eds.), *Principles and Practice of Infectious Diseases*, 3rd ed., Churchill Livingstone, New York, 1990, page 1426.
5 FRAIZ and JONES, *Ann. Rev. Med.*, **39**, 357 (1988).
6 DAROUGAR et al., *CRC Crit. Rev. Microbiol.*, **16**, 369 (1989).
7 Report of a WHO Scientific Group, *Wld Hlth Org. techn. Rep. Ser.*, No. 660 (1981).
8 WHO Expert Committee on Venereal Diseases and Treponematoses, *Wld Hlth Org. techn. Rep. Ser.*, No. 736 (1986).
9 SCHRYVER and MEHEUS, *Bull. Wld Hlth Org.*, **68**, 639 (1990).
10 BOWIE, W. R., *Med. Clin. N. Amer.*, **74**, 1543 (1990).
11 SMITH et al., *Brit. med. J.*, **302**, 82 (1991).
12 MARTIN, D. H., *Med. Clin. N. Amer.*, **74**, 1367 (1990).
13 BARNES, R. C., *Clin. Microbiol. Rev.*, **2**, 119 (1989).
14 BOBO et al., *J. Clin. Microbiol.*, **28**, 1968 (1990).
15 *Med. Lett. Drug. Ther.*, **33**, No. 860 (1991).
16 TOOMEY and BARNES, *Rev. infect. Dis.*, **12**, Suppl. 6, S645 (1990).

Infections caused by Chlamydia trachomatis[2–5]

Biovar	Serovar	Clinical disease or syndrome	Geographic distribution
Trachoma	A, B, Ba, C	Trachoma	Endemic in Asia and Africa
	D, Da, F, G, H, Ia, J, K	Inclusion conjunctivitis (paratrachoma) in neonates, children and adults Pneumonia in infants Otitis media in children Myocarditis in children Nongonococcal urethritis in men Epididymitis Reactive arthritis Urethral syndrome in women Mucopurulent cervicitis Salpingitis, endometritis Proctitis Perihepatitis and peritonitis	Worldwide
Lymphogranuloma venereum	L_1, L_2, L_2a, L_3	Lymphogranuloma venereum (lymphogranuloma inguinale, climatic bubo, NICOLAS–FAVRE disease, poradenitis)	Worldwide

No.	**Bacterium** *Synonyms* Common names	Characteristics	Habitat Host Transmission	Associated disease
135	**Mycoplasma pneumoniae** SOMERSON et al.	GRAM-negative, coccoid to short filamentous organisms. No cell wall. Nonmotile. Aerobic, facultatively anaerobic. Requires cholesterol and lipoproteins for growth. Can be cultured in media containing serum and yeast extract. Optimal growth at 36 to 38 °C. No arginine hydrolysis. Highly sensitive to erythromycin	Oropharynx and respiratory tract in man. Transmission by respiratory secretions	Mycoplasma pneumonia (formerly called primary atypical pneumonia)[1]. Worldwide distribution. Infections range from mild upper respiratory tract symptoms to pneumonia (important cause of community-acquired pneumonia[2]); arthritis, central nervous system disease[3]. Incubation period 2–3 weeks *Remark*. A tetracycline or a macrolide such as erythromycin are the recommended drugs for treatment[2,4]
135a	**Mycoplasma hominis** (FREUNDT) EDWARD	As for *M. pneumoniae*. Arginine hydrolysis. Not sensitive to erythromycin	Very common in mucosa of the lower urogenital tract in females, more rarely found in oropharynx	Postpartum fever. Wound infections, pyelonephritis, septicemia, arthritis, endocarditis[5,6] *Remark*. Clindamycin or a tetracycline (possibly in combination) are suggested for treatment[6]
136	**Ureaplasma urealyticum** SHEPARD et al.	GRAM-negative, pleomorphous organisms. No cell wall. Nonmotile. Microaerophilic. Require cholesterol for growth. Can be cultured in media containing serum and yeast extract. Optimal growth at 37 °C. Urea hydrolysis with production of ammonia	Oropharynx, respiratory tract and urogenital tract in man and animals	Nongonococcal urethritis (see also page 49), epididymitis, prostatitis (?), arthritis (?). Infection of the female genital tract, neonatal infections[5,7] *Remark*. Erythromycin, clindamycin or a tetracycline may be effective for treatment[4,5]
136a	**Stomatococcus mucilaginosus** BERGAN and KOCUR	GRAM-positive, spherical organisms, 0.9–1.3 µm in diameter. Mostly in clusters. Nonmotile. Facultatively anaerobic. Catalase-negative or weakly positive	In man, part of normal flora of mouth and respiratory tract	Endocarditis, septicemia (often catheter-related)[8]
137	**Staphylococcus aureus** ROSENBACH Staphylococcus	GRAM-positive, spherical organisms, 0.5–1.0 µm in diameter. Single, in pairs or in irregular clusters. Nonmotile. Good growth on ordinary media. Many strains form a golden-yellow pigment. Aerobic, facultatively anaerobic. Coagulase-positive. Incomplete or complete hemolysis on blood agar. For further differential characteristics, see Table 1 on next page. Formation of several exotoxins (all strains), of leucocidin (many strains) and of enterotoxins (some strains)[9]	In man, common saprophyte of the nasal mucosa and skin. Ubiquitous	Common pathogen of inflammation and suppuration of widely different types. For review, see WALDVOGEL[10] and also text on pages 51, 52
138	**Staphylococcus epidermidis** (WINSLOW and WINSLOW) SCHLEIFER and KLOOS *Albococcus epidermidis*	GRAM-positive, spherical organisms, 0.5–1.5 µm in diameter. Single, in pairs and tetrads. Whitish or yellowish colonies on usual media. Aerobic, facultatively anaerobic. Coagulase-negative. Hemolysis, when present, usually weak. For further differential characteristics, see Table 1 on next page	Ubiquitous	Occasionally isolated from superficial skin lesions. Male cystitis. Principle cause of nosocomial septicemia[11,12]. For review, see ARCHER[13] and also text on pages 51, 52

[1] COUCH, R. B., in MANDELL et al. (Eds.), *Principles and Practice of Infectious Diseases*, 3rd ed., Churchill Livingstone, New York, 1990, page 1446.
[2] Editorial, *Lancet*, **337**, 651 (1991).
[3] WAITES et al., in STANEK et al. (Eds.), *Recent Advances in Mycoplasmology*, Fischer, Stuttgart, 1990, page 379.
[4] *Med. Lett. Drug. Ther.*, **32**, No. 817 (1990).
[5] TAYLOR-ROBINSON, D., in MANDELL et al. (Eds.), *Principles and Practice of Infectious Diseases*, 3rd ed., Churchill Livingstone, New York, 1990, page 1458.
[6] MCMAHON et al., *Amer. J. Med.*, **89**, 275 (1990).
[7] O'LEARY, W. M., *CRC Crit. Rev. Microbiol.*, **17**, 161 (1990).
[8] ASCHER et al., *Rev. infect. Dis.*, **13**, 1048 (1991).
[9] LENTNER, C. (Ed.), *Geigy Scientific Tables*, 8th ed., Volume 4, Ciba-Geigy Ltd., Basel, 1986, page 201.
[10] WALDVOGEL, F. A., in MANDELL et al. (Eds.), *Principles and Practice of Infectious Diseases*, 3rd ed., Churchill Livingstone, New York, 1990, page 1489.
[11] STILLMAN et al., *Infect. Control*, **8**, 108 (1987).
[12] MARTIN et al., *Ann. intern. Med.*, **110**, 9 (1989).
[13] ARCHER, G. L., in MANDELL et al. (Eds.), *Principles and Practice of Infectious Diseases*, 3rd ed., Churchill Livingstone, New York, 1990, page 1511.

No.	Bacterium Synonyms Common names	Characteristics	Habitat Host Transmission	Associated disease
139	**Staphylococcus saprophyticus** (FAIRBROTHER) SCHLEIFER and KLOOS *Peptococcus saccharolyticus*	GRAM-positive, spherical organisms. Single, in pairs and tetrads. Unpigmented or yellowish colonies on usual media. Aerobic, facultatively anaerobic. Coagulase-negative. Usually no hemolysis. For further differential characteristics, see Table 1 below	Ubiquitous	Urinary tract infections in young women[1]. In other aspects similar to *S. epidermidis*. For review, see ARCHER[2] and also text below
139a	Other *Staphylococcus* species of clinical importance: see text below			

[1] LATHAM et al., *J. Amer. med. Ass.*, **250**, 3063 (1983); BEUTH et al., *Dtsch. med. Wschr.*, **117**, 687 (1992).

[2] ARCHER, G. L., in MANDELL et al. (Eds.), *Principles and Practice of Infectious Diseases*, 3rd ed., Churchill Livingstone, New York, 1990, page 1511.

Staphylococci

All staphylococci are catalase-positive, but can be divided into 2 groups on the basis of coagulase production (Table 1); 23 species of staphylococci have been identified, 21 species are coagulase-negative[1]. Three species – *S. aureus*, *S. epidermidis* and *S. saprophyticus* – are of major clinical importance. For uncommon staphylococci, see Table 2.

Differentiation of strains of *S. aureus* by phage typing is widely used. *S. aureus* typing phages in the international basic set include phage group I: 29, 52, 52A, 79, 80; phage group II: 3A, 3C, 55, 71; phage group III: 6, 42E, 47, 53, 54, 75, 77, 83A, 84, 85; and not allocated: 81, 94, 95, 96. Some strains are untypable by these phages[2].

Of all bacterias, staphylococci most frequently accompany man and affect him sporadically throughout his life. About 90% of neonates discharged from hospital are staphylococcal carriers, and 30–40% of adults are carriers of the organism[3,4]. Serious staphylococcal infections occur mainly in debilitated persons.

S. aureus is responsible for most staphylococcal infections; the latter can be either invasive (furuncles, septicemia, endocarditis, osteomyelitis, pneumonia, deep abscesses) or toxic (see below)[5].

Coagulase-negative staphylococci. All species listed in Table 2 – with the exception of *S. aureus* – are coagulase-negative. They are the most common cause of nosocomial septicemia, especially following major surgery, such as heart valve replacement (see Table 4 on page 27), *S. epidermidis* is the single most common organism infecting intravenous catheters and cerebrospinal fluid shunts[6]. Two distinct populations of patients develop urinary tract infection due to *S. epidermidis* or *S. saprophyticus* (Table 3).

Staphylococcus toxins

A number of staphylococcal strains (coagulase-positive, occasionally coagulase-negative) can form single-chain polypeptide enterotoxins. Based on immunological reactions several individual enterotoxins have been identified (A, B, C_1, C_2, C_3, D, E). The consumption of toxin-containing foodstuffs can cause food poisoning in man (see Table 4). It is in many respects difficult to determine the time and circumstances in which a particular food item became contaminated with enterotoxin-forming staphylococci. The incubation period is 2–6 hours[5]. The first manifestations are vomiting, abdominal cramps and diarrhea; these normally subside quickly (within 1–3 days). A search for staphylococci must be carried out on every suspect food item. The diagnosis of staphylococcal food poisoning can be established fairly accurately on the basis of finding a high number of staphylococci. In the USA, 131 outbreaks of staphylococcal food poisoning were recorded between 1977 and 1981[7].

Table 2 *Common habitation sites and pathogenicity of staphylococci that are part of the normal flora in man*[1]

	Habitation sites	Pathogenicity
S. aureus	Nasal mucosa	Common
S. epidermidis	Nasal mucosa; axillae; skin of head, arms and legs	Common
S. saprophyticus	Skin (occasionally)	Common
S. haemolyticus	Skin of head, arms and legs	Uncommon
S. hominis	Axillae; skin of head, arms and legs	Uncommon
S. simulans	Skin (occasionally)	Uncommon
S. cohnii	Skin (occasionally)	Uncommon
S. warneri	Skin (occasionally)	Uncommon
S. saccharolyticus	Skin (rarely)	Uncommon
S. capitis	Skin of head, face, ear and arms	Rare
S. auricularis	Ear	Rare
S. xylosus	Skin (occasionally)	Rare

Common: isolated from > 20% of staphylococcal infections.
Uncommon: isolated from 5–20% of staphylococcal infections.
Rare: isolated from < 5% of staphylococcal infections.

(Continued on next page)

Table 1 *Differential characteristics of the common* Staphylococcus *species*[2]

	S. aureus	*S. epidermidis*	*S. saprophyticus*
Coagulase activity	+	–	–
Phosphatase activity	+	+	–
Acid production (aerobically) from sucrose	+	+	+
– from mannitol	+	–	d
Novobiocin resistance	–	–	+
Hemolysis	+	–/w	–

+ 90% or more strains are positive.
– 90% or more strains are negative.
d 11–89% strains are positive.
–/w Negative or weak reaction.

Table 3 *Urinary tract infections caused by* Staphylococcus epidermidis *and* Staphylococcus saprophyticus[6]

	S. epidermidis	*S. saprophyticus*
Gender of patients	Men and women equally	Women (95%)
Age of patients	Usually > 50 years	16–35 years
Population at risk	Hospitalized patients with urinary tract complications	Healthy outpatients
Incidence	Uncommon (3.5% or less of all urinary tract infections in hospitalized patients)	Common (20% or more of all urinary tract infections in this age group)
Presentation	90% asymptomatic	90% symptomatic; indistinguishable from *E. coli* urinary tract infections

Table 4 *Staphylococcal toxin syndromes*[9]

	Food poisoning	Scalded skin syndrome	Toxic shock syndrome
Predominant phage group	III (others)	II (I)	I (others)
Toxin(s)			
– designation	Enterotoxin	Epidermolytic toxins	Toxic shock syndrome toxin-1 (probably others)
– types	A–E	A, B	Several
Production site	Food	Nasopharynx; focal infection	Vagina (menstruation, tampon use); focal infection
Exposure	Ingestion	Systemic absorption or local	Systemic absorption
Site of action	Intestine	Epidermis	Unknown (possibly endothelium)
Mode of action	Vagus nerve reflex	Splitting of the desmosomes in the stratum granulosum	Capillary leakage (?)
High-risk groups	Any age	Children	Children; menstruating women

Several membrane-damaging (cytolytic) toxins produced by staphylococci are known: α toxin, β toxin, γ toxin, δ toxin and leucocidin[8]:

- Staphylococcus β toxin damages susceptible membranes probably through altering membrane permeability, with consequent major disruption of cellular activity. It is particularly active against erythrocyte membranes and is therefore a hemolytic toxin. The toxin has the property of Mg^{2+}-requiring sphingomyelin phosphodiesterase, which splits sphingomyelin into ceramide and choline phosphate
- Staphylococcus δ toxin likewise attacks cell membranes, but in a less specific manner than the β toxin. It is a complex protein with a high proportion of hydrophobic amino acids that seem to be able to penetrate, disrupt and produce lysis of some cell membranes. It also has the effect of stimulating the adenylate-cyclase system in a manner not unlike that of cholera toxin
- Staphylococcus α toxin has a similar but obviously more specific effect than the δ toxin. It probably consists of a binding fragment, which reacts with specific membrane receptors, and hydrophobic fragment, which penetrates and disrupts the integrity of the membrane. No enzymatic activity is definitely associated with this action
- Leucocidin. The activity of this cytolytic toxin is restricted to polymorphonuclear leukocytes and macrophages

Several epidermolytic toxins (also referred to as 'exfoliatin'), produced mainly by phage-group II *S. aureus*, are responsible for exfoliative dermatitis (scalded skin syndrome, see Table 4). Proteins isolated with toxic activity have been designated ETA (M_r 30000) and ETB (M_r 29500).

The toxic shock syndrome toxin, produced mainly by phage-group I *S. aureus*, has some similarity to staphylococcal enterotoxins. The clinical syndrome associated with this toxin – the toxic shock syndrome (see Table 4) – is known since 1978[10]. The disease is characterized by sudden onset of fever, hypotension, vomiting, diarrhea, as well as scarlet-fever-like exanthema. The pathogenesis of the syndrome is still not known[11]. For a review published in 1991, see FREEDMAN and BEER[19].

Remarks. In treating *S. aureus* or *S. epidermidis* infections, resistance is often a problem and susceptibility tests should be performed. Treatment depends on whether the organism is non-penicillinase producing, penicillinase-producing or methicillin-resistant[12]. The increase of methicillin-resistant *S. aureus* is well documented[13-16]. Resistance to vancomycin may be an emerging clinical problem[17,18].

References

1 PATRICK, C. C., *J. Pediat.*, **116**, 497 (1990).
2 KLOOS and SCHLEIFER, in SNEATH et al. (Eds.), *Bergey's Manual of Systematic Bacteriology*, Vol. 2, Williams & Wilkins, Baltimore, 1986, page 1013.
3 MORSE, S. I., in BRAUDE et al. (Eds.), *Infectious Diseases and Medical Microbiology*, 2nd ed., Saunders, Philadelphia, 1986, page 236.
4 COHEN, J. O., in BARON, S. (Ed.), *Medical Microbiology*, 2nd ed., Addison-Wesley, Menlo Park, CA, 1986, page 360.
5 WALDVOGEL, F. A., in MANDELL et al. (Eds.), *Principles and Practice of Infectious Diseases*, 3rd ed., Churchill Livingstone, New York, 1990, page 1489.
6 ARCHER, G. L., in MANDELL et al. (Eds.), *Principles and Practice of Infectious* Diseases, 3rd ed., Churchill Livingstone, New York, 1990, page 1511.
7 HOLMBERG and BLAKE, *J. Amer. med. Ass.*, **251**, 487 (1984).
8 LENTNER, C. (Ed.), *Geigy Scientific Tables*, 8th ed., Vol. 4, Ciba-Geigy Ltd., Basel, 1986, page 201.
9 TODD, J. K., *Ann. Rev. Med.*, **36**, 337 (1985).
10 TODD et al., *Lancet*, **2**, 1116 (1978).
11 EYKYN, S. J., *Lancet*, **1**, 100 (1988).
12 *Med. Lett. Drug. Ther.*, **32**, No. 817 (1990).
13 BRUMFITT and HAMILTON-MILLER, *New Engl. J. Med.*, **320**, 1188 (1989).
14 MAPLE et al., *Lancet*, **1**, 537 (1989).
15 REBOLI et al., *Amer. J. Dis. Child.*, **143**, 34 (1989).
16 SAHAI, J., *New Engl. J. Med.*, **321**, 1342 (1989).
17 JOHNSON et al., *Clin. Microbiol. Rev.*, **3**, 280 (1990).
18 VEACH et al., *J. clin. Microbiol.*, **28**, 2064 (1990).
19 FREEDMAN and BEER, *Advanc. intern. Med.*, **36**, 363 (1991).

No.	**Bacterium** *Synonyms* Common names	Characteristics	Habitat Host Transmission	Associated disease
140	**Streptococcus pyogenes** ROSENBACH *Streptococcus haemolyticus*	GRAM-positive, spherical, coccal-like organisms, 0.5–1.0 µm in diameter. In pairs or chains of various lengths (usually 10 or more cocci). Nonmotile. LANCEFIELD group A. Poor growth in first cultures on ordinary media. Addition of blood or serum enhances growth. β-Hemolysis on blood agar. Also atypical forms showing α- or γ-hemolysis; some strains show α-hemolysis when aerobic, β-hemolysis when anaerobic. Sensitive to bacitracin. Aerobic, facultatively anaerobic. See also Table 1 on page 55	Respiratory tract in man. Dust in hospitals. Occasionally in udders and milk of cows infected by man	Various kinds of inflammation and suppuration; panaris, phlegmon, erysipelas, scarlet fever, pharyngitis, tonsillitis, otitis, pneumonia, empyema, nephritis, meningitis, puerperal fever, septicemia. Streptococcal toxic shock syndrome includes deep-seated infection associated with shock and multiorgan failure[1]. For review, see BISNO[2] and also text on pages 54–56
141	**Streptococcus agalactiae** LEHMANN and NEUMANN	GRAM-positive, spherical or ovoid coccal-like organisms, 0.6 to 1.2 µm in diameter. In chains, seldom less than 4 cocci, frequently very long. LANCEFIELD group B. 30–50% of strains produce β-hemolysis on blood agar. Aerobic, facultatively anaerobic. See also Table 1 on page 55	Nasopharynx of healthy persons. Commonest cause of mastitis in cows	Pharyngitis, pneumonia, empyema, wound infections, puerperal fever, urinary tract infections, peritonitis, meningitis, endocarditis. Infections are similar to those caused by group D streptococci (*S. faecalis*, *S. faecium*), but differentiation is important since benzylpenicillin is effective in streptococcus B infections. For review, see EDWARDS and BAKER[3]
142	**Streptococcus pneumoniae** (KLEIN) CHESTER *Micrococcus pneumoniae* Pneumococcus	GRAM-positive, oval or spherical coccal-like organisms, 0.5 to 1.25 µm in diameter. In pairs, occasionally single or in short chains; the distal ends of each pair is lance shaped. Capsulated on primary isolation, but not in cultures. Nongroupable or LANCEFIELD group O. Aerobic, facultatively anaerobic. Growth enhanced by the addition of blood, serum or ascitic fluid to culture media. α-Hemolysis on blood agar. Colonies on blood agar appear smooth, glistening, and flat or dome-shaped, 0.5 to 1.5 µm in diameter. 84 different serovars have been identified[3]. See also Table 1 on page 55	Respiratory tract in man	Often saprophytic. Pathogenic types cause lobar pneumonia, bronchitis, bronchopneumonia, empyema, conjunctivitis, meningitis, otitis media, peritonitis, mastoiditis. For review, see MUFSON[4] and also text on pages 54–56
143	**Streptococcus equisimilis** FROST and ENGELBRECHT	Similar to *S. pyogenes*. LANCEFIELD group C. β-Hemolysis. Aerobic, facultatively anaerobic. See also Table 1 on page 55	Upper respiratory tract of normal and diseased man and animals	Endocarditis, septicemia, pneumonia, meningitis, mild upper respiratory infection, skin and wound infections
144	**Streptococcus salivarius** ANDREWES and HORDER	GRAM-positive, spherical or ovoid coccal-like organisms. In short to very long chains. Nongroupable or LANCEFIELD group F, H, K. Slow growth. No β-hemolysis. Aerobic, facultatively anaerobic. See also Table 1 on page 55	Pharynx, mouth, tonsils in man	Dental abscesses, caries, nephritis, arthritis, pneumonia, empyema, septicemia; isolated from blood in endocarditis
145	**Streptococcus sanguis** WHITE and NIVEN *Streptococcus sanguis I*	GRAM-positive, spherical or ovoid coccal-like organisms, 0.8 to 1.2 µm in diameter. In medium-long or long chains. Nongroupable or LANCEFIELD group F, H, K. α-Hemolysis. See also Table 1 on page 55	Dental plaque and other parts of mouth, intestinal tract in man	Caries, endocarditis

[1] STEVENS, D. L., *Clin. infect. Dis.*, **14**, 2 (1992).
[2] BISNO, A. L., in MANDELL et al. (Eds.), *Principles and Practice of Infectious Diseases*, 3rd ed., Churchill Livingstone, New York, 1990, page 1519.
[3] EDWARDS and BAKER, in MANDELL et al. (Eds.), *Principles and Practice of Infectious Diseases*, 3rd ed., Churchill Livingstone, New York, 1990, page 1554.
[4] MUFSON, M. A., in MANDELL et al. (Eds.), *Principles and Practice of Infectious Diseases*, 3rd ed., Churchill Livingstone, New York, 1990, page 1539.

No.	Bacterium *Synonyms* Common names	Characteristics	Habitat Host Transmission	Associated disease
146	**Streptococcus mitis** ANDREWES and HORDER	GRAM-positive, spherical or ovoid cocci, 0.6–1.0 µm in diameter. Single, in pairs or in long chains. Nongroupable or LANCEFIELD group K, M, O. Most strains show α-hemolysis on blood agar, some produce zones of β-hemolysis. See also Table 1 on next page	Upper respiratory tract in man	Caries, endocarditis
147	**Streptococcus sanguis II** FACKLAM	Similar to *S. mitis*. Nongroupable or LANCEFIELD group F, H, K, O. α-Hemolysis. See also Table 1 on next page	Upper respiratory tract, intestinal tract in man	Caries, endocarditis
148	**Streptococcus anginosus** ANDREWES and HORDER *Streptococcus milleri* Minute haemolytic streptococcus	GRAM-positive, spherical or ovoid coccal-like organisms. Single, in pairs or in short chains. Nongroupable or LANCEFIELD group F, G, K. On blood agar pin-point colonies with β-hemolysis. Aerobic, facultatively anaerobic. See also Table 1 on next page	Pharynx, vagina, skin and feces of healthy persons, dogs	Tonsillitis, septicemia, septic foci, abscesses, glomerulonephritis, rheumatic disorders, mild upper respiratory tract infection. For review, see RUOFF[1]
149	**Streptococcus mutans** CLARKE	GRAM-positive cocci, 0.5 to 0.75 µm in diameter. In pairs, short or medium-long chains. Nongroupable or LANCEFIELD group E, K. Most strains show α-hemolysis. See also Table 1 on next page	Dental plaque, intestinal tract in man	Caries, endocarditis
150	**Streptococcus faecalis** ANDREWES and HORDER Enterococcus	GRAM-positive, ovoid cocci, 0.5 to 1.0 µm in diameter. Usually in pairs or in short chains. Morphologically similar to pneumococci. Some strains motile. LANCEFIELD group D. Tellurite-positive. Most strains nonhemolytic, but a few show β-hemolysis. Aerobic, facultatively anaerobic. Resistance to heat (60 °C for 30 min) in neutral media. See also Table 1 on next page	Intestinal tract in man and animals. Common in nonsterile foods	Urinary tract infections, endocarditis, septicemia
151	**Streptococcus faecium** ORLA-JENSEN *Enterococcus faecium*	GRAM-positive, spherical or ovoid coccal-like organisms. In pairs or short chains. LANCEFIELD group D. α-Hemolysis on blood agar. Aerobic, facultatively anaerobic. Resistance to heat (60 °C for 30 min) in neutral media. See also Table 1 on next page	Intestinal tract in man and animals. Common in nonsterile foods	Urinary tract infections, endocarditis, septicemia

[1] RUOFF, K. L., *Clin. Microbiol. Rev.*, **1**, 102 (1988).

Streptococci

29 species have been identified[1]. The streptococci may be classified by at least 4 schemes based on:

- Clinical presentation (pyogenic, oral, enteric streptococci)
- Biochemical characteristics
- Hemolysis (complete hemolysis [β], incomplete hemolysis [α] and no hemolysis)
- Serologic properties

The serologic grouping system by LANCEFIELD is based on antigens that are either polysaccharides associated with the cell wall, as in the groups A, B, C, E, F and G, or teichoic acids situated in the region between the cell membrane and the inner surface of the cell wall (groups D and N)[1]. Serogroups A to H and K to V have been recognized; some streptococci are nongroupable by the LANCEFIELD grouping system that was initially devised for the identification of pathogenic β-hemolytic streptococci, but certain α-hemolytic and nonhemolytic species also contain group-specific antigens (Table 1). In addition to the major group antigens, type-specific surface antigens are recognized; such antigens are commonly proteins, but polysaccharide type antigens also occur (Table 2).

Streptococcal infections have been comprehensively reviewed by PARKER[4] and by various authors in MANDELL et al.[5].

Pneumococcal disease

84 capsular types of *Streptococcus pneumonia* have been detected (Table 3). The most frequent pathogens in severe disease in children are the types 6, 14, 19 and 23 (Table 4). In adults, types 1, 3, 4, 7, 8, 9, 12 and 14 are those most commonly associated with pneumococcal septicemia[6], types 3, 4, 6, 14, 19, 23 and 26 are those most commonly recognized in respiratory isolates[7]. The organisms who do not possess a capsular polysaccharide are called 'rough' pneumococci and are not pathogenic in man.

Pneumococcal disease remains a problem in very young children,

Table 1 *Differential characteristics of medically important species of the genus* Streptococcus[1–3]

	Hemolysis	Growth at 45 °C	Bile solubility	Growth in 6.5% NaCl	Esculin hydrolysis	Acid production from: Lactose	Sucrose	Mannitol	Salicin	LANCEFIELD group antigen
S. pyogenes . . .	β*	−	−	−	−	+	+	−	+	A
S. agalactiae . .	α/β	−	−	−	−	v	+	−	+	B
S. equisimilis . .	β	−	−	−	v	v	+	−	v	C
S. faecalis	−/β	+	−	+	+	+	v	+	+	D
S. faecium	−/α	+	−	+	+	+	−◊	+	+	D
S. mutans	−/α	v	v	−	+	+	+	+	+	−/E, F, K
S. anginosus . . .	−/α	−	−	−	v	−	+	−	+	−/F, G, K†
S. salivarius . . .	−/α	+	−	−	+	+	+	−	+	−/F, H, K†
S. sanguis I . . .	α	v	v	−	v	+	+	−	+	−/F, G, H, K
S. sanguis II . . .	α	v	v	−	−	+		−		−/F, G, H, K, M, O†
S. mitis	α	v	v	−	−	+	−	−	−	−/K, M, O†
S. pneumoniae .	α	−	+	−	−	+	+	−	−	−/O

\+ Typically positive.
− Typically negative.
v Variable.
* Some strains show α-hemolysis when aerobic, β-hemolysis when anaerobic.
◊ Mostly negative, seldom positive.
† Strains may possess antigens of group A and/or C.

the elderly and persons with high-risk conditions (see below under prophylaxis). Pneumococcal pneumonia causes over 1 million deaths every year in children under 5 years of age in developing countries[9]. In the USA, pneumococci cause 10–25% of all pneumonia cases (with an estimated 40000 deaths annually); the estimated rate of pneumococcal septicemia is 15–19 persons per 100000, that for pneumococcal meningitis 1–2 persons per 100000 every year[10].

Prophylaxis. The commercial pneumococcus vaccine now available includes (in a single dose of 0.5 mL) 25 µg of each of 23 different capsular polysaccharides (US nomenclature: 1, 2, 3, 4, 5, 8, 9, 12, 14, 17, 19, 20, 22, 23, 26, 34, 43, 51, 54, 56, 57, 68, 70)[6,9,10]. In the USA, vaccination has been recommended for a wide range of conditions[10]:

Table 3 *Designation of* Streptococcus pneumonia *serovars*[6]

USA	Denmark	USA	Denmark	USA	Denmark
1	1	29	29	57	19A
2	2	30	15A	58	19B
3	3	31	31	59	19C
4	4	32	32F	60	24B?
5	5	33	9A	61	35C
6	6A	34	10A	62	35A
7	7A	35	35F	63	22A
8	8	36	36	64	23B
9	9N	37	37	65	24A
10	10F	38	41F	66	35B
11	11F	39	33C	67	32A
12	12F	40	33A	68	9V
13	13	41	34	69	39
14	14	42	33B	70	33F
15	15F	43	11A	71	38
16	16	44	18A	72	45
17	17	45	40	73	46
18	18F	46	23A	74	41A
19	19F	47	35A	75	43
20	20	48	7B	76	11B
21	21	49	9L	77	15C
22	22F	50	7C	78	17A
23	23F	51	7F	79	28A
24	24F	52	47F	80	42
25	25	53	11C	81	44
26	6B	54	15B	82	48
27	27	55	18B	83	12A
28	28	56	18C	84	47A

- Children ⩾2 years old with chronic illnesses specifically associated with increased risk of pneumococcal disease or its complications (e.g. anatomic or functional asplenia [including sickle cell disease], nephrotic syndrome, cerebrospinal fluid leaks, and conditions associated with immunosuppression)
- Children ⩾2 years old with asymptomatic or symptomatic human immunodeficiency virus (HIV) infection
- Immunocompetent adults who are at increased risk of pneumococcal disease or its complications because of chronic illnesses (e.g. cardiovascular disease, pulmonary disease, diabetes mellitus, alcoholism, cirrhosis, or cerebrospinal fluid leaks) or who are ⩾65 years old
- Immunocompromised adults at increased risk of pneumococcal disease or its complications (e.g. persons with splenic dysfunction or anatomic asplenia, Hodgkin's disease, lymphoma, multiple myeloma, chronic renal failure, nephrotic syndrome, or conditions such as organ transplantation associated with immunosuppression)
- Adults with asymptomatic or symptomatic HIV infection

(Continued on next page)

Table 2 *Antigenic and chemical properties of pyogenic hemolytic streptococci pathogenic in man*[1]

	LANCEFIELD group antigen: Symbol	Major chemical constituents	Type antigen(s): Symbol	Chemical nature	Location	Other major cell antigens
Streptococcus pyogenes	A	N-Acetylglucosamine, rhamnose	M SOF T	Protein Protein Protein	Fimbriae Cell wall Cell wall	LTA MAP R protein
Streptococcus agalactiae	B	Rhamnose, galactose, N-acetylglucosamine	I–IV Ib, c, R, X	Polysaccharides Proteins	Capsule Capsule	
Streptococcus spp. group C	C	N-Acetylgalactosamine, rhamnose		Proteins	Capsule	R protein
Streptococcus spp. group G	G	Rhamnose, galactosamine		Proteins	Cell wall	R protein
Streptococcus spp. group L	L	N-Acetylglucosamine, N-acetylgalactosamine, galactose, rhamnose		Proteins	Cell wall	R protein
Streptococcus spp. group M	M	Not known		Proteins		
Streptococcus pneumoniae		Ribitol teichoic acid, choline phosphate	SSS	Polysaccharides	Capsule	M-like proteins

SOF Serum opacity factor. LTA Lipoteichoic acid.
SSS Specific soluble substance. MAP M-associated protein.

No.	**Bacterium** *Synonyms* Common names	Characteristics	Habitat Host Transmission	Associated disease
152	**Leuconostoc mesenteroides** (TSENKOVSKII) VAN TIEGHEM	GRAM-positive, spherical organisms, occurring in pairs and chains. Facultatively anaerobic. Optimal growth at 20–30 °C. Catalase-negative. Gas production from glucose. No hemolysis	Plants, milk, milk products	Septicemia, meningitis, peritonitis in patients with underlying disease reported[1]
153	**Leuconostoc paramesenteroides** GARVIE	Similar to *L. mesenteroides*	As for *L. mesenteroides*	See *L. mesenteroides*
154	**Aerococcus viridans** WILLIAMS et al.	GRAM-positive, spherical organisms, 1.0–2.0 µm in diameter; tendency toward tetrad formation. Nonmotile. Microaerophilic. Acid production from glucose, fructose, galactose, mannose, maltose. Catalase activity absent or weak. α-Hemolysis	Widely distributed in dust and on raw and processed vegetables	Implicated in urinary tract infection, septicemia, endocarditis, and meningitis in children[2]
155	**Peptostreptococcus magnus** (PRÉVOT) EZAKI et al. *Diplococcus magnus* *Peptococcus magnus*	GRAM-positive cocci, 0.7–1.2 µm in diameter, occurring singly, in pairs, tetrads and clusters. Anaerobic	Mouth, respiratory tract, intestinal tract and vagina	Orodental, face and neck infections, uterine infections, bone and joint infections, abscesses of the buttock and breast[3]
156	Other *Peptostreptococcus* species: **Peptostreptococcus anaerobius** **Peptostreptococcus asaccharolyticus** **Peptostreptococcus prevotii** **Peptostreptococcus micros**	GRAM-positive cocci, smaller than *P. magnus*	As for *P. magnus*	See *P. magnus*

[1] HANDWERGER et al., *Rev. infect. Dis.*, **12**, 602 (1990).
[2] NATHAVITHARANA et al., *Brit. med. J.*, **286**, 1248 (1983).
[3] BOURGAULT et al., *Ann. intern. Med.*, **93**, 244 (1980).

Table 4 Streptococcus pneumoniae *serovars isolated most frequently in infected children (Alabama and Papua New Guinea)*[8]

Serovar	Alabama, 1986 ($N = 1310$)					Papua New Guinea, 1984 ($N = 25$)
	Meningitis	Septicemia	Otitis media	Pneumonia*	Total	Pneumonia◊
	% of total isolates					
3	7	2	8	4	6	–
6	32	17	15	21	17	24
14	14	29	14	9	15	12
18	9	11	3	3	4	–
19	7	7	28	22	23	12
23	7	11	11	16	12	8

* Cultures from miscellaneous sites, mainly the respiratory tract in patients with putative pneumonia.
◊ Cultures from lung aspirates and blood.

Children under 2 years of age have a poor antibody response to many of the serotypes in the pneumococcus vaccine[9]. In the USA, vaccination is not recommended for recurrent upper respiratory tract infection or otitis media in children[10]. The efficacy of pneumococcus vaccine in the high-risk group is still under discussion[6, 9–11]. Immunity, as measured by antibody levels, seems to persist for 5 years in young healthy adults[12].

Remarks. Increasing resistance of pneumococcal strains (particularly to penicillin, tetracyclines, chloramphenicol, trimethoprim–sulfamethoxazole, as well as multiple drug resistance[6, 13, 14]) is often a problem and susceptibility tests should be performed.

For treatment of pneumococcal infections, benzylpenicillin and phenoxymethylpenicillin are still the drugs of choice; erythromycin, a cephalosporin, chloramphenicol, a tetracycline, or vancomycin may be effective[6, 15]. In meningitis, as well as in septicemia, prompt treatment is essential and antimicrobial drugs should not be withheld until laboratory tests are performed[15].

References

1 ROTTA, J., in SNEATH et al. (Eds.), *Bergey's Manual of Systematic Bacteriology*, Vol. 2, Williams & Wilkins, Baltimore, 1986, page 1047.
2 HARDIE, J. M., in SNEATH et al. (Eds.), *Bergey's Manual of Systematic Bacteriology*, Vol. 2, Williams & Wilkins, Baltimore, 1986, page 1054.
3 MUNDT, J. O., in SNEATH et al. (Eds.), *Bergey's Manual of Systematic Bacteriology*, Vol. 2, Williams & Wilkins, Baltimore, 1986, page 1063.
4 PARKER, M. T., *Pathogenic Streptococci*, Reedbooks, Chertsey, 1979.
5 MANDELL et al. (Eds.), *Principles and Practice of Infectious Diseases*, 3rd ed., Churchill Livingstone, New York, 1990, pages 1519–1572.
6 MUFSON, M. A., in MANDELL et al. (Eds.), *Principles and Practice of Infectious Diseases*, 3rd ed., Churchill Livingstone, New York, 1990, page 1539.
7 JORGENSEN et al., *J. infect. Dis.*, **163**, 644 (1991).
8 JOHNSTON, R. B., *Rev. infect. Dis.*, **13**, Suppl. 6, S509 (1991).
9 SHANN, F., *Lancet*, **335**, 898 (1990).
10 *Morb. Mort. wkly Rec.*, **38**, 64 (1989).
11 Health and Public Policy Committee, *Ann. intern. Med.*, **104**, 118 (1986).
12 MUFSON et al., *Amer. J. med. Sci.*, **30**, 279 (1987).
13 SPIKA et al., *J. infect. Dis.*, **163**, 1273 (1991).
14 ALLEN, K. D., *J. Hosp. Infect.*, **17**, 3 (1991).
15 *Med. Lett. Drug. Ther.*, **32**, No. 817 (1990).

No.	**Bacterium** *Synonyms* Common names	Characteristics	Habitat Host Transmission	Associated disease
157	**Bacillus subtilis** (EHRENBERG) COHN *Vibrio subtilis* Hay bacillus	GRAM-positive, slender rods, 0.7 to 0.8 µm wide and 2–3 µm long, occurring singly, seldom in chains. Motile, with peritrichous flagella. Ellipsoidal, central endospores. Growth on minimal media. Aerobic. See also table below	Soil, dust, water, hay, water, milk	Occasional cause of eye infections, urinary tract infection, septicemia, meningitis, otitis[1] *Remark.* Spore strips of *B. subtilis* are used to test the efficiency of sterilizers[2]
158	**Bacillus anthracis** COHN Anthrax bacillus DAVAINE's bacillus	GRAM-positive, plump rods, 1.0 to 1.2 µm wide and 3–5 µm long, occurring in chains. Nonmotile. Glutamyl polypeptide capsule formation *in vivo* and on serum plates. Ellipsoidal, central endospores. Aerobic, facultatively anaerobic. Thiamine and amino acids required in a minimal medium. See also table below. Produces toxin (protective antigen, edema factor, lethal factor)	Soil; cattle, sheep and other animals, also man. Transmission by contact with infected brushes or when handling and depilating skins; rarely by inhalation of material containing spores or consumption of infected meat	Anthrax in man (milzbrand, woolsorters' disease)[3,4]: cutaneous, pulmonary or intestinal anthrax, depending on portal of entry. Rare complications: septicemia and meningitis. Incubation period 1–10 days[4]. Skin anthrax predominates (95%). Anthrax is extremely rare in the USA and western Europe, small epidemics may occur[5]
			Remarks. Vaccination of professionally exposed persons is recommended (veterinarians, leather workers, brushmakers, etc.)[4]. Treatment with benzylpenicillin recommended[3,6]	
159	**Bacillus cereus** FRANKLAND and FRANKLAND	GRAM-positive. Similar to *B. anthracis*, but motile with peritrichous flagella. Strains of *B. cereus* have been classified into 23 serovars[7]. See also table below. Produces 2 enterotoxins	Soil, dust, water, foodstuffs (corn, milk)	Often reported to cause food poisoning; eye infections (panophthalmitis), wound infections, septicemia, endocarditis, meningitis, pneumonia, musculoskeletal infections[1,8–11]
160	**Bacillus licheniformis** (WEIGMANN) CHESTER *Clostridium lichiniformis*	GRAM-positive. Similar to *B. subtilis*. Glutamyl polypeptide capsule formation. Spores may survive severe heat treatment. See also table below	Soil, foodstuffs	Implicated in food poisoning, eye infections, wound infections, septicemia, pneumonia[1,11,12]
161	**Bacillus stearothermophilus** DONK	GRAM-positive. Similar to *B. subtilis*. Optimal growth 45–65 °C. See also table below	Soil, dust, water, foodstuffs (corn, milk)	Not pathogenic in man *Remark.* Spore strips of *B. stearothermophilus* are used to test the efficiency of sterilizers and autoclaves[2]

[1] TUAZON, C. U., in MANDELL et al. (Eds.), *Principles and Practice of Infectious Diseases*, 3rd ed., Churchill Livingstone, New York, 1990, page 1595.
[2] PERKINS, J. J., *Principles and Methods of Sterilization Health Sciences*, 2nd ed., Thomas, Springfield, IL, 1978, page 494.
[3] LAFORCE, F. M., in MANDELL et al. (Eds.), *Principles and Practice of Infectious Diseases*, 3rd ed., Churchill Livingstone, New York, 1990, page 1593.
[4] BRACHMAN, P. S., in WARREN and MAHMOUD (Eds.), *Tropical and Geographical Medicine*, 2nd ed., McGraw-Hill, New York, 1990, page 877.
[5] PFISTERER, R. M., *Schweiz. med. Wschr.*, **121**, 813 (1991).
[6] *Med. Lett. Drug. Ther.*, **32**, No. 817 (1990).
[7] WILLIAMS, R. P., in BRAUDE et al. (Eds.), *Infectious Diseases and Medical Microbiology*, 2nd ed., Saunders, Philadelphia, 1986, page 270.
[8] SLIMAN et al., *Medicine (Baltimore)*, **66**, 218 (1987).
[9] DRYDEN, M. S., *J. roy. Soc. Med.*, **80**, 480 (1987).
[10] ÅKESSON et al., *Scand. J. infect. Dis.*, **23**, 71 (1991).
[11] BARON and FINEGOLD (Eds.), *Bailey & Scott's Diagnostic Microbiology*, 8th ed., Mosby, St. Louis, 1990.
[12] THURN and GOODMAN, *Amer. J. Med.*, **85**, 708 (1988).

Differential characteristics of some species of the genus Bacillus

	B. subtilis	*B. anthracis*	*B. cereus*	*B. licheniformis*	*B. stearothermophilus*
Motility	+	–	+	+	+
Growth at 45 °C	+	–	d	+	+
Growth at 65 °C	–	–	–	–	+
Growth at pH 5.7	+	+	+	+	–
Growth in 7% NaCl	+	+	d	+	–
Utilization of citrate	+	d	+	+	d
Anaerobic growth in glucose broth	–	+	+	+	+
Acid production from glucose	+	+	+	+	+
– from arabinose	+	–	–	+	d
– from mannitol	+	–	–	+	d
– from xylose	+	–	–	+	d
Nitrate reduction	+	+	+	+	d
Catalase activity	+	+	+	+	d

\+ 90% of strains are positive.
– 90% of strains are negative.
d 11–89% of strains are positive.

Reference

CLAUS and BERKELEY, in SNEATH et al. (Eds.), *Bergey's Manual of Systematic Bacteriology*, Volume 2, Williams & Wilkins, Baltimore, 1986, page 1105.

No.	Bacterium *Synonyms* Common names	Characteristics	Habitat Host Transmission	Associated disease
162	**Clostridium botulinum** (VAN ERMENGEM) BERGEY et al. *Bacillus botulinus*	GRAM-positive, straight rods, 0.5–2.4 µm wide, up to 22 µm long, occurring singly and in pairs. Motile, with peritrichous flagella. Oval, subterminal spores. Obligately anaerobic. Eight distinct toxin types (A, B, C_1, C_2, D, E, F, G) are known: a given strain produces only a single type of toxin	Soil, etc. (see text on page 60). Toxin types associated with human disease generally follow the geographical distribution of types; type E is usually associated with fish products[3]	Botulism with neurological disorder is most commonly caused by toxin types A, B and E[1–3] (1) Ingestion by preformed toxin (food poisoning). Incubation period 12–36 hours, but may range from 6 hours to 8 days[3] (2) Production of the toxin *in vivo*: (a) wound botulism (very rare); (b) infant botulism[4,5] recognized in the USA since 1976 with 70 cases reported in 1991[6] (often suggested in association with honey consumption). A few cases resembling infant botulism have been reported in adults[1]
163	**Clostridium difficile** (HALL and O'TOOLE) PRÉVOT *Bacillus difficilis*	GRAM-positive, straight rods, 0.5–1.9 µm wide and 3–17 µm long, occurring singly, in pairs or in short chains. Motile, with peritrichous flagella. Oval, subterminal (rarely terminal) spores. Obligately anaerobic. Produces toxins	Soil, etc. (see text on page 60). Very common fecal organism in infants and young children, seldom in healthy adults. Detected in the environment of patients with antibiotic-associated diarrheal syndrome	Pseudomembranous colitis; usually associated with colitis and diarrhea due to antibiotic therapy[7–10]. Diarrhea usually begins 4–9 days after starting antibiotic therapy *Remarks.* Improvement when antimicrobial agent is discontinued. Vancomycin or metronidazole are recommended for treatment in persistent or severe cases[7,11]
164	**Clostridium histolyticum** (WEINBERG and SÉGUIN) BERGEY et al. *Bacillus histolyticus*	GRAM-positive, straight rods, 0.5–0.9 µm wide and 1.3–9.2 µm long, occurring singly, in pairs or in short chains. Motile, with peritrichous flagella. Oval, central to subterminal spores. Anaerobic and microaerophilic. Produces 5 toxins, the combination of which causes complete tissue destruction	Soil, etc. (see text on page 60)	Rare cause of clostridial myonecrosis (gas gangrene), possibly as a component of a mixture of *Clostridium* species[1]
165	**Clostridium novyi** (MIGULA) BERGEY et al. *Clostridium pedematiens* *Bacillus novyi* NOVY's bacillus	GRAM-variable, straight rods, 0.6–2.5 µm wide and 1.6–22 µm long, occurring singly or in pairs. Motile, with peritrichous flagella. Oval, central or subterminal spores. Anaerobic. Types A, B, and C are distinguished; types A and B produce several toxins, type C none	Soil, etc. (see text on page 60)	Types A and B rare cause of clostridial myonecrosis (gas gangrene)[1,12–14]
166	**Clostridium perfringens** (VEILLON and ZUBER) HAUDUROY et al. *Bacillus perfringens* *Bacterium welchii* ACHALME's bacillus Gas bacillus WELCH's bacillus WELCH–FRAENKEL gas bacillus	GRAM-positive, long rods, 0.6 to 2.4 µm wide and 1.3–19 µm long, occurring singly or in pairs. Nonmotile. Spores rarely seen; when present, they are large, oval, central or subterminal. Obligately anaerobic. Types A, B, C, D, and E are distinguished according to the toxin types produced	Soil, etc. (see text on page 60). Food contamination (meat products) may be of importance	Type A most frequent cause of clostridial myonecrosis (gas gangrene)[1,13,14], also common cause of food poisoning as well as enterotoxin-associated diarrhea[1,12]. Endocarditis reported[15]. Incubation period of clostridial myonecrosis is 1–4 days, rarely longer[13,14]. Incubation period of food poisoning 8–24 hours[12]. Type C causes necrotizing enterocolitis[1,12]

1 HATHEWAY, C. L., *Clin. Microbiol. Rev.*, **3**, 66 (1990).
2 DONTA, S. T., in BRAUDE et al. (Eds.), *Infectious Diseases and Medical Microbiology*, 2nd ed., Saunders, Philadelphia, 1986, page 892.
3 SCHAFFNER, W., in MANDELL et al. (Eds.), *Principles and Practice of Infectious Diseases*, 3rd ed., Churchill Livingstone, New York, 1990, page 1847.
4 ARNON, S. S., *Ann. Rev. Med.*, **31**, 541 (1980).
5 SCHREINER et al., *Pediatrics*, **87**, 159 (1991).
6 *Morb. Mort. wkly Rep.*, **40**, No. 52, 898 (1991).
7 FEKETY, R., in MANDELL et al. (Eds.), *Principles and Practice of Infectious Diseases*, 3rd ed., Churchill Livingstone, New York, 1990, page 863.
8 GERDING, D. N., *Ann. intern. Med.*, **110**, 255 (1989).
9 TABAQCHALI, S., *Rev. infect. Dis.*, **12**, Suppl. 2, S 192 (1990).
10 BARTLETT, J. G., *Rev. infect. Dis.*, **12**, Suppl. 2, S 243 (1990).
11 *Med. Lett. Drug. Ther.*, **31**, 93 (1989).
12 HOBBS, B. C., in BRAUDE et al. (Eds.), *Infectious Diseases and Medical Microbiology*, 2nd ed., Saunders, Philadelphia, 1986, page 407.
13 BORNSTEIN, D. L., in BRAUDE et al. (Eds.), *Infectious Diseases and Medical Microbiology*, 2nd ed., Saunders, Philadelphia, 1986, page 1490.
14 BARTLETT, J. G., in MANDELL et al. (Eds.), *Principles and Practice of Infectious Diseases*, 3rd ed., Churchill Livingstone, New York, 1990, page 1850.

No.	**Bacterium** *Synonyms* Common names	Characteristics	Habitat Host Transmission	Associated disease
167	**Clostridium septicum** (MACÉ) FORD *Bacillus septicus* GHON–SACHS bacillus	GRAM-positive, straight or curved pleomorphous rods, 0.6 to 1.9 µm wide and 1.9–35 µm long, occurring singly or in pairs. Motile, with peritrichous flagella. Forms long filaments on the peritoneal surface of the liver in infected animals. Oval, subterminal spores. Anaerobic. Produces 4 major toxins	Soil, etc. (see text on next page)	Rare cause of clostridial myonecrosis (gas gangrene)[1,2], septicemia, necrotizing enterocolitis[3]
168	**Clostridium sordellii** (HALL and SCOTT) PRÉVOT *Bacillus sordellii* SORDELLI's bacillus	GRAM-positive, straight rods, 0.5 to 1.7 µm wide and 1.6–21 µm long, occurring singly or in pairs. Oval, central or subterminal spores, often occurring as free spores. Motile, with peritrichous flagella. Anaerobic. Urease-positive. A lethal factor (β-toxin) is responsible for the pathogenicity of *C. sordellii*	Soil, etc. (see text on next page)	Rare cause of clostridial myonecrosis (gas gangrene). *C. sordellii* infections in association with obstetrical surgical incisions[3]. Endocarditis reported[4]
169	**Clostridium tetani** (FLÜGGE) BERGEY et al. *Bacillus tetani* NICOLAIER's bacillus	GRAM-positive, slender rods, 0.5 to 1.7 µm wide and 2.1–18 µm long, occurring singly or in pairs. Motile, with peritrichous flagella; some strains are nonflagellated and nonmotile. Round, terminal spores (drumstick-shaped organisms). Obligately anaerobic. Colonies often swarm on agar medium. Exotoxin (tetanolysin and tetanospasmin) production	Especially cultivated soil; intestinal tract in man and animals (particularly horses). See also text on next page	Tetanus[5–7]: local, cephalic and generalized (about 80% of cases) forms. Worldwide distribution. Very common disease in developing countries, with high mortality in neonates[7]; rare in developed countries (49 cases in the USA 1991[8], about 15 cases in FRG yearly[9]). Incubation period usually less than 2 weeks, with a range from a few days to months[5] *Remarks.* Active immunization with tetanus toxoid is a routine prophylactic practice[10]; protective levels of serum antitoxin persist for 10 or more years[11]. For antimicrobial therapy, benzylpenicillin is the drug of choice[7,12]
170	**Clostridium baratii**	GRAM-positive, straight rods, 0.5 to 1.9 µm wide and 1.6–10 µm long, occurring singly. Round subterminal to terminal spores. Nonmotile	Soil, etc. (see text on next page). Usually nonpathogenic in man	Infant botulism type F reported[13]
170a	**Clostridium bifermentas**	Similar to *C. sordellii*. Urease-negative	As for *C. baratii*	Rare cause of clostridial myonecrosis (gas gangrene)[1,2]; endocarditis reported[4]
170b	**Clostridium butyricum**	GRAM-positive, straight rods, 0.5 to 1.7 µm wide and 2.4–7,6 µm long, occurring singly, in pairs, or in short chains, occasionally long filaments. Oval, central to subterminal spores. Motile	As for *C. baratii*	Infant botulism type E reported[14]

[1] BORNSTEIN, D. L., in BRAUDE et al. (Eds.), *Infectious Diseases and Medical Microbiology*, 2nd ed., Saunders, Philadelphia, 1986, page 1490.
[2] BARTLETT, J. G., in MANDELL et al. (Eds.), *Principles and Practice of Infectious Diseases*, 3rd ed., Churchill Livingstone, New York, 1990, page 1850.
[3] HATHEWAY, C. L., *Clin. Microbiol. Rev.*, **3**, 66 (1990).
[4] KOLANDER et al., *Arch. intern. Med.*, **149**, 455 (1989).
[5] CATE, T. R., in MANDELL et al. (Eds.), *Principles and Practice of Infectious Diseases*, 3rd ed., Churchill Livingstone, New York, 1990, page 1842.
[6] VERONESI and FOCACCIA, in BRAUDE et al. (Eds.), *Infectious Diseases and Medical Microbiology*, 2nd ed., Saunders, Philadelphia, 1986, page 1168.
[7] GORBACH, S. L., in WARREN and MAHMOUD (Eds.), *Tropical and Geographical Medicine*, 2nd ed., McGraw-Hill, New York, 1990, page 872.
[8] *Morb. Mort. wkly Rep.*, **40**, No. 52, 898 (1991).
[9] MÜLLER et al., *Dtsch. med. Wschr.*, **113**, 1326 (1988).
[10] HINMAN and ORENSTEIN, *Lancet*, **335**, 707 (1990).
[11] FRENKEL, L. D., *Pediat. Clin. N. Amer.*, **37**, 531 (1990).
[12] *Med. Lett. Drug. Ther.*, **32**, No. 817 (1990).
[13] HALL et al., *J. clin. Microbiol.*, **21**, 654 (1985).
[14] AURELI et al., *J. infect. Dis.*, **154**, 207 (1986).

No.	**Bacterium** *Synonyms* Common names	Characteristics	Habitat Host Transmission	Associated disease
170c	**Clostridium fallax**	GRAM-positive rods, 0.5–1.4 µm wide and 1.6–15.4 µm long, occurring singly or in pairs. Oval, central to subterminal spores. Motile	As for *C. baratii*	Rare cause of clostridial myonecrosis (gas gangrene)[1,2]
170d	**Clostridium sporogenes**	GRAM-positive, straight rods, 0.3 to 1.4 µm wide and 1.3–16.0 µm long, occurring singly. Oval subterminal spores. Motile	As for *C. baratii*	Capable of increasing the pathogenicity of other anaerobes, such as *C. perfringens*, in polymicrobial infections. Endocarditis reported[3]

[1] BORNSTEIN, D. L., in BRAUDE et al. (Eds.), *Infectious Diseases and Medical Microbiology*, 2nd ed., Saunders, Philadelphia, 1986, page 1490.
[2] BARTLETT, J. G., in MANDELL et al. (Eds.), *Principles and Practice of Infectious Diseases*, 3rd ed., Churchill Livingstone, New York, 1990, page 1850.
[3] KOLANDER et al., *Arch. intern. Med.*, **149**, 455 (1989).

Clostridia

Of the 83 species of *Clostridium* listed in *Bergey's Manual of Systematic Bacteriology*[1], about 20 are pathogenic or otherwise encountered in clinical or environmental specimens pertaining to infections in man or animals[2].

Members of the genus are found in soil, sewage, marine sediments, and the intestinal tract of man and animals, and in decaying animal and plant products[1]. Because of the ubiquity of these organisms, they find their way into wounds, foods, and feeds and are often responsible for serious disease, usually (if not always) mediated by their toxins[2].

Biochemical characteristics of selected *Clostridium* species affecting man are given in the table below. Associated diseases are mentioned in *Nos. 162–170d*, pages 58–60.

References

[1] CATO et al., in SNEATH et al. (Eds.), *Bergey's Manual of Systematic Bacteriology*, Volume 2, Williams & Wilkins, Baltimore, 1986, page 1141.
[2] HATHEWAY, C. L., *Clin. Microbiol. Rev.*, **3**, 66 (1990).

Differential characteristics of Clostridium *species affecting man*[1,2]

	Motility	Indole production	Lecithinase activity	Lipase activity	β-Hemolysis	Acid production from Glucose	Acid production from Lactose	Gelatine hydrolysis	Esculin hydrolysis	Meat digested
C. botulinum										
– group I (toxin types A, B, F)	(+)	–	–	+	+	+	–	+	+	+
– group II (toxin types B, E, F)	+	–	–	+	+	+	–	+	–	–
– group III (toxin types C_1, C_2, D)	(+)	(–)	+	+	+	+	–	+	+	(+)
– group IV (*C. argentinense*, toxin type G)	+	–	–	–	+	–	–	+	–	(+)
C. difficile	(+)	–	–	–	–	+	–	+	+	–
C. histolyticum	(+)	–	–	–	+	–	–	+	–	+
C. novyi										
– type A	(+)	–	+	+	+	+	–	+	–	–
– type B	(+)	(+)	+	–	+	+	–	+	–	+
– type C	+	+	–	–	+	+	–	+	–	+
C. perfringens	–	–	+	–	+	+	+	+	(+)	(+)
C. septicum	(+)	–	–	–	+	+	+	+	+	–
C. sordellii	(+)	+	+	–	+	+	–	+	(–)	+
C. tetani	(–)	(+)	–	–	+	–	–	+	–	(–)

+ All strains are positive.
(+) Most strains are positive.
– All strains are negative.
(–) Most strains are negative.

No.	**Bacterium** *Synonyms* Common names	Characteristics	Habitat Host Transmission	Associated disease
171	**Lactobacillus** spp. 'Döderlein bacillus'	GRAM-positive rods varying from long and slender rods to short coccobacilli. Chain formation is common. Nonmotile. No spores are produced. Microaerophilic. Catalase-negative. Growth enhanced by the addition of glucose, yeast extract or blood to culture media. Optimal growth at pH 5.5–6.2. For differentiation from *Listeria* and *Erysipelothrix*, see table below	Found in the mouth, vagina, and intestinal tract in man and animals. Widely distributed in nature: dairy products, grain and meal products, water, sewage, beer, wine, fruits, etc.	Common in dental caries. Very seldom involved in human infections (pleuropulmonary infections[1], endocarditis[2,3])
172	**Listeria monocytogenes** (MURRAY et al.) PIRIE *Bacterium monocytogenes*	GRAM-positive, short rods, 0.4 to 0.5 µm wide and 0.5–2 µm long, occurring singly, in short chains, in V-shaped groups or in groups lying parallel along an axis. In older cultures, filaments of 6 to 20 µm may develop. Motile at 20–25 °C, with few peritrichous flagella. Do not form spores. Aerobic, facultatively anaerobic. Special cold enrichment may be needed to isolate the organism from specimens with mixed flora. β-Hemolysis on blood agar. Esculin is hydrolyzed. At least 16 serovars have been distinguished[4,5]. Listeriolysin D, a hemolytic and cytolytic toxin, is produced[6]. For differentiation from *Lactobacillus* and *Erysipelothrix*, see table below	Found in organs, blood, spinal fluid, placenta in man and animals. Widely distributed in nature, e.g. soil, dust, water, sewage, decaying vegetation, animal feeds, silage. Gastrointestinal tract is the most likely source of infection after ingestion of contaminated foodstuffs[5,7,8]. Foods which are often contaminated with *L. monocytogenes*[5,7]: milk from cows with *Listeria* mastitis, cheese, raw vegetable products, raw meat and uncooked sausages, uncooked seafood, ready cooked chicken, chilled foods (*L. monocytogenes* can multiply in refrigerators at 4–6 °C[7]). Invasion of the eye and the skin after direct exposure has been reported[9]. Transplacental transmission[8]	Listeriosis in animals (worldwide). In man, incubation period varies from 1–70 days[2]. All age groups may be affected, especially neonates, infants, and the aged, also pregnant women and immunocompromised persons[5,7–10]. Clinical features range from influenza-like illness to meningitis and meningo-encephalitis; septicemia, endocarditis, septic arthritis, etc., have been reported. Infection of the fetus can lead to abortion, stillbirth or an ill infant[11] *Remark*. Treatment with ampicillin with or without gentamicin; as an alternative trimethoprim–sulfamethoxazole has been recommended[12]
173	**Listeria seeligeri** ROCOURT and GRIMONT	Morphologically similar to *L. monocytogenes*. Weak β-hemolysis on blood agar	Probably widely distributed in nature, e.g. soil, decaying vegetation, animal feces	Usually nonpathogenic. A case of purulent meningitis reported[13]
173a	**Listeria ivanovii** SEELIGER et al.	Morphologically similar to *L. monocytogenes*. Pronounced β-hemolysis on blood agar	Found in healthy animals and human carriers. Probably widely distributed in nature	Pathogenic in animals, especially in pregnant sheep. Very rarely pathogenic in man[4]

[1] BARTLETT, J. G., *Chest*, **91**, 901 (1987).
[2] SUSSMAN et al., *Rev. infect. Dis.*, **8**, 771 (1986).
[3] ATKINS et al., *J. Infect.*, **21**, 322 (1990).
[4] SEELIGER and JONES, in SNEATH et al. (Eds.), *Bergey's Manual of Systematic Bacteriology*, Volume 2, Williams & Wilkins, Baltimore, 1986, page 1235.
[5] JONES, D., *Lancet*, **336**, 1171 (1990).
[6] GEOFFREY et al., *Infect. Immun.*, **55**, 1641 (1987).
[7] WHO Working Group on Foodborne Listeriosis, *Bull. Wld Hlth Org.*, **66**, 421 (1988).
[8] SCHUCHAT et al., *Clin. Microbiol. Rev.*, **4**, 169 (1991).
[9] ARMSTRONG, D., in MANDELL et al. (Eds.), *Principles and Practice of Infectious Diseases*, 3rd ed., Churchill Livingstone, New York, 1990, page 1587.
[10] GELLIN and BROOME, *J. Amer. med. Ass.*, **261**, 1313 (1989).
[11] SPENCER, J. A., *Brit. med. J.*, **295**, 349 (1987).
[12] *Med. Lett. Drug. Ther.*, **32**, No. 817 (1990).
[13] ROCOURT et al., *Schweiz. med. Wschr.*, **116**, 248 (1986).

Differential characteristics of the genera Lactobacillus, Listeria *and* Erysipelothrix

	Lactobacillus	*Listeria*	*Erysipelothrix*
Motility	–*	+◊	–
Catalase activity	–	+	–
H_2S production	–	–	+
Acid production from glucose	+	+	+
MK-7 as major menaquinone	–	+	–
L-Lysine in cell wall	–	–	+

\+ 90% or more of strains are positive.
– 90% or less of strains are negative.
* Most strains nonmotile, but a few motile strains occur.
◊ All strains motile at 20–25 °C, poorly or nonmotile at 37 °C.

Reference

SEELIGER and JONES, in SNEATH et al. (Eds.), *Bergey's Manual of Systematic Bacteriology*, Volume 2, Williams & Wilkins, Baltimore, 1986, page 1235.

No.	Bacterium *Synonyms* Common names	Characteristics	Habitat Host Transmission	Associated disease
174	**Erysipelothrix rhusiopathiae** (MIGULA) BUCHANAN *Erysipelothrix insidiosa* *Bacterium rhusiopathiae* Bacillus of swine erysipelas	GRAM-positive, slender rods, 0.2 to 0.4 µm wide and 0.8–2.5 µm long, occurring singly, in pairs to give V-forms, or in groups. Filaments may be 60 µm or more in length. Nonmotile. Aerobic, facultatively anaerobic. Acid, but no gas production from glucose. Catalase-negative. Esculin not hydrolyzed. α-Hemolysis, no β-hemolysis on blood agar. *E. rhusiopathiae* may be divided into 22 serovars. For differentiation from *Listeria* and *Lactobacillus*, see table on page 61	Mucosa and tonsils of healthy pigs. In feces of affected animals and in fish. Transmission by contact with animals, fish and animal products. Sites of entry: small skin lesions or bites of animals or fish. Direct transmission from swine to man appears to be uncommon	Erysipeloid in man[1,2]. Incubation period usually less than 4 days, may be as long as 7 days[1]. A localized cutaneous form is usually self-limiting, averaging 3 weeks. The septicemic form is often associated with endocarditis
175	**Corynebacterium diphtheriae** LEHMANN and NEUMANN *Bacillus diphtheriae* LOEFFLER bacterium	GRAM-positive, straight or slightly curved rods, 0.3–0.8 µm wide and 1.0–8.0 µm long, frequently swollen at one or both ends. Often contain metachromatic granules. V-shaped or palisade arrangement of cells. Nonmotile. Aerobic, facultatively anaerobic. Complex media required for growth. Optimal growth at 30 to 37°C. Most strains produce a highly lethal exotoxin. See also text on next page	Man is the only known reservoir. In nasopharyngeal mucosa of diphtheria patients, also of healthy carriers. In superficial wounds, rarely on other mucous membranes (e.g. external ear, genitalia). Transmission by airborne respiratory droplets and/or direct contact with respiratory secretions or exudate from infected skin; fomites can play a role. Epidemics have been caused by contaminated milk	Respiratory tract diphtheria, cutaneous diphtheria. See text on next page
176	**Corynebacterium jeikeium** *Corynebacterium* group JK	GRAM-positive, coccoid rods. Nonmotile. Obligately aerobic. Slow growth on sheep blood agar. See also text on next page	Skin (healthy carriers)[3]	Usually nosocomial infections in immunocompromised patients[4,5]. Septicemia, endocarditis, pneumonia *Remarks*. Multiple antibiotic resistance reported[6,7]. Vancomycin may be effective[8]
177	Other *Corynebacterium* species of clinical importance[4,5]:			
	Corynebacterium ulcerans	Similar to *C. diphtheriae*. Produces exotoxin. See also text on next page	Pharyngeal mucosa and skin in man	Pharyngitis, diphtheria[9]
	Corynebacterium pseudotuberculosis *Corynebacterium ovis*	Similar to *C. diphtheriae*. Produces exotoxin. See also text on next page	Animal products	Suppurative granulomatous lymphadenitis (very rare in man)
	Corynebacterium pseudodiphtheriticum *Corynebacterium hofmannii*	Similar to *C. diphtheriae*. Club forms and metachromatic granules minimal or absent. See also text on next page	Pharyngeal mucosa in man	Respiratory tract infections, endocarditis[10]
	Corynebacterium minutissimum	Similar to *C. diphtheriae*. Metachromatic granules. See also text on next page	Skin in man	Erythrasma
	Corynebacterium xerosis	Similar to *C. diphtheriae*. Occasionally club forms and metachromatic granules. See also text on next page	Skin and mucous membranes in man	Endocarditis[11]
	Corynebacterium urealyticum *Corynebacterium* group D-2	Similar to *C. jeikeium*. Strongly urease-positive. No acid production from glucose	Skin and mucous membranes in man	Urinary tract infections[12]; septicemia, endocarditis[13] *Remark*. Multiple antibiotic resistance reported[6,7]

[1] MCCLAIN, J. B., in MANDELL et al. (Eds.), *Principles and Practice of Infectious Diseases*, 3rd ed., Churchill Livingstone, New York, 1990, page 1599.
[2] FRELAND, C., in BRAUDE et al. (Eds.), *Infectious Diseases and Medical Microbiology*, 2nd ed., Saunders, Philadelphia, 1986, page 1512.
[3] WICHMANN et al., *Europ. J. clin. Microbiol. infect. Dis.*, **4**, 502 (1985).
[4] BROWN, A. E., in MANDELL et al. (Eds.), *Principles and Practice of Infectious Diseases*, 3rd ed., Churchill Livingstone, New York, 1990, page 1581.
[5] COYLE and LIPSKY, *Clin. Microbiol. Rev.*, **3**, 227 (1990).
[6] PHILIPPON and BIMET, *Europ. J. clin. Microbiol. infect. Dis.*, **9**, 892 (1990).
[7] DE BRIEL et al., *J. Hosp. Infect.*, **17**, 35 (1991).
[8] *Med. Lett. Drug. Ther.*, **32**, No. 817 (1990).
[9] GUBLER et al., *Schweiz. med. Wschr.*, **120**, 1812 (1990).
[10] COLT et al., *Rev. infect. Dis.*, **13**, 73 (1991).
[11] RØDER and FRIMODT-MØLLER, *Europ. J. clin. Microbiol. infect. Dis.*, **9**, 233 (1990).
[12] SORIANO et al., *Rev. infect. Dis.*, **12**, 1019 (1990).
[13] ENA et al., *J. Infect.*, **22**, 95 (1991).

No.	**Bacterium** *Synonyms* Common names	Characteristics	Habitat Host Transmission	Associated disease
178	**Arcanobacterium haemolyticum** (MACLEAN et al.) COLLINS et al. *Corynebacterium haemolyticum*	GRAM-positive, slender, irregular rods. Coccoid forms in older cultures. Nonmotile. Not acid-fast. Facultatively anaerobic, growth enhanced by CO_2. Acid production from glucose. Catalase-positive, nitrate reduction. Urease-negative. β-Hemolysis	Pharyngeal mucosa and skin in man	Pharyngeal and skin infections (pharyngitis often accompanied with rash)[1,2]. Rarely endocarditis, meningitis *Remark.* Usually sensitive to penicillins, erythromycin and tetracyclines[1]

[1] BROWN, A. E., in MANDELL et al. (Eds.), *Principles and Practice of Infectious Diseases*, 3rd ed., Churchill Livingstone, New York, 1990, page 1581.
[2] COYLE and LIPSKY, *Clin. Microbiol. Rev.*, **3**, 227 (1990).

Corynebacteria

The genus *Corynebacterium* has been redefined on the basis of structural chemical criteria. This definition means that many organisms traditionally assigned to it now belong to other genera: the anaerobic or microaerophilic skin coryneforms (anaerobic diphtheroids) to *Propionibacterium*; *Corynebacterium pyogenes* and *Corynebacterium haemolyticum* are assigned to *Actinomyces* and *Arcanobacterium*, respectively; and *Corynebacterium equi* has been transferred to the genus *Rhodococcus*[1]. See also Table 1.

Diphtheria

The species *C. diphtheriae* is subdivided into 3 cultural types – gravis, intermedius and mitis – based on colonial morphology on blood tellurite agar (Table 2). Many strains isolated cannot be placed in any one type. Most strains produce a highly lethal exotoxin; the toxin produced by the cultural types is identical[1]. Toxin production by *C. diphtheriae* depends upon the presence of a lysogenic β-phage which carries the gene (tox^+) for toxin liberation. Toxigenicity of individual *C. diphtheriae* strains can be determined by ELEK's test[4].

Current reservoirs for disease are obscure. In endemic conditions, 3% of healthy individuals may harbor the organism in their throats[5], but in highly developed countries isolation of the organism from healthy individuals has become extremely rare. Diphtheria incidence is decreasing worldwide, though the disease remains endemic in some parts of the world[4]. Small epidemics have been reported in western Europe and the USA in the last decade[6]; *C. diphtheriae* from these outbreaks were investigated by phagelysis typing[7] and DNA hybridization[8]. In the USA, only 2 cases of diphtheria were reported in 1991[9].

Respiratory tract diphtheria. Average incubation period 2–4 days[4]. Systemic complications are due to effects of the diphtheria toxin on heart and nervous system[4].

Cutaneous diphtheria. Occurs most frequently in tropical and subtropical climates – especially in young children. In adults, the disease is known as 'tropical ulcers' and 'desert ulcers'[3]. Systemic complications are rare[4].

Remarks. Active immunization with diphtheria toxoid is a routine prophylactic practice[10], but the duration of full immunity lasts only 3 years with partial immunity lasting 10 years[11]. Once a tentative diagnosis of diphtheria has been made, diphtheria antitoxin should be administered as quickly as possible. As cultures take 24 to 72 hours, antitoxin treatment should be given on the basis of clinical and epidemiological evidence[3].

Although antibiotics do not alter the clinical course of diphtheria, all patients should be treated to eradicate *C. diphtheriae* and group A β-hemolytic streptococci, which are frequently found in both respiratory and cutaneous diphtheria infections[3]. The antibiotics of choice are erythromycin or benzylpenicillin[12].

References

[1] COLLINS and CUMMINS, in SNEATH et al. (Eds.), *Bergey's Manual of Systematic Bacteriology*, Volume 2, Williams & Wilkins, Baltimore, 1986, page 1266.
[2] COYLE and LIPSKY, *Clin. Microbiol. Rev.*, **3**, 227 (1990).
[3] HALSEY and SMITH, in WARREN and MAHMOUD (Eds.), *Tropical and Geographical Medicine*, 2nd ed., McGraw-Hill, New York, 1990, page 860.
[4] MACGREGOR, B. R., in MANDELL et al. (Eds.), *Principles and Practice of Infectious Diseases*, 3rd ed., Churchill Livingstone, New York, 1990, page 1574.
[5] KALAPOTHAKI et al., *Infection*, **12**, 387 (1984).
[6] HARNISCH et al., *Ann. intern. Med.*, **111**, 71 (1989).
[7] NAUMANN et al., *Dtsch. med. Wschr.*, **111**, 288 (1986).
[8] RAPPUOLI et al., *New Engl. J. Med.*, **318**, 12 (1988).
[9] *Morb. Mort. wkly Rep.*, **40**, No. 52, 898 (1991).
[10] HINMAN and ORENSTEIN, *Lancet*, **335**, 707 (1990).
[11] FRENKEL, L. D., *Pediat. Clin. N. Amer.*, **37**, 531 (1990).
[12] *Med. Lett. Drug. Ther.*, **32**, No. 817 (1990).

Table 1 *Differential characteristics of* Corynebacterium *species pathogenic in man*[1,2]

	C. diphtheriae	*C. jeikeium*	*C. ulcerans*	*C. pseudotuberculosis*	*C. pseudodiphtheriticum*	*C. minitissimum*	*C. xerosis*
Catalase activity	+	+	+	+	+	+	+
Urease activity	–	–	+	+	+	–	–
Acid production from glucose	+	+	+	+	–	+	+
– from maltose	+	d	+	+	–	+	+
– from sucrose	–	–	–	–	–	d	+
– from starch	d	–	+	–	–	–	–
Nitrate reduction	+	–	–	d	+	–	+
Gelatine hydrolysis	–	–	–/+*	–	–	–	–
β-Hemolysis	+	–	+	+	–	–	–

+ 90% or more strains are positive within 4 days.
– 90% or more strains are negative.
d 11–89% of strains are positive.
* Negative or weak reaction at 37 °C, positive reaction at 25 °C.

Table 2 *Characteristics of* Corynebacterium diphtheriae *cultural types*[3]

	Shape of colonies	Pigment on tellurite agar	Hemolysis	Acid production from Starch	Acid production from Glycogen
Mitis	Smooth, convex	Black	Weak	–	–
Gravis	Semirough, flat	Gray to black	–	+	+
Intermedius	Smooth, small	Black center	–	–	–

No.	**Bacterium** *Synonyms* Common names	Characteristics	Habitat Host Transmission	Associated disease
179	**Arachnia propionica** (BUCHANAN and PINE) PINE and GEORG *Actinomyces propionicus*	Similar to *Actinomyces israelii*. Most strains require anaerobic conditions for isolation	Oral cavity, dental plaque, tonsillar crypts in man	Actinomycosis (disease similar to that caused by *Actinomyces israelii*)[1]
180	**Propionibacterium acnes** (GILCHRIST) DOUGLAS and GUNTER *Corynebacterium acnes*	GRAM-positive, pleomorphic rods, 0.5–0.8 µm wide and 1 to 5 µm long, often with clubbed ends. Cells may be coccoid, bifid or branched, occurring singly, in pairs, short chains or clusters. No spore formation. Nonmotile. Anaerobic to aerotolerant. Propionic and acetic acid production. Catalase- and indole-positive. Sometimes β-hemolysis on blood agar	Dairy products; skin of man and intestinal tract of man and animals	Related to acne vulgaris[2]; septic arthritis, endocarditis, meningitis[3]
180a	**Eubacterium** spp.	GRAM-positive, straight or slightly curved rods, 0.2–1.6 µm wide, of varying length. No spore formation. Obligately anaerobic	Oral cavity and intestinal tract of man and animals	Some strains may be pathogenic[4]
181	**Actinomyces israelii** (KRUSE) LACHNER-SANDOVAL *Streptothrix israeli*	GRAM-positive, straight or slightly curved rods, 0.2–1.0 µm wide, of varying length, and slender filament with true branching. Short rods with or without clubbed ends, occurring singly, in pairs, short chains or small clusters. No spore formation. Nonmotile. Not acid-fast. Anaerobic, microaerophilic. Growth enhanced by CO_2. Catalase- and urease-negative. No β-hemolysis on blood agar	Worldwide distribution. Common in oral cavity, especially the tonsillar crypts in man. Invasion of the tissues favored by traumata. Mode of transmission unknown	Actinomycosis; affects mainly the cervicofacial, pulmonary and abdominal regions[1,5,6]. Rare cause of mycetoma[7] *Remark*. Benzylpenicillin or a tetracycline have been recommended for treatment[8]
182	**Actinomyces pyogenes** (GLAGE) REDDY et al. *Bacillus pyogenes* *Corynebacterium pyogenes*	GRAM-positive to GRAM-variable, short rods, 0.2–1.0 µm wide and 1.5–5.0 µm long, sometimes coccoid forms or short filaments. Rods occur with or without clubbed ends. No spore formation. Nonmotile. Not acid-fast. Anaerobic, microaerophilic. Requires addition of blood or serum for growth. Catalase- and urease-negative. β-Hemolysis on blood agar	Domestic animals, especially cattle, goats and pigs. Transmission probably by flies[9]	Cutaneous infections; systemic complications possible (small epidemics reported from Denmark and Thailand)[9,10]
183	Other *Actinomyces* species of clinical importance[1,11,12]: **Actinomyces naeslundii** **Actinomyces odontolyticus** **Actinomyces viscosus** **Actinomyces meyeri**	Similar to *A. israelii*		
184	**Bifidobacterium adolescentis** REUTER *Actinomyces eriksonii*	GRAM-positive rods of various shapes. No spore formation. Nonmotile. Not acid-fast, 4 biovars (a, b, c, d). Catalase-negative. Optimal growth at 37 to 41 °C	Sewage; intestinal tract in man	Lung abscess reported[11]

[1] LERNER, P. I., in MANDELL et al. (Eds.), *Principles and Practice of Infectious Diseases*, 3rd ed., Churchill Livingstone, New York, 1990, page 1932.
[2] CUMMINS and JOHNSON, in SNEATH et al. (Eds.), *Bergey's Manual of Systematic Bacteriology*, Volume 2, Williams & Wilkins, Baltimore, 1986, page 1346.
[3] YOCUM et al., *J. Amer. med. Ass.*, **248**, 1740 (1982).
[4] MOORE and MOORE, in SNEATH et al. (Eds.), *Bergey's Manual of Systematic Bacteriology*, Volume 2, Williams & Wilkins, Baltimore, 1986, page 1353.
[5] STANLEY and QUALE, *J. roy. Soc. Med.*, **81**, 667 (1988).
[6] MEIER et al., *Schweiz. med. Wschr.*, **120**, 509 (1990).
[7] ELLNER and MORRISSEY, in WARREN and MAHMOUD (Eds.), *Tropical and Geographical Medicine*, 2nd ed., McGraw-Hill, New York, 1990, page 975.
[8] *Med. Lett. Drug. Ther.*, **32**, No. 817 (1990).
[9] COYLE and LIPSKY, *Clin. Microbiol. Rev.*, **3**, 227 (1990).
[10] BROWN, A. E., in MANDELL et al. (Eds.), *Principles and Practice of Infectious Diseases*, 3rd ed., Churchill Livingstone, New York, 1990, page 1581.
[11] PINE, L., in BRAUDE et al. (Eds.), *Infectious Diseases and Medical Microbiology*, 2nd ed., Saunders, 1986, page 391.
[12] SCHAAL, K. P., in SNEATH et al. (Eds.), *Bergey's Manual of Systematic Bacteriology*, Volume 2, Williams & Wilkins, Baltimore, 1986, page 1383.

No.	Bacterium *Synonyms* Common names	Characteristics	Habitat Host Transmission	Associated disease
185	**Mycobacterium tuberculosis** (ZOPF) LEHMANN and NEUMANN *Bacterium tuberculosis* Human tubercle bacillus KOCH's bacillus MUCH's bacillus	GRAM-positive, straight or slightly curved rods, 0.3–0.6 μm wide and 1–4 μm long. Single, occasionally in threads. Nonmotile. Stain uniformly or irregularly. Strongly acid-fast and acid–alcohol-fast. Aerobic. Slow growth: generation time *in vitro* under optimal condition 14 to 15 hours. Optimal growth at 37 °C and pH 6.4–7.0. See also table on page 66	Man. Strictly parasitic. Transmission by respiratory droplets and dust	Pulmonary and extrapulmonary tuberculosis in man. Pathogenic in guinea pigs, cattle, rabbits, mice. See text on page 67
186	**Mycobacterium bovis** KARLSON and LESSEL Bovine tubercle bacillus	Morphologically similar to *M. tuberculosis*, but rods a little plumper, with weak or granular staining. Microaerophilic. See table on page 66	Cattle. Transmission to man through raw milk	Bovine tuberculosis. Pulmonary and extrapulmonary tuberculosis in man. Pathogenic in rabbits, guinea pigs, mice
187	**Mycobacterium africanum** CASTETS et al.	Morphologically similar to *M. tuberculosis*. See table on page 66	Man	Tuberculosis in man in tropical Africa
188	**Mycobacterium kansasii** HAUDUROY	Morphologically similar to *M. tuberculosis*. See table on page 66	Aquatic environment, cattle, pigs, deer	Pulmonary disease, disseminated infections in various organs[1]
189	**Mycobacterium marinum** ARONSON	Morphologically similar to *M. tuberculosis*, but rods somewhat longer. Often end-to-end or in chains. Best growth on LÖWENSTEIN–JENSEN medium at 32 °C in 2–4 weeks[2], also on ordinary media. Aerobic. See also table on page 66	Aquatic environment; walls of swimming-pools; occasionally tropical fish aquaria	Benign but protracted skin infection when exposed to contaminated fish or water (swimming-pool granuloma, fish-tank granuloma)[2]
190	**Mycobacterium avium** CHESTER Avian tubercle bacillus	Morphologically similar to *M. bovis*. Optimal growth at 42 °C. Growth in 3–4 weeks on either ordinary or special media. See also table on page 66	Soil; poultry and other birds. Transmissible also to cattle, pigs, horses, dogs and cats	Avian tuberculosis. Pulmonary disease mainly in patients with other pulmonary disorders[3], disseminated infections reported in immunocompromised persons (especially AIDS)[4]; in children cervical lymphadenopathy[5]
190a	**Mycobacterium intracellulare** (CUTTINO and MCCABE) RUNYON	Closely related to *M. avium*. Difficult to distinguish from *M. avium* by cultural and biochemical tests[6]. See table on page 66		
191	**Mycobacterium ulcerans** MACCALLUM et al.	Morphologically similar to *M. tuberculosis*. Good growth on special media at 30–33 °C. No growth at 37 °C. See table on page 66	Reservoir unknown (aquatic environment suggested[7]). Human skin lesions	Skin ulcers in Australia, Africa, Mexico, Central and South America
192	**Mycobacterium leprae** (HANSEN) LEHMANN and NEUMANN *Bacillus leprae* HANSEN's bacillus Leprosy bacillus	GRAM-positive rods, 0.3–0.5 μm wide and 4.0–7.0 μm long, with rounded ends. Obligately intracellular. When numerous, generally arranged in clumps, rounded masses (globi) or groups. Acid- and alcohol-fast. No confirmed growth on artificial media. Can be grown in armadillos, mouse foot-pads and thymectomised rats[8]. Only mycobacterium with an affinity for nerve tissue; even small numbers cause a characteristic cellular infiltration	Infected humans, armadillos (*Dasypus novemcinctus*). Transmission most probably through inhalation of bacilli-laden droplets of nasal or nasopharyngeal secretions of an untreated leprosy patient. A scratched, abraded or insect-bitten skin may facilitate the entry of bacilli in the droplets into the skin	Leprosy in man. See text on pages 68–70

[1] LILLO et al., *Rev. infect. Dis.*, **12**, 760 (1990).
[2] BAILEY et al., *J. Amer. med. Ass.*, **247**, 1314 (1982); GRAY et al., *Brit. med. J.*, **300**, 1069 (1990).
[3] ISEMAN, M. D., *New Engl. J. Med.*, **321**, 896 (1989).
[4] HORSBURGH et al., *Medicine (Baltimore)*, **64**, 36 (1985); FRIEDMAN et al., *Amer. J. Med.*, **85**, 257 (1988); BENSON et al., *Arch. intern. Med.*, **151**, 582 (1991); ELLNER et al., *J. infect. Dis.*, **163**, 1326 (1991).
[5] LAI et al., *J. Amer. med. Ass.*, **251**, 1286 (1984); NUNN and MCADAM, *Brit. med. Bull.*, **44**, 801 (1988).
[6] SAITO et al., *J. clin. Microbiol.*, **28**, 1694 (1990).
[7] HAYMAN, J., *Lancet*, **2**, 1015 (1984); BARKER, D. J. P., *Lancet*, **2**, 1277 (1984).
[8] MYERS and MARTY, *Drugs*, **41**, 832 (1991).

No.	**Bacterium** *Synonyms* Common names	Characteristics	Habitat Host Transmission	Associated disease
193	**Mycobacterium chelonae** BERGEY et al.	GRAM-positive, pleomorphic organisms. Long narrow rods to short thick rods with coccoidal forms. Strongly acid-fast. Aerobic. Good growth on most media at 37 °C. See also table below	Aquatic environment, soil	Soft-tissue infections (e.g. surgical invasive procedures), occasionally osteomyelitis, keratitis, disseminated infections[1]
194	**Mycobacterium fortuitum** DA COSTA CRUZ	GRAM-positive, pleomorphic organisms. Rods, 1–3 µm long, short or coccoidal forms; also long rods. Strongly acid-fast. Aerobic. Good growth on most media at 37 °C. 3 biovars recognized. See also table below	Aquatic environment, soil	Soft-tissue infections (e.g. surgical invasive procedures), occasionally osteomyelitis, disseminated infections[2]
195	Other *Mycobacterium* species of clinical importance:	Morphologically similar to other *Mycobacterium* species		
	Mycobacterium malmonese			Pulmonary disease, lymphadenopathy[3]
	Mycobacterium gordonae		Hospital water supply	Pulmonary disease, occasionally disseminated infections[4]
	Mycobacterium asiaticum			Pulmonary disease[5]
	Mycobacterium szulgai			Pulmonary disease, skin infections[3], disseminated infections reported[6]
	Mycobacterium simiae		Primates, possibly water	Pulmonary disease[3]
	Mycobacterium scrofolaceum		Soil, water, foodstuffs	Lymphadenopathy, especially in young children[3]
	Mycobacterium xenopi		Hospital water supply	Pulmonary disease[3,7], disseminated infections[3,8]
	Mycobacterium haemophilum			Skin and subcutaneous lesions in immunocompromised persons[3]

[1] LAU, J. H., *Brit. med. J.*, **292**, 444 (1986); COOPER et al., *Amer. J. Med.*, **86**, 173 (1989); SAFRANEK et al., *New Engl. J. Med.*, **317**, 197 (1987); WENGER et al., *J. Amer. med. Ass.*, **264**, 373 (1990).
[2] SUBBARAO et al., *Amer. J. Dis. Child.*, **141**, 1018 (1987); NOLAN et al., *J. infect. Dis.*, **163**, 1150 (1991); SCHLOSSBERG and AARON, *Arch. intern. Med.*, **151**, 1010 (1991).
[3] SANDERS and HOROWITZ, in MANDELL et al. (Eds.), *Principles and Practice of Infectious Diseases*, 3rd ed., Churchill Livingstone, New York, 1990, page 1914.
[4] STINE et al., *J. Amer. med. Ass.*, **258**, 809 (1987); LONDON et al., *Amer. J. Med.*, **85**, 703 (1988).
[5] TAYLOR et al., *Tubercle*, **71**, 303 (1990).
[6] GUR et al., *Arch. intern. Med.*, **144**, 1861 (1984).
[7] DWYER et al., *Amer. J. Med.*, **74**, 161 (1983).
[8] WEINBERG et al., *Lancet*, **1**, 1033 (1985); WILKS and GEORGE, *J. roy. Soc. Med.*, **83**, 401 (1990).

Differential characteristics of several species of the genus Mycobacterium

	M. tuberculosis	*M. bovis*	*M. africanum*	*M. kansasii*	*M. marinum*	*M. avium*	*M. intracellulare*	*M. ulcerans*	*M. fortuitum*	*M. chelonae*
Growth rate	Slow	Slow	Slow	Slow	Slow	Slow	Slow	Slow	Rapid	Rapid
Growth at 25 °C	–	–	–	+	+	(–)	+	(+)	+	+
Growth at 45 °C	–	–	–	–	–	–	(+)	–	–	–
Growth in media with 5% NaCl	–	–	–	–	d	–	–	–	+	+/–*
Growth on MACCONKEY agar	–	–	–	–	–	–	–	–	+	+
Urease activity	+	+	+	+	+	–	–	n.d.	+	+
Catalase activity	–	–	–	+	(–)	–	–	+	+	+
Nitrate reduction	+	–	(–)	+	–	–	–	–	+	d
Niacin accumulation	+	–	(–)	–	–	–	–	(–)	n.d.	n.d.
Photochromogenic pigment formation	–	–	–	+	+	–	–	–	–	–
Scotochromogenic pigment formation	–	–	–	–	–	(–)	(+)	(+)	–	–
Pathogenicity in guinea pigs	+	+	+	–	–	–	+	–	+	–
– in chicken	–	–	–	–	–	+	+	–	–	–
– in rabbits	–	+	+	+	+	+	–	+	+	–
– in mice	+	+	n.d.	+	+	+	+	+	+	+

\+ 85% or more of strains are positive.
(+) 51–84% of strains are positive.
– 85% or more of strains are negative.
(–) 50–84% of strains are negative.
d Variable.
n.d. No data available.

* *M. chelonae* subsp. *chelonae* are negative.

Reference

WAYNE and KUBICA, in SNEATH et al. (Eds.), *Bergey's Manual of Systemic Bacteriology*, Volume 2, Williams & Wilkins, Baltimore, 1986, page 1436.

Tuberculosis

Tuberculosis remains common throughout most parts of the world, about half the world population being infected with *Mycobacterium tuberculosis*. An estimated 10 million new cases and 3 million deaths from tuberculosis occur every year – most of them in developing countries[1]. In developed countries, there have been considerable reductions in both the incidence and the mortality of tuberculosis since the turn of the century[2]. In England and Wales, for example, the death rate of 25 per 100000 in 1950 had fallen to 1 per 100000 by 1980[3]. In the USA, the incidence of pulmonary tuberculosis – also decreasing over recent decades – shows a slight resurgence in the last few years (Fig. 1). This seems to be due, at least in part, to the spread of acquired immunodeficiency syndrome (AIDS)[4,5].

Fig. 1 *Incidence of pulmonary tuberculosis in the USA, 1982–1990*[5]

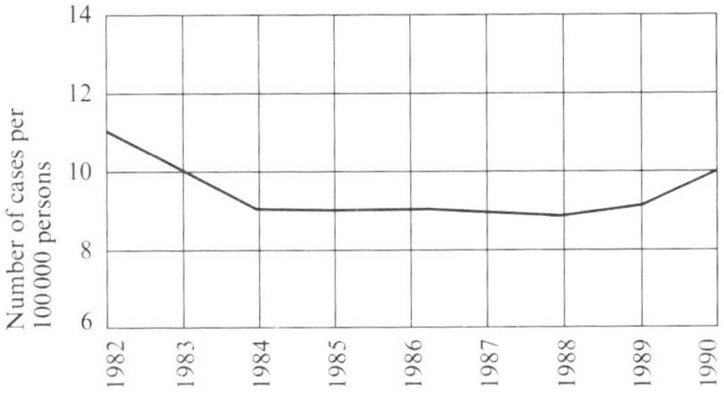

The most important determinants of contagion are the closeness of contact and the infectiousness of the source, which may vary widely among individuals. Age, poverty, urban living and malnutrition are factors associated with the prevalence of tuberculosis.

Following primary infection, which rarely causes significant symptoms (although the primary focus in children sometimes becomes an area of advancing pneumonia), healing occurs in about 85–95% of individuals, leaving the characteristic GHON complex in a few cases and causing tuberculin reactivity. Only 5–15% of individuals with primary infections develop active tuberculosis[1]. Dissemination from the primary pulmonary focus may occur via lymphatic, hematogenous or tubular routes – either during primary or during reactivated tuberculosis: late reactivation may occur at distant sites of dissemination[1,6–14].

Diagnosis. Chest X-rays showing characteristic patterns are highly suggestive of active tuberculosis, as are strongly positive tuberculin skin tests (e.g. +++ or ++++ in the HEAF test). The diagnosis must however rest upon the identification of *M. tuberculosis* in sputum or other material from the patient.

Bacteriological diagnosis can be made by 3 different methods for demonstrating *M. tuberculosis*, provided suitable material is available for investigation (e.g. sputum, laryngeal smear, pleural effusion, or biopsies of lymph nodes, liver, etc.):

- *Smear examination*, direct or after digestion and concentration, either by ZIEHL–NEELSEN staining and normal microscopy, or by auramine staining and fluorescence microscopy
- *Cultures* (special media are required) with radiometric detection of CO_2 produced by growing organisms or with antigen detection by immunoassay[15], or occasionally
- *Animal tests* (guinea pigs)

If any of these are positive, the diagnosis of tuberculosis is established. However ZIEHL–NEELSEN and auramine stains lack sensitivity, only half of the patients with pulmonary tuberculosis and a quarter of patients with extrapulmonary tuberculosis being identified by these means[16]. Failure to demonstrate *M. tuberculosis* does not exclude the diagnosis.

Most serological tests (e.g. hemagglutination, gel diffusion, bentonite flocculation test, fluorescent antibody test), are not in general use because of the high number of false positive and false negative results[17]. The value of *M. tuberculosis* antigen detection by enzyme-linked immunosorbent assay (ELISA) is being discussed[15,16].

Polymerase chain reaction may be a useful tool in rapid detection of extrapulmonary tuberculosis (e.g. tuberculous meningitis)[15,18,19]. It has a high degree of sensitivity and specificity, but the technology is too complex for routine application[15].

Prophylaxis. The sole vaccine available, BCG, contains the bacillus CALMETTE–GUERIN and was first used against human tuberculosis in 1921. It is applicable only to tuberculin-negative persons. Vaccination does not prevent infection, but limits its proliferation, usually to such a degree that clinical disease does not develop[1].

Most countries of the world (exceptions are the Netherlands and the USA) recommend routine BCG vaccination of children for prevention of tuberculosis. The policies differ between countries – from a single dose at birth, as recommended by the WHO Expanded Programme on Immunization[20], via a single dose at age 10–14 years, as recommended in England and Wales[21], to repeated doses throughout childhood, as recommended in many countries (particularly eastern Europe). These policy differences are related as much to differences of opinion about the mechanism of action and the effectiveness of the vaccines as to local differences in the epidemiology of tuberculosis[22].

From clinical trials of the efficacy of BCG, vaccination does not substantially influence the chain of transmission. Only a small fraction of the total number of sources of infection present in a population, mainly cases with smear-positive pulmonary tuberculosis, can be prevented by BCG vaccination[23].

Neonatal BCG vaccination is highly protective against severe disseminated ('miliary') tuberculosis[24]. And chemoprophylaxis appears to reduce the risk of overt tuberculosis developing in children, adolescents or adults with a strongly positive tuberculin test (+++ or ++++) but no other evidence of active disease (see under treatment).

Treatment. The principal chemotherapeutic agents used in treatment of tuberculosis and their mode of action are listed in the table below.

Tuberculosis is generally treated with a combination of drugs to enhance efficacy and reduce the risk of resistance developing. As standard treatment, a combination of isoniazid (INH) with rifampin with or without pyrazinamide has been recommended[25], depending on the sensitivities of the organisms, local conditions, and target cure rates. Three drugs are preferred, at least until the sensitivities are known or where they cannot be routinely obtained. One or more other drugs, such as streptomycin, ethambutol, ethionamide, cycloserine, kanamycin or capreomycin, may be used in 3- or 4-drug combinations, usually with INH and/or rifampin, to overcome problems of bacterial resistance or drug intolerance. For drug regimens, see References[1,26,27,30].

Rifampin used concurrently with other drugs helps to prevent the emergence of resistance; it should always be included in regimens for treatment of INH-resistant *M. tuberculosis* infections and is generally used in combination with isoniazid in the treatment of cavitary and far-advanced pulmonary tuberculosis as well as for extrapulmonary tuberculosis[25].

Chemoprophylaxis with isoniazid is increasingly used in those aged 21–35 years found to have +++ or ++++ responses to tuberculin testing, without clear evidence of infection. Isoniazid has been demonstrated to be active as prophylactic therapy at a daily dose of 300 mg (5–10 mg/kg in children) for 6–12 months[26]. Prophylaxis of 2 month's duration with daily administration of isoniazid, rifampin and pyrazinamide may be as effective as prophylactic therapy with isoniazid for 12 months[26]. Immunocompromised persons, e.g. patients with AIDS, are at such high risk for tuberculosis reactivation that isoniazid chemoprophylaxis is indicated[28,29].

Table 1 *Action of chemotherapeutic agents*[1]

Isoniazid (isonicotinoyl-hydrazine, INH)	Bactericidal against both intracellular and extracellular organisms
Rifampin (RMP)	Bactericidal against both intracellular and extracellular organisms; maintains activity against very slowly metabolizing bacilli
Pyrazinamide (PZA) ..	Bactericidal only at acidic pH such as within cells; greatest activity in first few months of therapy
Streptomycin (STM) ..	Excluded from the intracellular environment; activity only against extracellular organisms
Ethambutol (EMB) ...	Bacteriostatic against both intracellular and extracellular organisms

(For References, see next page)

References (tuberculosis)

[1] DES PREZ and HEIM, in MANDELL et al. (Eds.), *Principles and Practice of Infectious Diseases*, 3rd ed., Churchill Livingstone, New York, 1990, page 1877.
[2] STYBLO, K., *Rev. infect. Dis.*, **11**, Suppl. 2, S339 (1989).
[3] HORNE, N. W., *Brit. med. J.*, **288**, 1249 (1984).
[4] COLLINS, F. M., *Rev. infect. Dis.*, **13**, 940 (1991).
[5] JEREB et al., *Morb. Mort. wkly Rep.*, **40**, No. SS-3 (1991).
[6] ALVAREZ and MCCABE, *Medicine (Baltimore)*, **63**, 25 (1984).
[7] GORSE et al., *Medicine (Baltimore)*, **62**, 178 (1983).
[8] TANG and SWASH, *J. roy. Soc. Med.*, **78**, 429 (1985).
[9] TRAUB et al., *Quart. J. Med.*, N.S. **53**, 209 (1984).
[10] KIM et al., *Rev. infect. Dis.*, **12**, 583 (1990).
[11] MACDONELL et al., *Rev. infect. Dis.*, **12**, 432 (1990).
[12] WELLS et al., *J. roy. Soc. Med.*, **79**, 149 (1986).
[13] COPE et al., *J. infect. Dis.*, **21**, 293 (1990).
[14] DINNING et al., *J. roy. Soc. Med.*, **78**, 576 (1985).
[15] DANIEL, T. M., *J. Lab. clin. Med.*, **116**, 277 (1990).
[16] WILKINS and IVANYI, *Lancet*, **336**, 641 (1990).
[17] Editorial, *Lancet*, **1**, 1024 (1983).
[18] SHANKAR et al., *Lancet*, **337**, 5 (1991).
[19] BÖTTGER, E. C., *Dtsch. med. Wschr.*, **116**, 777 (1991).
[20] World Health Organization, *Expanded Programme on Immunization*, Update, August 1989.
[21] GOODWIN, S., *Pediatrics*, **86**, Suppl., 1056 (1990).
[22] FINE and RODRIGUES, *Lancet*, **335**, 1016 (1990).
[23] PIO, A., *Rev. infect. Dis.*, **11**, Suppl. 2, S360 (1989).
[24] Editorial, *Lancet*, **336**, 1479 (1990).
[25] *Med. Lett. Drug. Ther.*, **34**, No. 863, 10 (1992).
[26] GROSSET, J. H., *Rev. infect. Dis.*, **11**, Suppl. 2, S347 (1989).
[27] SCHABERG and LODE, *Dtsch. med. Wschr.*, **115**, 1799 (1990).
[28] SELWYN et al., *New Engl. J. Med.*, **320**, 545 (1989).
[29] JORDAN et al., *J. Amer. med. Ass.*, **265**, 2987 (1991).
[30] American Academy of Pediatrics, Committee on Infectious Diseases, *Pediatrics*, **89**, 161 (1992).

Leprosy*

Leprosy is one of the major public health problems in developing countries. More than 1.6 billion people live in countries where the estimated prevalence rate of leprosy is greater than 1 per 1000[1]. Currently, the World Health Organization estimates the total number of leprosy cases in the world to be 10–12 million[1,2]. The exact number is unknown, because leprosy is greatly underreported[3]. Leprosy is most prevalent in tropical and subtropical countries (Central Africa, India, South-East Asia, Central and South America), but climate does not play an important role in the epidemiology of this disease[3]. Over 83% of all registered leprosy cases in the world are found in only 5 countries (India, Brazil, Nigeria, Myanmar and Indonesia; in descending order of magnitude)[4].

Leprosy may to a great extent be considered an immunological disease; the causative organism being virtually nontoxic, and most symptoms of the disease are due to immune reactions against antigenic constituents of *Mycobacterium leprae*[5].

Transmission. In general, prolonged and/or close contact has been regarded as necessary in order to contract leprosy, but in susceptible persons it is likely that even a short period of exposure may be enough to acquire the disease. Close contact with a person suffering from multibacillary leprosy, within the family, is more risky than occasional non-familial contact. The contact does not need to be 'skin to skin', as previously believed, because the nose is the main route of exit of bacilli from untreated persons with leprosy. The inhalation of bacilli-laden droplets of nasal and/or nasopharyngeal secretions is at present regarded as the most likely mode of entry of bacilli into contact persons[3].

Incubation period. After entry of bacilli into the human body, a susceptible person may develop leprosy after about 5 (±2) years. The exact incubation period is, however, not known; extremes of 2 months and 40 years have been recorded. To date, the youngest recorded case of leprosy is a 2 month old female infant reported from India in 1989[6].

Evolution of leprosy lesions. Most individuals who have been in contact with persons suffering from multibacillary leprosy develop a subclinical infection. However, in 90–95% of such persons, the infection fails to establish itself and they never develop any manifestation of the disease[5,7]. The remaining cases usually develop a single macule or a few hypopigmented or faintly erythematous patches of indeterminate leprosy as initial manifestation of disease. For further evolution of leprosy lesions, see Figure 1. The central defect in lepromatous leprosy is lack or absence of cell-mediated immune response to *M. leprae*[8].

Clinical features of leprosy. Leprosy is not an easily communicable disease. Therefore only a few of those in contact with leprosy sufferers develop recognizable signs and symptoms of leprosy. Depending on the infected person's resistance to the disease, leprosy presents a broad spectrum of clinical signs, ranging from one or few small hazy patches to widespread multiple shiny nodules or tumors (Table 1)[3,6]. An important diagnostic characteristic of leprosy lesions is that they are symptomless.

In persons with fairly good resistance the invading leprosy bacilli can be destroyed to a great extent and such individuals develop paucibacillary leprosy. On the other hand persons having very poor or no resistance cannot contain the infection and develop multibacillary leprosy. In such persons bacilli multiply almost unchecked. They are found in large numbers in the skin, peripheral nerves, inner lining of the nose, liver, spleen, lymph nodes, testes, eyes, muscles and blood vessel walls. Multibacillary leprosy is a generalized disease affecting the liver, spleen, bones, muscles, kidneys, lymph glands, upper respiratory tract, etc. Nose, testes and eyes are frequently affected. Leprosy bacilli prefer the relatively cooler parts of the human body, such as the face, ears, the front of the eye, fingers, etc.[3,6].

Signs of leprosy may include[6]:

- Single or few, well-demarcated, non-itching, flat, pale (lighter in color) or raised reddish patches on the skin in which sensations of touch, heat and/or pain are impaired. The surface is rough, lustreless and dry due to decreased sweating, and may be hairless
- Non-itching and non-irritating, diffuse shiny redness of the face without sensory loss, becoming worse on exposure to sunlight
- Non-itching, smooth, shiny, reddish diffuse thickening of the skin prominent on the face, ears and hands, especially after exposure to sunlight. The eyebrows are lost, starting in the lateral third. Sensory loss is slight or negligible in the affected areas
- Multiple, shiny, glossy, reddish or skin-coloured, symptomless papules or nodules in the skin of exposed parts, e.g. ears and face
- A feeling of 'pins and needles', shooting pain or tingling sensation, especially in the hands and feet, clumsiness of fine movements of fingers and dropping of small objects
- Burns resulting from contact with hot articles, which at the time of contact do not cause any pain or discomfort, and therefore go unnoticed
- Spontaneous painless blisters or wounds, especially on the fingers
- In some cases there are no patches on the skin, but the only sign of leprosy is the loss of sensation (numbness) in the hand or foot, associated with enlargement and tenderness of the related peripheral nerve
- Nasal discharge, with or without blood, and stuffiness in the nose may in rare cases be the first indication of multibacillary leprosy

Diagnosis. The 3 cardinal diagnostic signs of leprosy are

(1) Inability to feel touch, heat and/or pain in the affected area. It is present in the majority of leprosy cases and often occurs in the order: heat, light touch, pain
Touch sensation can be tested easily by using a wisp of cotton-wool, a nylon or cotton thread or a feather. It can also be tested by touching lightly with the tip of a ballpoint pen. Heat sensation is tested with 2 test tubes – one containing hot and the other cold water – and pain sensation is determined by pinprick. The diagnosis of paucibacillary cases depends on detecting sensory loss
(2) Enlargement and/or tenderness of peripheral nerves, associated with signs of nerve damage, such as sensory loss in the corresponding skin area and/or paralysis
(3) Finding of non-cultivable bacilli in skin smears taken from the affected areas. This is very important for the diagnosis of multibacillary type of leprosy. In paucibacillary leprosy, skin smears are usually negative. Skin smears should be taken from all patients suspected of having leprosy in any form. In patients with active lesions 6 smears should be taken, one from each ear lobe and 4 from active lesions[3].

Evaluation of smears. The bacteriological (or bacterial) index (BI) indicates the density of leprosy bacilli in smears and includes both

* In collaboration with S. J. Yawalkar, Medical Department, Ciba-Geigy Limited, Basel.

Table 1 *Characteristic features of the main types of leprosy*[6]

	Paucibacillary (PB) leprosy	Multibacillary (MB) leprosy
Prevalence	More common, especially among Indians and Africans. It accounts for about 80% of the total leprosy cases worldwide	Less common, but Americans, Europeans, Chinese, Japanese, Koreans and Burmese are more prone to develop MB leprosy
Body's resistance to the disease	Fairly good	Poor or none
Leprosy bacilli	Leprosy bacilli are extremely few in the patches of PB leprosy. Skin smears taken from the affected area are usually negative for these bacilli	Leprosy bacilli are present in enormous numbers in the affected areas. Skin smears are always positive for these bacilli
Skin lesions		
– Number	Usually single, maximum 3. The higher the body's resistance, the fewer and better demarcated the lesions	Many
– Distribution	Asymmetrical	Mostly symmetrical
– Description	Usually well-demarcated, non-itching, pale or reddish, flat or raised patches with a distinct edge	Shiny, reddish, poorly demarcated areas, papules, nodules, tumors and raised patches with sloping edges. The margin merges imperceptibly with the surrounding skin
– Surface	Rough, dry, hairless	Smooth and shiny
Sensory loss in lesions	Marked; patients do not feel touch, heat or pain in the affected area	Slight or none
Diagnostic criteria	Presence of sensory loss in the affected area	Presence of bacilli in skin smears
Infectiousness	Nil or negligible	Highly infectious (principal source of infection)
Outlook	Good	Poor if untreated

living (solid-staining) and dead (fragmented or granular) bacilli. According to RIDLEY's logarithmic scale, it ranges from 0 to 6+ and is based on the number of bacilli seen, on average, in microscopic fields of the smear using an oil-immersion objective.

- 0 No bacilli in any of 100 oil-immersion fields
- 1+ 1–10 bacilli, on average, in 100 oil-immersion fields
- 2+ 1–10 bacilli, on average, in 10 oil-immersion fields
- 3+ 1–10 bacilli, on average, in each oil-immersion field
- 4+ 10–100 bacilli, on average, in each oil-immersion field
- 5+ 100–1000 bacilli, on average, in each oil-immersion field
- 6+ More than 1000 bacilli, on average, in each oil-immersion field

The BI of the patient is calculated by adding up the index from each site examined and dividing the total by the number of sites examined.

Skin biopsy. Histopathological evaluation is essential for accurate classification of leprosy lesions. Skin biopsy is advisable if multibacillary leprosy is considered likely, but no acid-fast bacilli are seen in the skin smears; the examiner's scalpel may not have penetrated pockets of bacilli located deep in the dermis. Skin biopsies should include the full depth of the dermis and should be taken from the most active edge of a lesion. In order to show the bacilli in sections, FITE–FARACOS method of staining is generally used, while sections are usually stained with hematoxylin and eosin for histology. Histological features of different types of leprosy are given in Table 2.

Sweat function tests, e.g. pilocarpine nitrate and acetylcholine tests, may be helpful in the diagnosis of non-lepromatous cases of leprosy, especially in children in whom sensory impairment cannot be determined with certainty[10].

The lepromin (MITSUDA) test is not of diagnostic help in leprosy. It may, however, serve to confirm an opinion (arrived at on clinical and bacteriological grounds) of the precise immunological classification of a patient with established leprosy. The lepromin test is helpful in indicating the prognosis. It is always negative in patients with lepromatous leprosy and is strongly positive in tuberculoid cases.

Serological assays can detect persons with early, subclinical lepromatous leprosy, who have high titers of antibody to phenolic glycolipid 1 and arabinomannan and may be useful for epidemiological

(Continued on next page)

Fig. 1 *The evolution of a leprosy infection*[9]

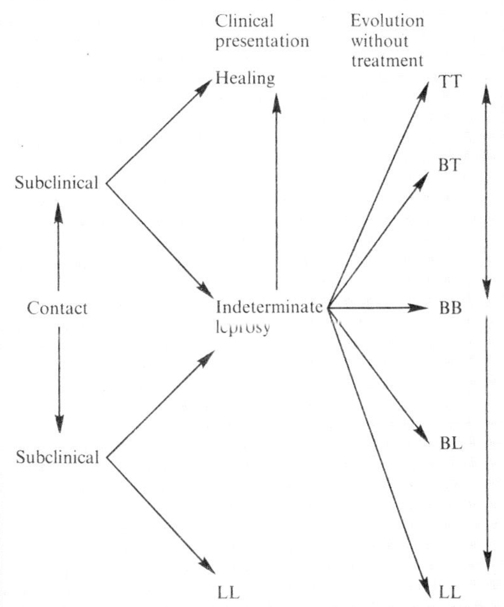

I Indeterminate leprosy TT Tuberculoid leprosy BT Borderline-tuberculoid leprosy	}	Paucibacillary leprosy
BB Mid-borderline leprosy BL Borderline-lepromatous leprosy LL Lepromatous leprosy	}	Multibacillary leprosy

Table 2 *Histological features of different types of leprosy*[9]

	TT	BT	BB	BL	LL
Epithelioid cells	++	++	++	±/−	−
Non-vacuolated giant cells	++/−	+/−	−	−	−
Histiocytes/foamy macrophages	−	−	−	++	++
Small vesicles	−	−	−	++/−	++/−
Vacuolated giant cells	−	−	−	−	±/−
Giant vacuoles	−	−	−	−	++/−
Lymphocytes	+±/+	+±/±	±	++/+	±/−
Dermal nerve, maximum diameter (μm)	1000	400	250	200	80
Onion-skin perineurium	−	±/−	+/−	++/±	−
Clear subepidermal zone	±/−	++/−	++	++	++
Erosion of epidermis	++/−	±/−	−	−	−
Acid-fast bacilli in granuloma (BI)	0 to 1+	0 to 2.5+	3+ to 4.5+	4+ to 5.5+	5.5+ to 6+

Table 3 *Recommended multidrug therapy for adult patients*[1,14]

	Paucibacillary leprosy	Multibacillary leprosy
Regimen	Dapsone 100 mg daily (self-administered) Rifampin 600 mg once a month (supervised)	Dapsone 100 mg daily (self-administered) Rifampin 600 mg once a month (supervised) Clofazimine 300 mg once a month (supervised) and 50 mg daily (self-administered)
Duration of treatment	6 months	At least 2 years, preferably until negative skin smears are obtained
Follow-up after cessation of treatment	At least 2 years	At least 5 years

studies[11]. An enzyme-linked immunosorbent assay which measures antibody against human nerve antigen appears to be promising for the early diagnosis of all types of leprosy[12].

Treatment. At present dapsone, rifampin and clofazimine are the principal antileprosy drugs. Rifampin is the most effective antileprosy drug, being bactericidal in action. High efficacy, good tolerability and practicability of the supervised once-monthly single-oral-dose rifampin regimen in the treatment of patients with multibacillary leprosy was first reported in 1982[13]. The overall antileprosy effect of clofazimine is about the same as that of dapsone. To date, only one case of possible resistance to clofazimine has been reported in 1982. This is the only antileprosy drug possessing an anti-inflammatory effect. Dapsone is the basic drug in the treatment of leprosy. Dapsone resistance was first reported from Malaysia in 1964 and was found on an increasing scale during the 1970s. Its threat to the control of leprosy worldwide was one of the most important factors leading to the WHO recommendations of 1982 on the use of multidrug therapy for leprosy[14] (Table 3). For implementation of multidrug therapy, careful bacteriological examination of skin smears is essential. By mid 1990, over 3 million leprosy patients had been put on multidrug therapy[2].

Vaccine against leprosy. BCG was the first vaccine to be considered against leprosy, but in general the protective effect of BCG against leprosy has been modest except in the trial carried out in Uganda[1]. The WHO-sponsored vaccine against leprosy contains armadillo-derived, heat-killed leprosy bacilli plus live BCG. Preliminary results showing that this vaccine could be useful in humans have been provided[15]. The WHO-sponsored field trial is under way in Venezuela and Malawi. Three vaccines against leprosy have been prepared in India from the Indian Cancer Research Centre (ICRC) bacilli, from '*Mycobacterium w*' and from *Mycobacterium habana*.

A comparative field trial of the first two Indian vaccines and the WHO-sponsored vaccine is being conducted since February 1991 by the Indian Council of Medical Research in Tamil Nadu in India[6]. About 300 000 people will be participating in this trial. The vaccinated population will have to be observed for at least 5 years before the results can be evaluated.

References

1 WHO Expert Committee on Leprosy, *Wld Hlth Org. techn. Rep. Ser.*, No. 768 (1988).
2 Noordeen et al., *Bull. Wld Hlth Org.*, **70**, 7 (1992).
3 Thangaraj and Yawalkar, *Leprosy for Medical Practitioners and Paramedical Workers*, 4th ed., Ciba-Geigy Ltd., Basel, 1989.
4 *Towards Elimination of Leprosy*, World Health Organization, Geneva, 1991.
5 Miller and Buchanan, in Warren and Mahmoud (Eds.), *Tropical and Geographical Medicine*, 2nd ed., McGraw-Hill, New York, 1990, page 851.
6 McDougall and Yawalkar, *Leprosy: Basic Information and Management*, 3rd ed., Ciba-Geigy Ltd., Basel, 1992.
7 Pettit and Parish, *Manual of Tropical Dermatology*, Springer, New York, 1984.
8 Cohn and Kaplan, *J. infect. Dis.*, **163**, 1195 (1991).
9 Ridley, D. S., *Bull. Wld Hlth Org.*, **51**, 451 (1974); *Skin Biopsy in Leprosy*, 3rd ed., Documenta Geigy, Ciba-Geigy Ltd., Basel, 1990.
10 Yawalkar and Sanjana, *Int. J. Leprosy*, **42**, 55 (1974).
11 Bryceson and Pfaltzgraff, *Leprosy*, 3rd ed., English Language Book Society/Churchill Livingstone, Edinburgh, 1990.
12 Meyers and Marty, *Drugs*, **41**, 832 (1991).
13 Yawalkar et al., *Lancet*, **1**, 1199 (1982).
14 WHO Study Group on Chemotherapy of Leprosy for Control Programmes, *Wld Hlth Org. techn. Rep. Ser.*, No. 675 (1982).
15 Convit et al., *Lancet*, **339**, 446 (1992).

No.	**Bacterium** *Synonyms* Common names	Characteristics	Habitat Host Transmission	Associated disease
196	**Nocardia asteroides** (EPPINGER) BLANCHARD *Cladothrix asteroides*	GRAM-positive to GRAM-variable, delicate branching hyphae, 0.5–1.2 μm wide. Fragmentation into bacteroid, rod-shaped to coccoid, nonmotile elements. Aerobic. Usually acid-fast. Catalase-positive	Soil, dust, plants, water, etc.	Nocardiosis (pulmonary, cerebral, subcutaneous, etc.)[1]. Rare cause of pseudomycetoma[2]. Eye infection reported[3]. Immunocompromised persons are at risk[4] *Remark.* A sulfonamide may be effective, but other antibiotic drugs alone or in combination may be necessary[5,6]
197	**Nocardia brasiliensis** (LINDENBERG) PINOY *Discomyces brasiliensis*	Similar to *N. asteroides*	Soil	Pseudomycetoma, particularly in Mexico, South America, India[2]
198	**Rhodococcus equi** (MAGNUSSON) GOODFELLOW and ALDERSON *Corynebacterium equi* *Corynebacterium hoagii* *Nocardia restricta*	GRAM-positive organisms. Rod-to-coccus morphologic variation during growth cycle. Obligately aerobic. Catalase- and urease-positive. Esculin not hydrolyzed. Growth on nonselective routine media	Soil, herbivore dung, intestinal tract in cattle, horses, sheep and pigs. Transmission by respiratory route (?)	Bronchopneumonia in foals. In man[7-10], infection mainly involves the lung; immunocompromised persons are at risk *Remarks.* Erythromycin and/or rifampin may be effective[8]. The organism is also susceptible to clindamycin, vancomycin, aminoglycosides and tetracyclines[7-10]
199	**Oerskovia** spp. PRAUSER et al.	GRAM-positive, extensively branching hyphae, 0.5 μm wide. Fragmentation into rod-shaped, motile, flagellate elements. Facultatively anaerobic. Not acid-fast. Catalase-positive. Oxidase-negative	Soil, decaying plants	Rarely pathogenic in man. Endocarditis, peritonitis[11]
200	**Capnocytophaga ochracea** LEADBETTER et al. *Bacteroides ochraceus* Dysgonic fermenter type 1	GRAM-negative, flexible rods or filaments, 0.4–0.6 μm wide and 2.5–5.7 μm long. Motile by gliding, no flagella. Facultatively anaerobic. Growth enhanced by CO_2, optimal temperature 35 to 37 °C. No growth on MACCONKEY agar. Oxidase-, catalase-, urease-, indole-negative. Acid production from glucose, sucrose and lactose	Oral cavity in man; indigenous to dental plaque	Periodontitis or other buccal lesions. Septicemia in immunocompromised persons[12,13]
200a	**Capnocytophaga canimorsus** sp. nov. Dysgonic fermenter type 2 DF-2 bacillus	GRAM-negative, slender rods, 1 to 3 μm long. Motile by gliding, no flagella. Microaerophilic. Growth enhanced by CO_2. Slow growth on blood agar at 35 °C. Oxidase- and catalase-positive. Urease-, indole- and citrate-negative. Acid production form glucose, maltose and lactose[14]	Oral cavity of dogs and cats[12]. Transmission to man by animal bites	Septicemia, meningitis, pneumonia, endocarditis, peripheral gangrene[12,15-17]

[1] LERNER, P. I., in MANDELL et al. (Eds.), *Principles and Practice of Infectious Diseases*, 3rd ed., Churchill Livingstone, New York, 1990, page 1926.
[2] ELLNER and MORRISSEY, in WARREN and MAHMOUD (Eds.), *Tropical and Geographical Medicine*, 2nd ed., McGraw-Hill, New York, 1990, page 975.
[3] KNOUSE and LORBER, *Rev. infect. Dis.*, **12**, 393 (1990).
[4] WILSON et al., *Medicine (Baltimore)*, **68**, 38 (1989).
[5] *Med. Lett. Drug. Ther.*, **32**, No. 817 (1990).
[6] RUPPERT et al., *Dtsch. med. Wschr.*, **113**, 1801 (1988).
[7] BROWN, A. E., in MANDELL et al. (Eds.), *Principles and Practice of Infectious Diseases*, 3rd ed., Churchill Livingstone, New York, 1990, page 1581.
[8] PRESCOTT, J. F., *Clin. Microbiol. Rev.*, **4**, 20 (1991).
[9] EMMONS et al., *Rev. infect. Dis.*, **13**, 91 (1991).
[10] DOIG et al., *Scand. J. infect. Dis.*, **23**, 1 (1991).
[11] RIHS et al., *J. clin. Microbiol.*, **28**, 1934 (1990).
[12] MCGOWAN and DEL RIO, in MANDELL et al. (Eds.), *Principles and Practice of Infectious Diseases*, 3rd ed., Churchill Livingstone, New York, 1990, page 1782.
[13] HAWKEY et al., *J. clin. Path.*, **37**, 1066 (1984).
[14] BRENNER et al., *J. clin. Microbiol.*, **27**, 231 (1989).
[15] ZUMLA et al., *Quart. J. Med.*, N.S. **68**, 741 (1988).
[16] MALINVERNI, R., *Schweiz. med. Wschr.*, **120**, 745 (1990).
[17] KULLBERG et al., *Medicine (Baltimore)*, **70**, 287 (1991).

No.	**Bacterium** *Synonyms* Common names	Characteristics	Habitat Host Transmission	Associated disease
201	**Streptomyces somaliensis** (BRUMPT) WAKSMAN and HENRICI *Indiella somaliensis*	GRAM-positive. Long, ramified, nonsegmented filaments. Yellowish colonies becoming downy white to cerebriform. In tissues, hard yellow grains 2 mm in diameter	Possibly soil	Occasional cause of pseudomycetoma prevalent in East Africa; also in West Africa and Mexico[1,2]
202	**Actinomadura madurae** (VINCENT) LECHEVALIER and LECHEVALIER *Nocardia madurae* *Streptothrix madurae*	GRAM-positive. Long, nonsegmented hyphae with true and spurious ramifications. Not acid-fast. Aerobic. Smooth, cerebriform colonies in cultures; in tissues, visible as yellowish granules 0.5–2 mm in diameter	Soil. Found in clinical specimens	Common cause of pseudomycetoma in warm climates[1]. Lesions mainly of the foot (madura foot) and hand
203	**Actinomadura pelletieri** (LAVERAN) LECHEVALIER and LECHEVALIER *Nocardia pelletieri* *Micrococcus pelletieri*	GRAM-positive. Long, ramified, nonsegmented hyphae. Coral-red to dark-red colonies. In tissues, red granules 0.5 mm in diameter	Found in clinical specimens	Occasional cause of pseudomycetoma in warm climates, especially in West Africa[1]

[1] ELLNER and MORRISSEY, in WARREN and MAHMOUD (Eds.), *Tropical and Geographical Medicine*, 2nd ed., McGraw-Hill, New York, 1990, page 975.

[2] LOCCI, R., in WILLIAMS et al. (Eds.), *Bergey's Manual of Systematic Bacteriology*, Vol. 4, Williams & Wilkins, Baltimore, 1989, page 2451.

Introduction

Classification

Fungi belong to the plant kingdom, but like bacteria they contain no chlorophyll. Assigned to the special class of thallophytes, they have an unusually wide morphological range – from single-cell structures to highly organized cell complexes with complicated processes of reproduction. The heterotrophic eumycetes can be subdivided on the basis of various criteria, namely morphological (botanical), ecological, biochemical, serological or pathogenic. There is a tendency among mycologists to regard fungi as representatives of an independent kingdom separate from the plants.

Morphological criteria, for instance, give a subdivision into species with septate or nonseptate mycelium (Figs. 1–3, page 97), species producing sexual endogenous spores (ascomycetes) (Fig. 24, page 99), and species in which only asexual spores have been observed. Most mycotic pathogens in man belong to the latter subdivision, the *fungi imperfecti*. When a perfect (sexual) stage of an imperfect fungus species is found, the taxonomic classification changes and with it the name (for instance *Monosporium apiospermum* becomes *Pseudoallescheria sheari*).

The fungi can also be divided into nonpathogens and (primary or facultative) pathogens. Primary pathogens such as *Coccidioides immitis*, *Histoplasma capsulatum*, *Paracoccidioides brasiliensis*, *Blastomyces dermatitidis* and *Sporothrix schenckii* cause diseases and symptoms. The many dermatophytes that affect the skin, hair and nails (see pages 89–95) can also be regarded as primary pathogens, though they do not invade living tissue. Facultatively pathogenic fungi, on the other hand, cause disease only under certain conditions such as various types of immunodeficiency. This group includes the budding fungi, like *Candida albicans* and species such as *Cryptococcus neoformans*, as well as molds like *Aspergillus fumigatus*, *Mucor* species, etc.

Another classification is afforded by the localized or disseminated character of the mycoses themselves: the obligate and facultative pathogenic fungi can be arranged according to the organ or system of organs they affect, for example the lungs ('pulmonary mycosis') or skin ('dermatophytosis'). In this connection it should be noted that treatment with antibiotics at high doses over a long period is an important cause of mycosis in that it brings about a shift in the flora of a mucous membrane in favor of fungi resistant to the chemotherapy used. There is also a significantly increased predisposition to mycosis in persons suffering from diseases such as leukemia, diabetes or HODGKIN's disease, as well as in patients under corticosteroid, immunosuppressive or radiation therapy; the same applies to victims of acquired immunodeficiency syndrome (AIDS).

The mode of infection also provides a basis for classification. Pityriasis versicolor, for instance, can be regarded as a mycosis connected with sweating, sun exposure, endogenously or exogenously administered corticosteroids, and lack of personal hygiene, and is especially prevalent in the tropics. Coccidioidomycosis and histoplasmosis are examples of exogenous inhalation mycoses, while sporotrichosis, maduromycosis and chromoblastomycosis are examples of mycoses preceded by trauma, for example from thorns or splinters in people habitually going barefoot in the tropics, where these fungi are especially common on plants and wood. These three forms of mycosis are always of exogenous origin, whereas secondary mycosis, such as thrush, is mainly of endogenous origin. Aspergillosis, and possibly cryptococcosis and others, can be either exogenous or endogenous in origin.

Another classification is based on the geographical distribution of the pathogen, for instance *Paracoccidioides brasiliensis* in South America. Many of the dematiaceous fungi produce yeast-like growth of black colonies which at a later stage of development or at subculture turn to dark, sometimes velvety, colonies producing different conidial structures. Others will produce moldy colonies and develop dark multicellular macroconidia.

Change of names – particularly among the so-called 'black fungi' – may lead to confusion. In a number of instances several names are listed for one species in this presentation.

The Actinomycetes, Streptomycetes and Maduromycetes, often still regarded as fungi, are in reality bacteria (*Nos. 181–183, 201–203*). The diseases they cause should not be confused with true mycoses.

Diagnosis

The diagnosis of mycosis calls absolutely for demonstration of the pathogen. Special attention must be paid to the morphological form of the pathogen in the material examined. In some of the dimorphic fungi, such as *Coccidioides immitis*, *Histoplasma capsulatum*, *Paracoccidioides brasiliensis*, *Blastomyces dermatitidis*, *Sporothrix schenckii*, as well as *Trichophyton* and *Microsporum* species, there are two distinct morphological forms corresponding to saprophytic (culture) and parasitic (tissue) phases.

The pathogenic importance of fungi for man and animals is difficult to assess owing to the frequent presence of harmless fungi on the skin as well as in the gastrointestinal tract.

Indirect evidence provided by intracutaneous tests and serological reactions (agglutination, precipitation, agar-gel diffusion, immunoelectrophoresis, complement fixation) is of value only in relatively few forms of mycosis (coccidioidomycosis, histoplasmosis, North and South American blastomycosis, sporotrichosis, aspergillosis, cryptococcosis and occasionally also candidosis).

Treatment

Former treatment of mycoses was very unsatisfactory owing to the lack of specific, internally active, antimycotic drugs. When given in time and in adequate dosage, amphotericin B has proved very effective in generalized mycosis (coccidioidomycosis, histoplasmosis, North and South American blastomycosis, also disseminated infections by budding fungi such as *Candida albicans* and *Cryptococcus neoformans*). Hydroxystilbamidine was found to be effective against *Blastomyces dermatitidis*, but is now hardly ever used because of its neurotoxic side effects. The polyene antibiotics have proved useful in local and inhalation treatment of candidosis of the respiratory tract. The latter can be treated successfully with flucytosine administered orally, but the cells of the fungus are sometimes resistant or become resistant after 10–14 days of treatment. The drug has been used in combination with amphotericin B to treat cryptococcosis and systemic candidosis.

Various imidazoles have been introduced for local and internal treatment of a great variety of mycotic infections because of their wide range of antifungal activity. Orally administered ketoconazole is being used for the therapy of local, internal and systemic mycosis, and is recommended for prophylactic use against secondary *Candida* infections in patients at risk. Vaginal *Candida* infections respond quickly to 1–2 days of local treatment with imidazoles or triazoles (see page 88).

Otomycosis (mycotic infection of the external auditory meatus) is often caused by *Aspergillus* species and can be cured by irrigation with antimycotic washes and thorough cleansing, together with treatment to eliminate bacterial infection.

Mycotic lung disease, caused by species of *Aspergillus* for instance, is difficult to treat, but amphotericin B may be tried. Itraconazole and flucytosine have been used with success in recent years. In patients with cavitation or granuloma formation (cryptococcosis), mycotic abscesses or destructive mycetoma of the lungs, extremities or eyes, surgical treatment is necessary and may be life-saving if carried out in time.

For zygomycosis, which is caused by species of the genera *Absidia*, *Mucor* and *Rhizopus*, amphotericin B remains the only proven effective therapy.

For treatment of dermatophytosis, see page 89.

Guideline for tables

Owing to the rather frequent name changes of pathogenic fungi, the differences in names of anamorphs and telemorphs, and the continued use of older designations, the listed fungi have been divided into several groups, depending on their distinguishing characteristics, and arranged alphabetically in these groups (with a few exceptions for logical reasons).

No.	**Fungus** *Synonyms*	Characteristics	Habitat Host Transmission	Associated disease
	Fungi causing zygomycosis (for references, see next page)			
204	**Absidia corymbifera** COHN *Mucor corymbifer* *Lichtheimia corymbifera*	Rapid growth at 37 °C. Branched, nonseptate mycelium. Abundant, woolly, aerial mycelium, white at first, later gray. Branching sporangiophores with terminal pyriform sporangia containing numerous endospores. Sporangiophores with long coniform apophysis along the stolon, not originating from the rhizoids. Details of *Mucorales* have been reviewed[1]	Worldwide distribution. Common on decaying vegetation, foodstuffs, etc. Occasionally found in human sputum, in the external auditory meatus, on the skin of horses and other animals	Facultatively pathogenic saprophyte, occasional cause of zygomycosis[2-4]. Infects the lungs and other internal organs (intravascular growth), the external auditory meatus (otomycosis), also the nose (rhinocerebral mycosis) and central nervous system. Similar disease is caused by the genera *Mucor*, *Rhizomucor* and *Rhizopus* (see below). Generalized infections are usually fatal. Predisposing factors are diabetes, malnutrition, amebiasis, burns, long-term corticosteroid therapy, intravenous drug use[5,6]
205	**Absidia ramosa** (LINDT) LENDNER	Possibly identical with *A. corymbifera*		
206	**Basidiobolus meristosporus** DRECHSLER *Basidiobolus haptosporus* *Basidiobolus ranarum*	Rapid growth of thin, pale-yellow to gray segmented mycelium, initially with smooth surface; later scanty white aerial mycelium. Mycelium with abundant chlamydospores and zygospores, also piriform sporangia with endospores	Saprophyte with worldwide distribution. Occasionally affects man (Indonesia, India, tropical Africa)	Rare cause of subcutaneous zygomycosis[7]
207	**Cunninghamella elegans** LENDNER	Rapid growth of floccose colony. White to gray with straight and vertically branched conidiophores. Spherical or oral echinulate conidia are formed on the surface of spherical vesicles. In tissue sections nonseptate hyphae. Does not grow at 40 °C	Worldwide distribution	Probably not pathogenic in man[8]
208	**Cunninghamella bertholletiae** MATRUCHOT 1903	Rapid growth of smooth hyaline hyphae, 7–11 µm in diameter, branched at acute and right angles, infrequent septa. Conidia spherical to ellipsoidal (7–14 µm)	Worldwide distribution	Occasional agent of zygomycosis in hematologic malignancies and in a liver transplant recipient[9]
209	**Entomophthora coronata** (CONSTANTIN) KEVORKIAN *Conidiobolus coronatus*	Rapid growth of flat, tough colonies with white aerial mycelium at 30 °C. Upright conidiophores with conidia 35–45 µm long ejected to a distance of up to 30 mm from the conidiophore. These are multigranular and sometimes form several asci. Fragments of hyphae and giant cells are found in affected tissues	In horses (nasal polyps) in Texas and Jamaica. Probably a primary saprophyte	Zygomycosis of the nose and nasal sinuses (rhino-entomophthoramycosis) in South America and tropical Africa[4]
210	**Mucor circinelloides** VAN TIEGHEM	Rapid growth at 22 °C and 37 °C, no growth at 45 °C. In 5–7 days abundant white downy aerial mycelium, later turning yellowish-gray to brown, usually not higher than 1 cm. Nonseptate mycelium with many chlamydospores. Erect single sporangiophores issue directly from the mycelium with terminal dark or brownish sporangium or branched with numerous sporangia containing endospores. Columellae are always present (see Fig. 12, page 97)	As for *Absidia*	As for *Absidia*. The only species of *Mucor* pathogenic in man

No.	**Fungus** *Synonyms*	Characteristics	Habitat Host Transmission	Associated disease
211	**Mucor mucedo** MICHELI ex FRIES	Rapid growth at 22 °C, abundant grayish-white fluffy aerial mycelium, usually much higher than 1 cm. Nonseptate mycelium ending in round terminal sporangia containing numerous endospores. Apophysis is always absent	As for *Absidia*	Nonpathogenic in man, but known to be a frequent contaminant of laboratory cultures and specimens
212	**Rhizopus** spp., e.g. **Rhizopus oryzae** **Rhizopus arrhizus** **Rhizopus rhizopodiformis**	Rapid growth at 22 °C (facultatively pathogenic species also at 37 °C). Abundant grayish-white wooly aerial mycelium after 2 days, changing to gray, yellowish, yellowish-brown or brown according to species, with brown or black dots (sporangia). Mycelium nonseptate and colorless, sporangiophores unbranched, 100–200 µm long and carrying dark-walled sporangia. These contain columellae and round endospores. Along the stolons, sporangia originate in tufts of 5 and more opposite the rhizoids, and can be seen with the naked eye	As for *Absidia*	Zygomycosis[2–4]. Hospital-acquired cutaneous infections may occur, especially by *R. rhizopodiformis*[12]
	Rhizopus stolonifer **Rhizopus nigricans**			These agents have not been found to be pathogenic, by contrast with other species of this genus, and should be regarded as saprophytes and laboratory contaminants
213	**Rhizomucor pusillus** (LINDT) SCHIPPER	Rapid growth at 22 °C. Even at 50 °C abundant growth in 5 to 7 days of a white downy aerial mycelium, later turning gray or brown. Nonseptate mycelium. Single sporangiophores issue directly from the mycelium and are either partly unbranched with terminal sporangium or branched with numerous round sporangia containing endospores. Columellae are brown and always present. Rhizoids are present, but not easily found with the magnifying glass	As for *Absidia*	As for *Absidia*. Occasional cause of mycotic abortion in mares, cows and other animals
214	**Saksenaea vasiformis** SAKSENA	Typical flask-shaped sporangia	Worldwide distribution	Occasional agent of zygomycosis following nosocomial infection, also in thalassemia. Rhinocerebral and disseminated infections usually fatal[10]
215	**Zygorhynchus heterogamus**		Saprophyte	Single case of cecal zygomycosis in acute myeloid leukemia[11]

1 SCHOLER et al., in HOWARD, D. H. (Ed.), *Fungi Pathogenic for Humans and Animals*, Part A, Dekker, New York, 1981, page 9.
2 BAKER, R. D., *J. Amer. med. Ass.*, **163**, 805 (1957).
3 RIPPON, J. W., *Medical Mycology*, 3rd ed., Saunders, Philadelphia, 1988, page 681.
4 SUGAR, A. M., in MANDELL et al. (Eds.), *Principles and Practice of Infectious Diseases*, 3rd ed., Churchill Livingstone, New York, 1990, page 1962.
5 DIEM and LENTNER (Eds.), *Pathogenic Organisms and Infectious Diseases*, Documenta Geigy, Basel, 1971, page 92.
6 STAVE et al., *Amer. J. Med.*, **86**, 115 (1989).
7 MUGERWA, J. W., in WARREN and MAHMOUD (Eds.), *Tropical and Geographical Medicine*, 2nd ed., McGraw-Hill, New York, 1990, page 1008.
8 WEITZMAN and CRIST, *Mycologia*, **71**, 1023 (1979).
9 NIMMO et al., *Postgrad. med. J.*, **64**, 82 (1988).
10 TANPHAICHITR et al., *Mycoses*, **33**, 303 (1990).
11 TOUBAS et al., *Rapport Soc. franç. de Mycol. méd.*, Séance du 16 nov. 1990.
12 MARCHEVSKY et al., *Hum. Path.*, **11**, 457 (1980).

No.	**Fungus** *Synonyms*	Characteristics	Habitat Host Transmission	Associated disease
	Fungi causing primarily mycetoma (for references, see next page)			
216	**Cephalosporium falciforme** CARRIÓN *Acremonium falciforme*	White to yellowish colony of hyaline hyphae and chlamydospores 12 µm in diameter. Seen in tissues as soft, white to yellowish granules. In cultures, sporulation is of *Cephalosporium* type (see Fig. 15, page 98)	Central and South America. Probably saprophytic, facultatively pathogenic	A cause of mycetoma (white form)
217	**Cephalosporium acremonium** CORDA	Smooth, rather tough colonies, pink-orange in color, later overgrown by loose, whitish mycelium (30–32 °C). Heads of one- or two-celled, small conidia on very thin, vertically arranged conidiophores. Coremia	Widely distributed in nature, usually saprophytic	A cause of mycetoma with white-yellowish grains
218	**Acremonium kiliense** GRÜTZ	Similar to *Cephalosporium acremonium*. Hyaline hyphae	As for *Cephalosporium acremonium*	A cause of mycetoma (hyalohyphomycosis); isolated from subcutis, bone, joints, pleural fluid
219	**Cephalosporium recifei** LEAO and LOBO *Acremonium recifei*	Rapid development of white mycelium, turning to pink and salmon color. On 10–15 µm long phialides development of clusters of elongated or sickle-shaped conidia		A cause of mycetoma
220	**Leptosphaeria senegalensis** SEGRETAIN, BAYLET, DARASSE and CAMAIN	Grayish-white, later brownish, colonies with black reverse, growing faster at 37 °C than at 30 °C. Vesicles and chlamydospores are rare; no conidia. Round, black perithecia (100 to 300 µm in diameter) with club-shaped asci containing 8 elongated hyaline or brown ascospores, each with 2–5 loculi. Seen in tissues as round or lobate, black granules about 1 mm in diameter	Presumably a soil fungus in West Africa. Human infections through injury	A cause of mycetoma (black form)
221	**Madurella grisea** MACKINNON, FERRADA and MONTEMAYOR	At 30 °C slow growth of gray, velvety, aerial mycelium on a brown base. Pale, thin, cylindric hyphae with adjacent thick hyphae made up of chains of budding cells. Secondary spore forms are rare. Seen in tissues as dark granules	Presumably soil. Infection through injuries from thorns, etc. Human infections mainly in South America	A cause of mycetoma (black form) *Remark*. Treatment as for *M. mycetomatis*
222	**Madurella mycetomatis** LAVERAN *Madurella americana* *Madurella ikedai*	At 37 °C slow growth of flat, plicate colonies with brown pigmentation and white aerial mycelium; chlamydospores, occasional microconidia on tiny bottle-shaped phialides; black sclerotia up to 750 µm in diameter. Seen in tissues as black granules	Soil and dust. Infection through injury from thorns. Widespread, especially in Africa, Asia, South and Central America	A common cause of mycetoma (black form)[1-3] *Remark*. Chemotherapy plus surgical treatment may be effective
223	**Neotestudina rosatii** SEGRETAIN and DESTOMBES *Zopfia rosatii*	Brown, slow-growing, flat colonies with grayish-brown surface mycelium with white patches. Grows on potatoes, carrots and cornflour, and forms round, black perithecia (350 µm in diameter) with round asci containing 8 bicameral, slightly arcuate, conical ascospores with rounded ends. Seen in tissues as soft brownish-white, rounded granules 0.5–1 mm in diameter	Somaliland, possibly also Central and West Africa	A cause of mycetoma (white form)

No.	Fungus *Synonyms*	Characteristics	Habitat Host Transmission	Associated disease
224	**Pseudoallescheria sheari** NEGRONI and FISCHER Anamorphs: *Glenospora boydii* *Indiella americana* *Monosporium apiospermum* *Scedosporium apiospermum* *Acremoniella lutzii* Teleomorphs: *Allescheria boydii* *Petriellidium boydii*	Seen in tissues as white to yellowish macroscopic granules composed of branched hyphae and large chlamydospores. Forms fast-growing white, later gray or grayish-green colonies with grayish-black reverse. Broad, hyaline, septate, branched mycelium. Numerous unicellular, ellipsoidal or piriform anelloconidia formed singly in dry chains at the apices of the annellides (see Fig. 18, page 98), occurring singly or in small numbers on upright short conidiophores. Occasional bundles of conidiophores. Perfect strains form cleistothecia with asci and ascospores. Homothallic. Urease-negative	Man and animals. Normally a saprophytic root fungus of privet hedges; also in sewage. Infection through injury (especially in persons going barefoot), occasionally by inhalation of dust. Human infection in tropical and subtropical India, occasionally also in temperate regions	A common cause of mycetoma (white form)[1-3], also known as allescheriasis or monosporiosis[4]. Occasionally localized infections of lung, cornea, bladder and meninges[5], also focally invasive infections of musculoskeletal tissues. Immunocompromised persons (corticosteroid treatment, transplant patients) are at risk *Remark*. Disseminated disease often fatal, but localized disease may be cured by chemotherapy plus surgical treatment[6]
225	**Scedosporium inflatum** MALLOCH and SALKIN 1984 Teleomorph: unknown	Culturally similar to *Scedosporium apiospermum*, but more rapid growth on nutrient agar media, formation of annelloconidia in clumps on cylindric annellides with swollen bases. Urease-positive	Isolated from soil in Canada	Isolated from mycetoma, sputum, peritoneal cavity (USA and Australia)[7]
226	**Pyrenochaeta romeroi** BORELLI	At 30°C rapid growth of dark-gray, woolly, white-edged colonies with a black reverse. Bright yellow pycnidia. Seen in tissues as black, soft, tubular granules	Venezuela. Saprophyte; human infection through injury	A cause of mycetoma (black form)

[1] MAHGOUB, E. S., in MANDELL et al. (Eds.), *Principles and Practice of Infectious Diseases*, 3rd ed., Churchill Livingstone, New York, 1990, page 1977.
[2] RIPPON, J. W., *Medical Mycology*, 3rd ed., Saunders, Philadelphia, 1988, page 80.
[3] ELLNER and MORRISSEY, in WARREN and MAHMOUD (Eds.), *Tropical and Geographical Medicine*, 2nd ed., McGraw-Hill, New York, 1990, page 975.
[4] GREEN and ADAMS, *Amer. J. clin. Path.*, **42**, 75 (1964); MOHR and MUCHMORE, *J. Amer. med. Ass.*, **204**, 355 (1968).
[5] DWORZACK et al., *Medicine (Baltimore)*, **68**, 218 (1989).
[6] PATTERSON et al., *Mycoses*, **33**, 297 (1990).
[7] SALKIN et al., *J. clin. Microbiol.*, **26**, 498 (1988).

No.	**Fungus** *Synonyms*	Characteristics	Habitat Host Transmission	Associated disease
	Dimorphic fungi causing systemic mycosis (for references, see next page)			
227	**Blastomyces dermatitidis** GILCHRIST and STOKES *Blastomycoides dermatitidis* *Glenospora brevis* *Mycoderma dermatitidis* *Monosporium tulanense* *Zymonema dermatitidis* Teleomorph: *Ajellomyces dermatitidis*	Dimorphic. Saprophytic form (at 24–30 °C): fairly slow growth of white tufty colonies, later turning dark-cream in color, with radial plication and concentric rings. Mycelium septate with aleuriospores (round, oval or pyriform) on short stalks. Tissue (yeast-like) form at 37 °C growth on enriched media of mesenteroid cream-colored colonies made up of spherical or ovoid yeast-like, budding cells 5 to 20 µm in diameter (single-budding forms only) possessing a thick, double-contoured membrane (see Fig. 28, page 99). Possibly two variants of different geographical occurrence[1]	Man and animals. Free existence in nature in connection with beaver lodges has been reported[6]. Infection mainly by inhalation of aleuriospores in dust from soil. Endemic only in North and Central America; sporadic occurrence in Tunisia and various parts of Central and South Africa, also reported from Asian countries	North American blastomycosis (GILCHRIST's disease)[2–5]. Primary site of infection is usually the lung, and disseminated lesions may develop involving almost any organ, e.g. skin, joints, urogenital tract, meninges (brain abscess), liver. Incubation periods between 20 and 100 days have been reported[4,6] *Remark*. Chemotherapy, as mentioned in the introduction
228	**Coccidioides immitis** RIXFORD and GILCHRIST	Dimorphic. Saprophytic form: culture whitish cotton-wool with brownish-black reverse. The hyphae are branched and septate, with barrel-shaped arthrospores 2–10 µm in diameter; the latter are highly infectious and develop from the 5th day after inoculation. Tissue form: spherules 5 to 200 µm in diameter, some thick-walled, which multiply by endosporulation (see Fig. 30, page 99)	Man and animals, mainly in southwestern USA, Mexico, Guatemala, Paraguay, Venezuela and Argentina. Infection by inhalation of arthrospores in dust from soil. Not transmissible from man to man or from animals to man	Coccidioidomycosis (San-Joaquin Valley fever)[7–9]: (a) acute bronchopneumonitis subsiding in 14 days, (b) generalized chronic form resembling pulmonary tuberculosis. Erythema nodosum or erythema multiforme are common; disseminated lesions may involve almost any organ (common cause of fungal meningitis[10]). Most human infections remain asymptomatic; only 0.5% of infected persons develop secondary or generalized coccidioidomycosis, with or without meningitis or coccidioidal granulomatosis[8,9]. Immunocompromised persons are at risk (frequent complication of AIDS[11,31]) *Remarks*. For severe or disseminated infections, chemotherapy as mentioned in the introduction. Surgical removal of pulmonary residuals may be necessary
229	**Histoplasma capsulatum** DARLING *Cryptococcus capsulatus* *Posadasia piriformis* Teleomorph[12]: *Emmonsiella capsulata* KWON-CHUNG	Dimorphic. Saprophytic form (at 25–30 °C): slow growth of white colonies with fine silky aerial mycelium, later beige-colored. Hyphae septate, with sessile or petiolate, round or pyriform microconidia and thick-walled round macroconidia 7 to 25 µm in diameter with spiny or finger-like projections. Tissue (yeast-like) form: on blood–cystine agar cream-colored colonies of budding cells, in tissues intracellular, ovoid cells, 1.5–2.0 µm by 3.0–3.5 µm (see Fig. 29a, page 99)	Typical geophilic species. Mainly found in droppings of birds (starlings, fowl) and bats; infects dogs, cats and man. Human infection by inhalation of dust from soil containing the conidia. Widespread in North, Central and South America; also reported in Italy, in former prisoners of war in the USA and in pilots undergoing training in endemic areas of the USA	Histoplasmosis (DARLING's disease)[13–15]. Portal of entry is the lung, with involvement of the regional lymph nodes; extrapulmonary primary lesions (skin, conjunctiva) are extremely rare. The primary lung infection is mostly benign and self-limiting. Clinical disease may be due to reinfection. Pulmonary and lymph-node lesions tend to calcify. Self-limiting hematogenous dissemination is common, with metastatic foci in liver and spleen; occasionally the gastrointestinal tract, adrenals, central nervous system[32], heart or eyes are involved with devastating impact. Pericarditis is a rare complication of the primary infection. Immunocompromised persons are at risk (frequent complication of AIDS[11,33]) *Remarks*. For severe or disseminated infections, chemotherapy as mentioned in the introduction

No.	**Fungus** *Synonyms*	Characteristics	Habitat Host Transmission	Associated disease
230	**Histoplasma capsulatum** var. **duboisii** VANBREUSEGHEM Teleomorph: *Emmonsiella capsulata* KWON-CHUNG	Dimorphic. Similar to *H. capsulatum*, but biochemically and serologically different. Tissue form: characteristic large budding cells (7–15 µm) with thick walls and numerous fat droplets; often intracellular (see Fig. 29b, page 99)	Probably soil and plants. Human infections in West and Central Africa; also infects monkeys. Primary inoculation via skin and mucous membranes suggested	Histoplasmosis duboisii (African histoplasmosis)[14,16–18]. Affects skin, bones, joints, regional lymph nodes, gastrointestinal tract and lungs
231	**Paracoccidioides brasiliensis** (CONANT and HOWELL) SPLENDORE *Lutziomyces histiosporocellularis* *Mycoderma brasiliense* *Blastomyces brasiliensis* *Zymonema brasiliense*	Dimorphic. Saprophytic form: similar to *Blastomyces dermatitidis*. Tissue form: in cultures similar to *Blastomyces dermatitidis*, cells up to 60 µm in diameter, but with multiple budding; daughter cells often very small (see Fig. 7, page 97)	Probably soil and plants, primary habitat not yet established. Infection by inhalation of aleuriospores in dust from soil. Limited to South and Central America and Mexico	Paracoccidioidomycosis (South American blastomycosis, paracoccidioidal granuloma)[19–21]. Primary site of infection seems to be the lung. Ulcerated lesions regularly on mouth, lips, tongue, nose, etc. (granulomatous appearance). Lymph nodes, adrenals, liver, spleen, gastrointestinal tract, bones and central nervous system may be involved *Remark*. Treatment as for *Histoplasmosis capsulatum*. This systemic mycosis is also treatable with sulfonamides
232	**Sporothrix schenckii** (HEKTOEN and PERKINS) MATRUCHOT *Rhinocladium schenckii* *Sporotrichum beurmannii* Teleomorph[22]: *Ceratocystis stenoceras* (sub judice) (ROBAK) MOREAU	Dimorphic. Saprophytic form: cultures initially bacteria-like, later with branched, scanty, aerial mycelium showing small ovoid conidia on short stalks, often dendroid in form (see Fig. 17, page 98) or arranged singly along slender hyphae; occasionally triangle-shaped, thick-walled 'macroconidia'. Colonies vary in color from cream to black. Tissue form: yeast-like growth on blood–cystine agar at 37 °C. These colonies and affected tissues contain fusiform bacteria-like, cigar-shaped cells 2–4 µm in length (see Fig. 31, page 99). Pus usually stains poorly on slides. Granular asteroid bodies are occasionally seen	Soil, plants, dead vegetation. Infection via injuries from thorns, etc. Worldwide distribution; common in Mexico, South America and South Africa, nearly non-existent in Europe. Occasionally epidemic (for instance miners); occupational disease of gardeners and seedling handlers[23]	Sporotrichosis[24–26], marked by skin ulceration and lymphadenitis; in rare cases affects lung, gastrointestinal tract, also joints and muscles. Meningitis seems to be very rare[27]. Incubation period for the cutaneous form 1 to 12 weeks[24] *Remarks*. Chemotherapy as for the other dimorphic fungi. Potassium iodide is recommended for the lymphocutaneous form[28]. Local heat treatment (40 to 41 °C)[28,34]
233	**Loboa loboi** (FILHO and LEAO) CIFERRI et al.	Not cultivated. Seen in tissue sections as round, elliptical or lemon-shaped cells in giant cells or macrophages. Unilocular or multilocular budding	Human infection in Central and South America; found in dolphins. Infection through skin injury	Lobomycosis (keloidal blastomycosis)[29,30]. Infection limited to subepidermal area. Regional lymph nodes are rarely involved. Incubation period 12 to 24 months[30]

1 Editorial, *Lancet*, **1**, 23 (1989).
2 FURCOLOW et al., *J. Amer. med. Ass.*, **198**, 115 (1966).
3 TENENBAUM et al., *CRC Crit. Rev. Microbiol.*, **9**, 139 (1982).
4 CHAPMAN, S. W., in MANDELL et al. (Eds.), *Principles and Practice of Infectious Diseases*, 3rd ed., Churchill Livingstone, New York, 1990, page 1999.
5 RIPPON, J. W., *Medical Mycology*, 3rd ed., Saunders, Philadelphia, 1988, page 474.
6 KLEIN et al., *New Engl. J. Med.*, **314**, 529 (1986).
7 FIESE, M. J., *Coccidioidomycosis*, Thomas, Springfield, 1958.
8 STEVENS, D. A., in MANDELL et al. (Eds.), *Principles and Practice of Infectious Diseases*, 3rd ed., Churchill Livingstone, New York, 1990, page 2008.
9 RIPPON, J. W., *Medical Mycology*, 3rd ed., Saunders, Philadelphia, 1988, page 433.
10 BOUZA et al., *Medicine (Baltimore)*, **60**, 139 (1981).
11 DIAMOND R. D., *Rev. infect. Dis.*, **13**, 480 (1991).
12 KWON-CHUNG, K. J., *Science*, **177**, 368 (1972).
13 SWEANY, H. C., *Histoplasmosis*, Thomas, Springfield, IL, 1960.
14 LOYD et al., in MANDELL et al. (Eds.), *Principles and Practice of Infectious Diseases*, 3rd ed., Churchill Livingstone, New York, 1990, page 1989.
15 RIPPON, J. W., *Medical Mycology*, 3rd ed., Saunders, Philadelphia, 1988, page 381.
16 GENTILINI et al., *Ann. Méd. interne*, **128**, 451 (1977).
17 RIPPON, J. W., *Medical Mycology*, 3rd ed., Saunders, Philadelphia, 1988, page 424.
18 SCHMIDT et al., *Schweiz. med. Wschr.*, **50**, 2016 (1987).
19 RESTREPO, A. M., in MANDELL et al. (Eds.), *Principles and Practice of Infectious Diseases*, 3rd ed., Churchill Livingstone, New York, 1990, page 2028.
20 RIPPON, J. W., *Medical Mycology*, 3rd ed., Saunders, Philadelphia, 1988, page 506.
21 GEER, D. L., in WARREN and MAHMOUD (Eds.), *Tropical and Geographical Medicine*, 2nd ed., McGraw-Hill, New York, 1990, page 981.
22 MARIAT, F., in IWATA, K. (Ed.), *Recent Advances in Medical and Veterinary Mycology*, University of Tokyo Press, 1977, page 265.
23 *Morb. Mort. wkly Rep.*, **37**, 652 (1988).
24 BENNETT, J. E., in MANDELL et al. (Eds.), *Principles and Practice of Infectious Diseases*, 3rd ed., Churchill Livingstone, New York, 1990, page 1972.
25 RIPPON, J. W., *Medical Mycology*, 3rd ed., Saunders, Philadelphia, 1988, page 325.
26 BENNETT, J. E., in WARREN and MAHMOUD (Eds.), *Tropical and Geographical Medicine*, 2nd ed., McGraw-Hill, New York, 1990, page 1007.
27 SCOTT et al., *New Engl. J. Med.*, **317**, 935 (1987).
28 *Med. Lett. Drug. Ther.*, **34**, No. 864, 14 (1992).
29 RIPPON, J. W., *Medical Mycology*, 3rd ed., Saunders, Philadelphia, 1988, page 353.
30 MCGINNIS, M. R., in WARREN and MAHMOUD (Eds.), *Tropical and Geographical Medicine*, 2nd ed., McGraw-Hill, New York, 1990, page 954.
31 FISH et al., *Medicine (Baltimore)*, **69**, 384 (1990).
32 WHEAT et al., *Medicine (Baltimore)*, **69**, 244 (1990).
33 WHEAT et al., *Medicine (Baltimore)*, **69**, 361 (1990).
34 MACKINNON, J. E., *El Torax*, **13**, 266 (1964).

No.	**Fungus** *Synonyms*	Characteristics	Habitat Host Transmission	Associated disease
	Fungi causing chromoblastomycosis, phaeohyphomycosis (black fungi) and tinea versicolor (for references, see page 83)			
234	**Aureobasidium pullulans** (DE BARY) ARNAUD 1918 *Pullularia pullulans* Teleomorph: *Guignardia pullulans*	Moderately rapid growth, turning from slimy cream- to pink-colored colonies to dark blackish color with tough consistency, on blood agar creamy, yeast-like growth of ovoid cells with bipolar budding	Saprophyte in soil, on higher plants causing dew-like 'sooty mold'	Occasionally associated with superficial infections; spleen abscess in a patient with lymphoma[1]
235	**Bipolaris spicifera** NELSON 1964 *Drechslera spicifera* (see also *Nos. 262, 263*)	Rapid growth of floccose, gray colonies, becoming dark brown. Sympodial conidiogenous cells, geniculate poroconidia broadly ellipsoidal to fusoid (9–14 µm by 20–40 µm), consistently 3 pseudosepta, very small hyaline zone. Maximum temperature 40 °C. Germ tube origin adjacent to hilum		Phaeohyphomycosis[2]. Sinusitis; most patients are immunocompetent[3]
235a	**Exserohilum mcginnisii**	Similar to *Bipolaris spicifera*		As for *Bipolaris spicifera*
236	**Cladosporium bantianum** (SACCARDO) BORELLI *Cladosporium trichoides* *Torula bantiana* *Xylohypha bantiana*	Slow growth of colonies about 3 cm in diameter (2 weeks' incubation) with a flat or raised velvety surface and radial folds. Color dark olive-green to black, reverse side black. Brown, septate mycelium. Long, sparsely branching chains of conidia on simple or septate conidiophores. Blastoconidia brown, ellipsoidal and separated by transverse dark areas. In pus appears as brown, branching, septate hyphae 1 to 2 µm in diameter with chlamydospores up to 8 µm. Grows even at 42–43 °C. Can be distinguished from *C. carrionii* by its rapid growth and extremely long chains of spores (see Fig. 16, page 98)	Probably primarily saprophytic, occasionally pathogenic in man	Subcutaneous phaeohyphomycosis, systemic infection possible (brain abscesses[4])
237	**Cladosporium carrionii** (EMMONS) BINFORD *Cladophialophora ajelloi*	Similar to *C. bantianum* but grows more slowly. Chains of conidia usually shorter	Wood and other vegetable matter; saprophyte in tropical and subtropical countries. Occasional human infections through injury; not transmissible from man to man	Chromoblastomycosis[5–7]; phaeohyphomycotic brain abscesses
238	**Dichotomophthoropsis nymphaearum** (RAND) ELLIS	Velvety, olivaceous-brown colonies on SABOURAUD glucose agar. Wide hyphae (2–6 µm) with conidophores up to 150 µm. Elongate, thick conidia, coiled 1 to 3.5 times	Saprophyte	A case of keratomycosis reported from Bangladesh[25]
239	**Exophiala jeanselmei** MCGINNIS and PADHYE 1977 *Phialophora jeanselmei* *Cadophora lignicola* *Torula jeanselmei*	Slow growth of black colonies, initially with a moist, skin-like surface, later a gray velvety aerial mycelium; reverse side black. Hyphae at first appear as chains of budding cells. Conidia develop as tube-shaped phialides. Nonproteolytic (unlike *Cladosporium*). Forms soft black grains of varying size consisting of brown hyphae and dark-brown chlamydospores. In affected tissues also seen as brownish sclerotia. Maximum temperature 37 °C	Probably saprophytic; widespread on wood. Human infection through injury. In tropical countries, also in the USA	Most common agent of subcutaneous phaeohyphomycosis; systemic infection possible[5,7]

No.	**Fungus** *Synonyms*	Characteristics	Habitat Host Transmission	Associated disease
240	**Exophiala pisciphila** McGinnis and Ajello 1974	Similar to *E. jeanselmei*, but larger conidia; slow growth of dark green to black fungus at 30 °C and 35 °C	Pathogen of fish	Chromoblastomycosis and phaeohyphomycosis possible[8]
241	**Exophiala spinifera** (Nielsen and Conant) McGinnis *Phialophora spinifera*	Primary colonies dark, moist, of yeast-like cells and segments of toruloid hyphae. Rigid, deeply pigmented, simple or spine-like tapering conidiophores (mature 36–60 µm long). Ovoid conidia, 1.0 µm by 1.0–1.5 µm, aggregated apiculately, unicellular. Short, urn-shaped phialides terminate in collarettes, conidia semiendogenously produced	Saprophyte	Subcutaneous phaeohyphomycosis[9]
242	**Fonsecaea compacta** Carrión *Phialophora compacta* *Hormodendrum compactum*	Similar to *F. pedrosoi* except that the conidia are not elongated but rounded and in short, compact chains	As for *F. pedrosoi*	Chromoblastomycosis (see *F. pedrosoi*)
243	**Fonsecaea pedrosoi** (Brumpt) Negroni *Phialophora pedrosoi* *Hormodendrum pedrosoi*	Mold-like cultures with formation of olive-green to black pigment; typical *Cladosporium*-type sporulation. On blood–cystine agar growth occasionally yeast-like. Seen in affected tissues as thick-walled cells (sclerotia), 6 to 12 µm in diameter, occurring singly or in groups, often divided but not budding (see Fig. 27, page 99)	Saprophyte of soil and decaying wood in South and Central America, Africa, the Antilles, southern CIS, Sumatra. Human infections through wound contamination, etc.	Commonest cause of chromoblastomycosis (dermatitis verrucosa)[5–7], a chronic infection mainly of the extremities, manifest initially as pustules, later as verrucous nodules or papillomata
244	**Hendersonula toruloidea** Nattrass Renamed *Nattrassia mangiferae* Sutton and Dyko 1989 Synanamorph: *Scytalidium dimidiatum* Sutton and Dyko 1989	Rapid growth at 25 °C. Floccose to strigose colonies with abundant aerial mycelium. Changing from white to pale gray and olive-gray within 10 days. Narrow hyaline and thick (4–7.5 µm in diameter) dematiaceous hyphae breaking up into one- or two-celled, barrel-shaped to oblong, dry arthroconidia (2 to 9.5 µm by 4–7.5 µm) with highly pigmented septa	Isolated in Africa, Canada	A rare cause of phaeohyphomycotic nail infections[10]
244a	**Onychocola canadensis** gen. et sp. nov. Sigler 1990	Slow growth of glabrous, light-grayish colonies at 28 °C, reverse side brownish-gray to yellowish-gray. Fluffy whitish aerial hyphae after 5–6 weeks. Abundant hyaline, 0–1 septate arthroconidia produced very slowly	Probably saprophyte	Hyphomycotic nail infections reported from Canada[26]
244b	**Phaeosklera dematioides** Sigler 1981	Very slow growth (1 cm in 4 weeks at 20–25 °C) of dark olive-brown and grayish-brown cerebriform colonies. Development of thick-walled dictyospores with longitudinal and transversal septa; typical cracks in the plating medium	Saprophyte of ligneous plants (*Pinus contorta*)	Pseudoepitheliomatous hyperplasia, secondary to chromoblastomycosis in an adult from Libya infected with *Fonsecaea compacta*. Duration 30 years[23] *Remark*. Healed under ketoconazole therapy
245	**Phialophora parasitica** Ajello, Georg, Steigbigel and Wang 1974	Felty colonies, gray or beige turning to maroon to grayish-black color. Short phialides with formation of ellipsoidal spores, 1 µm by 3 µm, later long phialides (30–40 µm) terminating in small collarettes; ellipsoidal spores in clusters	Saprophyte of decaying wood	Subcutaneous phaeohyphomycosis; septic arthritis in the knee of a kidney transplant patient[11]

No.	**Fungus** *Synonyms*	Characteristics	Habitat Host Transmission	Associated disease
246	**Phialophora repens** (DAVIDSON) CONANT 1937 *Cadophora repens*	Moderate growth of flat colonies (6 cm in diameter at 25 °C in 4 weeks). Velvety surface, light brown turning to dark brown. Reverse side nearly black. Light brown septate hyphae, often arranged in strands. Phialospores singly or in groups, often branched, tapering to 1 to 1.5 µm at the apex. Short, but distinct, collarette with phialospores in balls (endogenously formed, hyaline, curved or cylindric)	Saprophyte of decaying wood (causes blueing of wood pulp)	Subcutaneous phaeohyphomycosis (granulomatous nodule in the scalp under prednisolone therapy in leprosy patient[12])
247	**Phialophora richardsiae** (MELIN and NANNFELDT) CONANT 1937 *Cadophora americana*	At 25 °C after 15 days slightly raised and radially folded colony, central area leathery, tufts of aerial hyphae. Center grayish-brown, reverse grayish-black. Primary phialides in young cultures hyaline to light brown, thin-walled with hyaline cup-shaped collarette. Secondary phialides with characteristic saucer-shaped, broadly flaring collarette. Phialoconidia from primary phialides hyaline, ellipsoidal, occasionally curved. Secondary phialoconidia light-brown, thick-walled, forming ball-like clusters at the apex. Urease-positive	Saprophyte of decaying wood (causes blueing of wood pulp)	Subcutaneous phaeohyphomycosis[13,14]
248	**Phialophora verrucosa** MEDLAR *Cadophora americana* *Fonsecaea pedrosoi* var. *phialophorica*	Similar to *Fonsecaea pedrosoi* except that cultures exhibit bottle-shaped *Phialophora* type sporulation (see Fig. 11, page 97)	Saprophyte of decaying wood, mainly in Central and South America, also Algeria. Occasional human infection through injury	Chromoblastomycosis (see *Fonsecaea pedrosoi, No. 243*)
249	**Pityrosporum ovale** BIZZOZERO *Pityrosporum malassezii* *Pityrosporum orbiculare* Saprophytic stage of *Malassezia furfur*	On suitable agar media with a superficial thin layer of olive oil smooth or rough colonies with irregular periphery develop at 25 °C within 3–5 days; fruity odor. Consist of small ellipsoidal or flask-like cells with a typical collarette. The organism has an absolute requirement for medium- and long-chain fatty acids for growth. For tissue phase, see *No. 249a*	Part of normal skin flora in 90% of adults[15]. Parasitic; worldwide distribution. Common in the tropics (South America)	A cause of tinea versicolor (pityriasis)[16,17]. See also introduction, page 73. Systemic infections associated with intravenous catheters (e.g. parenteral nutrition)[15,18,19]
249a	**Malassezia furfur** (ROBIN) BAILON *Microsporon furfur*	Infected skin scales are yellow to brownish in color and contain many hyphae and clumps of globular spores	See *Pityrosporum ovale*	See *Pityrosporum ovale*
250	**Rhinocladiella** sp. nov. related to *Rhinocladiella aquaspersa* (BORELLI) SCHELL et al. 1983	Strains grow better at 37 °C than at 26 °C. Relatively large, ovoid conidia, 2.5–5 µm by 6–8 µm, with a distinct protruding hilum. The conidiophores are poorly differentiated from the mycelium, tending to unilateral sympodial growth	Saprophyte	Isolated in 4 cases of brain abscess in countries of the Middle East[24]
250a	**Tetraploa aristata** BERKELEY and BROOME 1950	Colonies on potato glucose agar after 2 weeks 22–25 mm in diameter; at 37 °C minimal growth. Septate branched mycelium, light to dark brown. On rough-walled conidiophores tetra-columnate dark conidia, 3–4 cells in each column, 2–4 dematiaceous appendages 10–60 µm in length	Saprophyte on leaves and stems of plants. Widely distributed	Isolated from phaeohyphomycotic cyst, also cause of keratomycosis[20] *Remark*. Surgical treatment of cyst

No.	**Fungus** *Synonyms*	Characteristics	Habitat Host Transmission	Associated disease
251	**Wangiella dermatitidis** (KANO) MCGINNIS 1977 *Fonsecaea dermatitidis* *Hormodendrum dermatitidis* *Phialophora dermatitidis* *Exophiala dermatitidis*	Initially the colony is moist, yeast-like and brownish-black. After 3–4 weeks a grayish mycelium starts to cover the surface. In the yeast-like phase the thallus consists of round to oval budding cells. In the mycelial phase the type of sporulation is not typical, usually aggregations at the site of production; also *Phialophora*-type seen. Maximum temperature 50 °C. Does not assimilate nitrate	Plants, wasp nests. Found in East Asia, Japan, Guatemala	Localized infection of skin and subcutis. Systemic disease reported[6,21]. Patients with cystic fibrosis are at risk[22]
252	**Wangiella mansonii** (CASTELLANI) MCGINNIS *Cladosporium mansonii* *Torula mansoni* Synanamorph: *Phaeococcomyces*	Greenish-black cultures with short dark hyphae. Sporangia have long chains of conidia springing from bottle-shaped annellides. Affected skin epithelium contains unbranched mycelium with round spores	Primarily saprophytic. Found in East Asia	Tinea nigra, a form of dermatomycosis with characteristic dark pigmentation[17]

[1] SALKIN et al., *J. clin. Microbiol.*, **23**, 828 (1986).
[2] ADAM et al., *Medicine (Baltimore)*, **65**, 203 (1986).
[3] MCGINNIS et al., *J. clin. Microbiol.*, **24**, 250 (1986).
[4] SEAWORTH et al., *Amer. J. clin. Path.*, **79**, 747 (1983).
[5] MCGINNIS et al., *J. Amer. Acad. Derm.*, **8**, 1 (1983).
[6] RIPPON, J. W., *Medical Mycology*, 3rd ed., Saunders, Philadelphia, 1988, page 276.
[7] MCGINNIS, M. R., in WARREN and MAHMOUD (Eds.), *Tropical and Geographic Medicine*, 2nd ed., McGraw-Hill, New York, 1990, page 954.
[8] SUGHAYER et al., *Rev. infect. Dis.*, **13**, 379 (1991).
[9] PADHYE et al., *Amer. J. trop. Med. Hyg.*, N.S. **32**, 799 (1983).
[10] KANE et al., *Mycoses*, **33**, 37 (1990).
[11] LAVARDE et al., *Bull. Soc. franç. Mycol. méd.*, **11**, 273 (1982).
[12] MEYERS et al., *Amer. J. clin. Path.*, **64**, 549 (1975).
[13] CORRADO et al., *Sabouraudia*, **18**, 97 (1980).
[14] TORSTRICK et al., *J. Bone Joint Surg.*, **61A**, 772 (1979).
[15] POWELL et al., *J. Pediat.*, **111**, 217 (1987).
[16] BENNETT, J. E., in MANDELL et al. (Eds.), *Principles and Practice of Infectious Diseases*, 3rd ed., Churchill Livingstone, New York, 1990, page 2031.
[17] RIPPON, J. W., *Medical Mycology*, 3rd ed., Saunders, Philadelphia, 1988, page 154.
[18] GARCIA et al., *Amer. J. Med.*, **83**, 790 (1987).
[19] ASCHNER et al., *Pediatrics*, **80**, 535 (1987).
[20] MARKHAM et al., *J. med. vet. Mycol.*, **28**, 147 (1990).
[21] VARTIAN et al., *Amer. J. Med.*, **78**, 703 (1985).
[22] HAASE et al., *Lancet*, **336**, 188 (1990).
[23] KREMPL-LAMPRECHT et al., *Mykosen*, **30**, 454 (1987).
[24] CAMPBELL, C. K., *Proc. XI Congress of ISHAM*, Montreal, 1991, Poster Session, PS2.68.
[25] WRIGHT et al., *Mycoses*, **33**, 477 (1990).
[26] SIGLER and CONGLY, *J. med. vet. Mycol.*, **28**, 405 (1990).

No.	Fungus *Synonyms*	Characteristics	Habitat Host Transmission	Associated disease
	Fungi causing secondary or opportunistic mycoses (for references, see page 86)			
253	**Alternaria tenuis** NEES 1817	Rapid growth of colonies forming a velvety black or dark green surface and black reverse, on short conidiophores club-shaped multicellular conidia in chains, arising as porospores	Saprophyte in soil or parasite on leaves and fruits. Worldwide distribution	Opportunistic pathogen, particularly after therapy, mainly involving the skin with formation of pustules; nodules, also erythematous, squamous lesions
254	Other *Alternaria* species of clinical importance[1-3]: **Alternaria alternata** **Alternaria chartarum** **Alternaria dianthicola** **Alternaria infectoria** **Alternaria brassicola** **Alternaria stemphylloides**			
255	**Aphanoascus** spp. CANO and GUARRO (12 species described)	Polymorphous colonies with smooth or folded thallus, covered with powdery or flaky aerial mycelium, usually white-greyish to creamy, reverse side yellow	Widely distributed in nature	Occasional cause of skin infection and possibly an internal opportunistic pathogen[4]
255a	Related to *Aphanoascus*: **Malbranchea** **Chrysosporium**			Possible agents of superficial mycosis in man
256	**Aspergillus fumigatus** FRESENIUS 1850	Rapid growth of colonies at 37 °C and 45 °C, white at first but after a few days acquiring a powdery, dark blue to green surface which later assumes a brownish or smoky-gray tinge. Conidiophores have a club-like pyriform terminal swelling (vesiculum) from which nearly parallel single rows of phialides bud; these carry chains of spherical conidia (see Fig. 13, page 98)	Ubiquitous; widespread on foodstuffs (corn, onions), dust, hay, wool and cotton wool. Infection by inhalation of spores. Not transmissible from man to man. Acute infections in man apparently require massive exposure (harvesting) or an existing pathological condition such as leukemia, BOECK's sarcoid, long-term corticosteroid therapy at high dosage, immunosuppressive therapy, carcinoma, agranulocytosis, tuberculosis; sometimes seen as occupational disease in threshers, cotton pickers and sorters, etc. Patients with asthma and cystic fibrosis are at special risk[5], whereas aspergillosis is unusual in patients with AIDS[6]	Commonest cause of aspergillosis[7-10]: pneumomycosis, bronchomycosis (filaments of fungus and spores demonstrated in sputum and bronchial secretion), otomycosis, eczema due to fungal toxin. Aspergillosis of the lungs may take an acute purulent, pneumonic form, a chronic granulomatous form with giant cells and cavities containing a fungus ball (aspergilloma), or a mycetoma form. Systemic infections may take a septic course. Corneal ulcers, endocarditis and brain aspergilloma also occur. Also associated with extrinsic allergic alveolitis (farmer's lung, bird fancier's lung) *Remarks.* Surgical treatment in localized infections. Intravenous amphotericin B is recommended for invasive aspergillosis[11]; itraconazole[6] or fluconazole may be an advance in therapy[12]
257	**Aspergillus flavus** LINK 1809	Rapid growth of yellowish-green colonies at 25–37 °C with close-textured basal mycelium. Conidiophores are thick-walled, have a round terminal swelling from which radial phialides bud; these carry chains of ellipsoidal to globose conidia. Forms hepatotoxic aflatoxins in some foodstuffs (groundnuts)[13,14]	Worldwide distribution. Mainly on decaying organic matter	Aspergillosis[7]; occasional cause of mycotic granuloma of nasal sinuses and lower respiratory tract. Brain aspergilloma has been reported[15] *Remark.* For treatment, see *A. fumigatus* (*No. 256*)
258	**Aspergillus nidulans** (EIDAM) WINT 1884	Rapid growth of colonies at 24 °C, usually none at 37 °C; white at first, later brownish-green. Phialides in double rows, perithecia with red ascospores, envelope cells	Worldwide distribution. Mainly on decaying organic matter; usually a saprophytic contaminant	Only exceptionally affects man (lungs, bones, abdomen); also subcutaneous infections[16]
259	**Aspergillus niger** VAN TIEGHEM 1867	Rapid growth of colonies, at first white, later yellow with small black sporing heads; after 4 to 5 days completely black powdery surface. Phialides in double rows	Worldwide distribution. Mainly on decaying organic matter; usually saprophytic contaminant	Aspergillosis[7]; otomycosis, rarely pulmonary infiltration

No.	**Fungus** *Synonyms*	Characteristics	Habitat Host Transmission	Associated disease
260	**Aspergillus terreus** THOM 1918	Rapid growth of cinnamon- to wood-brown colonies at 25 °C with floccose to velvety texture. Conidophores have a hemispherical terminal swelling. Phialides in double rows, ovoid conidia	Worldwide distribution. Mainly in soil and on decaying organic matter. Rarely pathogenic in man	Aspergillosis, particularly meningitis and pulmonary infiltration[17]
261	**Chaetomium globosum** KUNZE ex FRIES 1829 **Chaetomium atrobrunneum** AMES 1949 (over 100 *Chaetomium* species are recognized)	Rapid growth of white to yellowish aerial mycelium with broadly ovoid or ellipsoidal, scattered superficial perithecia, 250–300 μm by 200–250 μm, olivaceous to dark brown with slender, flexuous hairs. Asci oblong-clavate, 8-spored, faintly apiculate dark ascospores, broadly ovoid	Saprophyte in soil. Worldwide distribution	Few cases of onychomycosis[18]; in immunocompromised persons, invasion of the thoracic cavity and the brain[19-22]; systemic infection in a case with acute lymphoblastic leukemia reported[22]
262	**Drechslera hawaiiensis** (BUGNICOURT 1955) SUBRAMANIAM and JAIN 1966 *Bipolaris hawaiiensis*	Cottony, dark moldy growth, velvety, blackish brown, septate mycelium. Cylindric, multiseptate macroconidia with dark pigmented walls. Porospores produced from a sympodially extending conidiophore (resembling those of *Helminthosporium*)	Saprophyte in soil. Isolated from plants in India, New Guinea, Australia	Rarely pathogenic in immunocompromised persons; invades the brain[23]
263	Other *Drechslera* species of clinical importance: **Drechslera rostrata** **Drechslera longirostrata** (see also *No. 235*)			Osteolytic infection of the foot reported[24] Endocarditis, spondylitis reported[25]
264	**Fusarium oxysporum** SCHLECHT 1924	Rapid growth of whitish aerial mycelium. Reverse side of floccose colonies reveal shades of purple. Abundant microconidia with short chains and false heads. Long, sickle-celled, thin-walled macroconidia. May produce toxin[36]	Saprophyte in soil, pathogen of plants. Worldwide distribution	Localized infections of skin, nails and cornea after trauma or glaucoma; subcutaneous granulomas in immunocompromised persons (especially in burn patients); rarely disseminated[26, 27]. Food-borne intoxication associated with bronchial asthma. Toxin effective against pasture-grazing animals[36]
265	Other *Fusarium* species of clinical importance: **Fusarium solani** **Fusarium moniliforme** **Fusarium napiforme**[28]	Similar to *F. oxysporum*	As for *F. oxysporum*	As for *F. oxysporum* Implicated in the etiology of esophageal cancer in man in southern Africa and China in connection with the mycotoxin fusarin C[76]
266	**Myceliophthora thermophila** (APINIS) VAN OORSCHOOT	At 30 °C white, woolly colonies with a well defined margin (6 to 7 cm in 7 days) – later pale-brown. Blastoconidia terminally or laterally on hyphae, occasionally secondary blastoconidia may be born. Conidia ovoid to pyriform (4.5–11.0 μm by 3.0 to 45 μm), hyaline, thick-walled, rough or smooth surface	Saprophyte in soil	Systemic infection in a case with acute myeloblastic leukemia reported[29]
267	**Paecilomyces javanicus** (FRIEDRICHS and BALLY) BROWN and SMITH 1957 *Spicaria javanica*	Rapid growth of colonies with no pigment or odor on SABOURAUD glucose agar at 24–30 °C, poor growth at 37 °C. Verticillate branches with cylindric to fusiform phialides, smooth-walled conidia in long, almost straight chains	Saprophyte in soil. Widely distributed. Found in pupae of butterflies in Java	A case of prosthetic valve endocarditis reported[30]

No.	**Fungus** *Synonyms*	Characteristics	Habitat Host Transmission	Associated disease
268	**Paecilomyces lilacinus** (THOM) SAMSON 1974	Velvety growth of colonies with vinaceous color. Tapering phialides in verticillate arrangement and tangled chains of ovoid conidia	Saprophyte in soil and decaying matter	Rare cause of cutaneous infection in immunocompromised persons, also found in ocular, lung and sinus infections[31] and in a renal transplant[37]. Hyalohyphomycosis
269	**Paecilomyces variotii** BAINIER 1907	Flat olive-green colonies, initially white, surface felty and powdery; smooth-walled chains of ovoid, unicellular microconidia on flask-like phialides	As for *P. lilacinus*	Occasional cause of prosthetic valve endocarditis, pyelonephritis and sinusitis
270	**Paecilomyces marquandii** (MASSEE) HUGHES 1951	Closely related to *P. lilacinus* (*No. 268*)	As for *P. lilacinus*	Rare cause of cellulitis and hyalohyphomycosis
271	**Penicillium marneffei** SEGRETAIN, CAPPONI and SUREAU 1959	Growth more rapid at 27–30 °C than at 22 °C; cultures are velvety, white, later grayish-green and finally pink, with characteristic brush-like conidiophores. At 37 °C, colonies resemble *Geotrichum*, are slow-growing and form arthrospores. In affected tissues there is intracellular multiplication in reticulum cells (as in histoplasmosis and leishmaniasis)	Saprophyte. Widely distributed. Occasionally pathogenic in man, also in bamboo rats, mice and domestic animals	Generalized reticulosis (penicilliosis) in rodents. Resembles *Histoplasma capsulatum* (*No. 229*) (with which it should not be confused) in respect of growth in liver cells of bamboo rats; in man causes subcutaneous mycosis with local involvement of glands. Opportunistic pathogen in immunocompromised persons and AIDS[32]
272	**Scopulariopsis brevicaulis** (SACCARDO) BAINIER 1907	Rapid growth at 20 °C, young colonies white to cinnamon-brown. Unicellular, thick-walled, round and ovoid conidia (2 to 3.5 µm wide) with a rough surface in chains	Saprophyte in soil. Widely distributed	Occasional cause of onychomycosis, rarely invasive agent in immunocompromised persons[33]
273	**Scopulariopsis brumptii** SALVANET-DURST 1935	Gray olivaceous colonies, reverse side olivaceous-black, 25 mm at 28 °C. Annellides singly or in groups on short stipes. Dark brown, obovoid conidia in chains	Saprophyte in soil	Possible cause of mycetoma, onychomycosis[34]
274	**Trichoderma viride** related to **Trichoderma koningi** OUDEMANS	Rapid growth of white, then turning to light-green colonies (32–37 °C). Producing one-celled smooth conidia, ball-like fruiting heads on nonseptate, sometimes branched conidiophores (up to 25 µm in length)	Saprophyte in soil and cellulose debris, contaminant of laboratory media	Peritonitis associated with peritoneal dialysis reported[35]

1 DE BIEVRE, C., *J. Mycol. méd.*, **1**, 50 (1991).
2 BADILLET, G., *J. Mycol. méd.*, **1**, 59 (1991).
3 KASPERLIK-ZALUSKA and BIELUNSKA, *Lancet*, **337**, 53 (1991).
4 CANO et al., *Mycoses*, **33**, 41 (1990).
5 SEATON and ROBERTSON, *Lancet*, **1**, 893 (1989).
6 DENNING et al., *New Engl. J. Med.*, **324**, 654 (1991).
7 LEVITZ et al., *Advanc. intern. Med.*, **30**, 153 (1984).
8 BENNETT, J. E., in MANDELL et al. (Eds.), *Principles and Practice of Infectious Diseases*, 3rd ed., Churchill Livingstone, New York, 1990, page 1958.
9 RIPPON, J. W., *Medical Mycology*, 3rd ed., Saunders, Philadelphia, 1988, page 618.
10 YOUNG, L. S., in WARREN and MAHMOUD (Eds.), *Tropical and Geographic Medicine*, 2nd ed., McGraw-Hill, New York, 1990, page 933.
11 *Med. Lett. Drug. Ther.*, **34**, No. 864, 14 (1992).
12 QUIST and TAURIS, *Scand. J. infect. Dis.*, **22**, 749 (1990).
13 AUSTWICK, P. K., *Brit. med. Bull.*, **31**, 222 (1975).
14 GARNER, R. C., *Brit. med. Bull.*, **36**, 47 (1980).
15 PARTRIDGE and CHIN, *Postgrad. med. J.*, **57**, 439 (1981); STAIB, F., *'Hautnah', Mycologie aus der Praxis*, **3**, 116 (1991).
16 JOSHI et al., *J. trop. Med. Hyg.*, **88**, 41 (1985).
17 HARA et al., *Mayo Clin. Proc.*, **64**, 770 (1989).
18 RIPPON, J. W., *Medical Mycology*, 3rd ed., Saunders, Philadelphia, 1988, page 169.
19 HOPPIN et al., *Cancer*, **52**, 555 (1983).
20 ANANDI et al., *J. clin. Microbiol.*, **27**, 2226 (1989).
21 BARALE et al., *Bull. Soc. franç. Mycol. méd.*, **19**, 43 (1990).
22 RINALDI et al., *Proc. XI Congress of ISHAM*, Montreal, 1991, Poster Session, PS2.69.
23 FUSTE et al., *Sabouraudia*, **11**, 59 (1973).
24 AJELLO et al., *Mycologia*, **72**, 1094 (1980).
25 ZIZA et al., *Ann. Méd. interne*, **136**, 393 (1985).
26 ANAISSIE et al., *Medicine (Baltimore)*, **67**, 77 (1988).
27 NUOVO et al., *Amer. J. clin. Path.*, **90**, 738 (1988).
28 MELCHER, G. P., *Mycology Observer*, **10**, 7 (1990).
29 MCGOUGH et al., *Proc. XI Congress of ISHAM*, Montreal, 1991, Poster Session, PS2.99.
30 ALLEVATO et al., *Amer. J. clin. Path.*, **82**, 247 (1984).
31 DIVEN, D. G., *Mycology Observer*, **10**, 3 (1990).
32 HULSHOF et al., *Europ. J. clin. Microbiol. infect. Dis.*, **9**, 370 (1990).
33 NEGLIA et al., *Amer. J. Med.*, **83**, 1163 (1987).
34 NAIDU et al., *Mycopathologia (Den Haag)*, **113**, 159 (1991).
35 LOEPPKY et al., *Sth. med. J. (Bgham, Ala.)*, **76**, 798 (1983).
36 FARBER and SCOTT, in CHELKOWSKI, J. (Ed.), *Fusarium Mycotoxins, Taxonomy and Pathogenicity*, Elsevier, Amsterdam, 1989, page 41.
37 CASTRO et al., *J. med. vet. Mycol.*, **28**, 15 (1990).

No.	**Fungus** *Synonyms*	Characteristics	Habitat Host Transmission	Associated disease
	Yeasts causing mycoses (for references, see next page)			
275	**Candida albicans** (ROBIN) BERKHOUT 1923 *Monilia albicans* *Oidium albicans*	Cream-colored, smooth colonies on SABOURAUD glucose agar at 25 °C. In glucose broth at 25 °C, globose (5–7 µm) or elongate (4–6 µm by 6–10 µm) budding cells (see Fig. 5, page 97). Mycelium and pseudomycelium on cornmeal agar. Masses of blastospores at internodes. Terminal chlamydospores with thick walls formed by most strains. Urease-negative. Produces adhesin	Worldwide distribution; in man and certain animals, common saprophyte of skin and mucosa of the mouth and throat, vagina and intestine. Facultatively pathogenic in certain conditions (nutritional disorders, disturbance of equilibrium of microflora due to antibiotics, diabetes, carcinoma, corticosteroid or immunosuppressive therapy, therapy with oral contraceptives, drug addiction, use of intravenous or bladder catheters, acquired immunodeficiency syndrome [AIDS], etc.[6])	Candidosis (candidiasis, not recommended: moniliasis)[1–4]: (a) candidosis of mucous membranes (thrush), marked by massive growth of the fungus as grayish-white membranes and particularly common in infants; (b) candidosis of the skin (intertrigo, paronychia, general forms); (c) generalized candidosis with involvement of respiratory passages and gastrointestinal tract. Endocarditis involving prosthetic devices. Invasive candidosis with circulating enolase – infection of visceral organs by hematogenous spread – increasingly reported in the last decades, especially in neutropenic patients[5], but also in neonates[21]
276	Other *Candida* species: see text on next page			Pathogenicity in man usually low
277	**Cryptococcus neoformans** (SAN FELICE) VUILLEMIN 1901 *Cryptococcus bacillisporus* *Torula histolitica* *Torulopsis neoformans* Teleomorph: *Filobasidiella neoformans* KWON-CHUNG 1975	Var. *neoformans.* Rapid growth of mucoid colonies at 25 °C and 37 °C. On SABOURAUD glucose agar at 1 month, cream-colored or pinky colonies. Globose or ovoid single budding yeast-like cells (2.5–8 µm) surrounded by a very thick capsule (see Fig. 6, page 97). Encapsulation may vary with strain and medium used. Very rare strains produce mycelium. No pseudomycelium on cornmeal agar	Worldwide distribution. Soil saprophyte, particularly where enriched with bird excreta (pigeons). Human infection mostly via the respiratory tract, possibly also via the skin, food and dirt; also infects animals (e.g. udders). Preexisting pathological conditions (HODGKINS's disease, leukemia, corticosteroid or immunosuppressive therapy, acquired immunodeficiency syndrome [AIDS][6,24], etc. favor infection)	Cryptococcosis (torulosis, European blastomycosis, BUSSE–BUSCHKE's disease)[7,8]. Affects the skin (ulcerating tumors with gelatinous content), marked predilection for the central nervous system (cryptococcal meningitis, brain abscess)[9], also occasionally eyes, mouth, lungs, bone marrow, kidneys and joints *Remark.* Treatment as for candidosis (see next page)
		Var. *gattii.* Growth similar to var. *neoformans.* Temperature-sensitive, larger ovoid cells (3–7 µm by 3.5–8.0 µm)	Natural habitat: *Eucalyptus camaldulensis*	Cryptococcosis. High incidence in Australian aborigines[10]
278	**Geotrichum candidum** LINK ex PERSOON 1822 *Oidium pulmoneum* Teleomorph: *Endomyces geotrichum* BUTLER and PETERSEN 1972	Fast growth of glabrous, flat, white to cream-colored colonies on SABOURAUD glucose agar at 25 °C. At 37 °C, growth is very slow. Hyaline, branched mycelium, hyphae fragmenting into rectangular arthroconidia (see Fig. 9, page 97). Urease-negative *Remark. Geotrichum* species are molds resembling yeast colonies on initial isolation; they do not produce blastospores	Common saprophyte on foodstuffs (e.g. milk, cheese, eggs)	Geotrichosis[11]. Secondary pathogen in patients with tuberculosis, chronic bronchitis. Also in infections of the skin and gastrointestinal tract *Remark.* Sensitive to amphotericin B[12]
279	**Geotrichum capitatum** WEIJMAN 1979 *Trichosporon capitatum* Considered as a separate genus: *Blastoschizomyces capitatus* (comb. nova)[22] SALKIN et al. 1985	Fast growth of white, dry colonies at 37 °C. Abundant hyphae with arthroconidia and geniculate sympodial conidia. Urease-negative. No blastospores (see *No. 278*)	Common saprophyte, found on cactus roots	Occasional secondary pathogen in patients with severe underlying disease[13,14,22]. Localization in the skin and systemic complications[23]
280	**Hansenula anomala** (HANSEN) SYDOW and SYDOW 1891	Rapid growth on high-sugar media. Typical hat-shaped, hemispheroidal or Saturn-shaped ascospores. Urease-negative	Common saprophyte	Septicemia in immunocompromised persons (catheter-related)[15]
280a	**Hansenula fabianii** WICKERHAM 1965	Similar to *H. anomala*		Septicemia in an immunocompromised person reported[16]

No.	**Fungus** *Synonyms*	Characteristics	Habitat Host Transmission	Associated disease
281	**Saccharomyces cerevisiae** HANSEN 1883	Ovoid, budding cells. No mycelium. On cornmeal agar, rudimentary pseudomycelium and ascospores. Urease-negative	Common saprophyte. Cultivated for thousands of years (brewer's yeast, baker's yeast). Part of normal mucosal flora in man	Implicated in pulmonary disease, especially in brewers[17]. Invasive infection by hematogenous spread reported[18]
282	**Torulopsis glabrata** (ANDERSON) LODDER and DE VRIES 1938 *Candida glabrata* *Cryptococcus glabratus*	Glabrous, soft, cream-colored colonies on SABOURAUD glucose agar at 25°C. Ovoid, budding cells, 2.5–4.5 µm by 4–6 µm. Contrary to *Candida* spp., no formation of pseudomycelium	Most common yeast on body surface[1]	Low pathogenicity in man. Immunocompromised persons are at risk
282a	Other *Torulopsis* species of clinical importance: **Torulopsis famata** **Torulopsis inconspicua**			Low pathogenicity in man
283	**Trichosporon beigelii** (KUCHENMEISTER and RABENHORST) VUILLEMIN 1902 *Trichosporum beigelii* *Geotrichum beigelii*	Grayish-white colonies of creamy consistency with wrinkled surface. Forms true hyphae, arthrospores and blastospores	Worldwide distribution. Part of normal human flora (cultures of feces, skin and urine). Sexual transmission discussed[19]	White piedra (white hair-nodule disease), affecting the hair shafts of the scalp, body or pubic hair[19]. Endocarditis involving prosthetic devices[20]. Invasive infections (trichosporonosis) mainly in immunocompromised persons[13]

[1] RIPPON, J. W., *Medical Mycology*, 3rd ed., Saunders, Philadelphia, 1988, page 532.
[2] EDWARDS, J. E., in MANDELL et al. (Eds.), *Principles and Practice of Infectious Diseases*, 3rd ed., Churchill Livingstone, New York, 1990, page 1943.
[3] ODDS, F. C., *Candida and Candidosis*, 2nd ed., Baillière Tindall, Philadelphia, 1988.
[4] TÜMBAY et al. (Eds.), *Candida and Candidamycosis*, FEMS Sympos. No. 50, Plenum Press, New York, 1991.
[5] LEW, M. A., *Ann. Rev. Med.*, **40**, 87 (1989).
[6] DIAMOND, R. D., *Rev. Infect. Dis.*, **13**, 480 (1991).
[7] RIPPON, J. W., *Medical Mycology*, 3rd ed., Saunders, Philadelphia, 1988, page 582.
[8] DIAMOND, R. D., in MANDELL et al. (Eds.), *Principles and Practice of Infectious Diseases*, 3rd ed., Churchill Livingstone, New York, 1990, page 1980.
[9] YU et al., *Quart. J. Med.*, N.S. **66**, 87 (1988).
[10] ELLIS and PFEIFER, *Lancet*, **336**, 923 (1990).
[11] RIPPON, J. W., *Medical Mycology*, 3rd ed., Saunders, Philadelphia, 1988, page 715.
[12] BUCHTA and OTČEVÁŠEK, *Mycoses*, **31**, 363 (1988).
[13] WALSH, T. J., *Medicine (Baltimore)*, **65**, 268 (1986).
[14] MAHUL et al., *Mycoses*, **32**, 573 (1989).
[15] KLEIN et al., *Arch. intern. Med.*, **148**, 1210 (1988); MUÑOZ et al., *Arch. intern. Med.*, **149**, 709 (1989).
[16] DOOLEY et al., *J. infect. Dis.*, **161**, 1040 (1990).
[17] RIPPON, J. W., *Medical Mycology*, 3rd ed., Saunders, Philadelphia, 1988, page 615.
[18] AUCOTT et al., *Rev. infect. Dis.*, **12**, 406 (1990); NIELSEN et al., *Scand. J. Infect.*, **22**, 581 (1990).
[19] BENNETT, J. E., in MANDELL et al. (Eds.), *Principles and Practice of Infectious Diseases*, 3rd ed., Churchill Livingstone, New York, 1990, page 2031.
[20] KEAY et al., *Rev. infect. Dis.*, **13**, 383 (1991).
[21] BUTLER and BAKER, *Pediat. Clin. N. Amer.*, **35**, 543 (1988).
[22] MARTINO et al., *Rev. infect. Dis.*, **12**, 570 (1990).
[23] ANAISSIE and BODEY, *Europ. J. clin. Microbiol. infect. Dis.*, **10**, 711 (1991).
[24] PETTOELLO-MANTOVANI et al., *Lancet*, **339**, 21 (1992).

Candidosis

The genus *Candida* comprises about 150 asporogenous yeast species[1]. The distinguishing feature of the *Candida* species is their ability to form pseudohyphae, the only exception being *C. glabrata*. *C. albicans*, *C. tropicalis* and *C. glabrata* are the most frequently isolated (more than 80%) from medical specimens[1]. Some other *Candida* species of medical importance are listed in Table 1 – *C. albicans* possessing all of the known virulence determinants[2]. *C. stellatoidea* is differentiated from *C. albicans* as a variant by its inability to utilize sucrose[3]. The spectrum of diseases associated with the major *Candida* species is given in Table 2.

Remarks. Topical treatment – e.g. vulvovaginitis[4] – involves a wide variety of antifungal agents, such as polyene antibiotics (e.g. nystatin) or imidazole compounds (e.g. clotrimazole, miconazole). For treatment of systemic infections, amphotericin B, eventually combined with flucytosine[5], but imidazoles (e.g. ketoconazole) or triazoles (e.g. fluconazole, itraconazole) are said to be effective[6,7]. See also the discussion on page 73.

Table 1 *Virulence determinants of* Candida *spp.**[2]

	Formation of true hyphae	Resistance to phagocytosis	Adherence to host surface	Secretion of proteinase
C. albicans	++	++	++	++
C. tropicalis	±	++	+	+
C. parapsilosis	–	+	+	±
C. pseudotropicalis	–	+	±	–
C. krusei	–	+	–	–
C. guilliermondii	–	–	–	–
C. glabrata◊	–	–	–	–

++ High ability. ± Little ability.
\+ Ability. – Very weak or no ability.

* The species are listed in their rank order of pathogenicity.
◊ For more information, see *Torulopsis glabrata* (*No. 282*).

Table 2 Candida *spp. associated with human disease and the sites involved in candidosis*[2]

	Mouth	Vagina	Endocardium	Nervous system	Bone and joints	Multiorgan involvement
C. albicans	+++	+++	+++	+++	+++	+++
*C. glabrata**	+	+	+	+	–	++
C. guilliermondii	+	+	++	–	+++	++
C. krusei	+	+	++	–	+	+
C. parapsilosis	+	+	+++	+	+	++
C. tropicalis	+	+	++	+++	+++	+++

+++ Major cause. + Rare cause.
++ Cause. – No cases known.

* For more information, see *Torulopsis glabrata* (*No. 282*).

References

[1] SHEPHERD, M.G., in SAMARANAYAKE and MACFARLANE (Eds.), *Oral Candidosis*, Wright, London, 1990, page 10.
[2] ODDS, F.C., *CRC Crit. Rev. Microbiol.*, **15**, 1 (1987).
[3] KWON-CHUNG et al., *Infect. Immun.*, **57**, 527 (1989).
[4] WHO Study Group on Management of Patients with Sexually Transmitted Diseases, *Wld Hlth Org. techn. Rep. Ser.*, No. 810 (1991).
[5] *Med. Lett. Drug. Ther.*, **34**, No. 864, 14 (1992).
[6] VISCOLI et al., *Antimicrob. Agents and Chemother.*, **35**, 365 (1991).
[7] SHARKEY et al., *Antimicrob. Agents and Chemother.*, **35**, 707 (1991).

Dermatophytosis

The dermatophytes are commonly identified by assignment to the anamorph genera *Epidermophyton*, *Microsporum* and *Trichophyton*[1-4]. The known sexual stages of species of the genera *Microsporum* and *Trichophyton* belong to the teleomorph genus *Arthroderma*[5]. A sexual stage of *Epidermophyton* species has not yet been discovered.

Although about 40 species of dermatophytes are recognized, most of them are rarely implicated in disease (e.g. in the USA, 7 species account for about 95% of clinical infections[3]). The dermatophytes are equipped with enzymes which enable them to grow on cornified skin, hair and nails. Even if tissue invasion is possible, the dermatophytes are almost always limited to non-living tissue.

Epidemiology and host response are predicted from categorization of dermatophytes by their primary reservoir[1,3]. Anthropophilic dermatophytes are generally acquired from man and do not usually induce marked inflammation in infected individuals. Zoophilic dermatophytes are acquired largely from animals and cause marked inflammatory reactions in infected man. Soil is the predominant reservoir for geophilic dermatophytes that cause an inflammatory response in infected hosts.

Dermatophytosis usually responds to oral treatment with griseofulvin. This drug acts not by killing the fungus but by inhibiting its further growth. Griseofulvin accumulates preferentially in the cells of the stratum corneum of the skin, hair and nails and thus inhibits the growth and spread of the fungus. The affected tissue is eventually cast off and replaced by fungus-free tissue. Treatment with griseofulvin should be accompanied by the classical local measure on the principle of 'moist-on-moist' and 'dry-on-dry', as well as by treatment of the bacterial mixed or superinfection; other measures include corticosteroids locally as required, removal of loose skin, opening of blisters, disinfectant baths, and reduction of excessive sweating by local application of salicylic acid and powders.

An alternative oral treatment is offered in the form of imidazoles (e.g. ketoconazole)[2]; like griseofulvin they deposit in the stratum corneum.

References

[1] RIPPON, J.W., *Medical Mycology*, 3rd ed., Saunders, Philadelphia, 1988, page 169.
[2] HAY, R.J., in MANDELL et al. (Eds.), *Principles and Practice of Infectious Diseases*, 3rd ed., Churchill Livingstone, New York, 1990, page 2017.
[3] SALATA, R.A., in WARREN and MAHMOUD (Eds.), *Tropical and Geographical Medicine*, 2nd ed., McGraw-Hill, New York, 1990, page 993.
[4] DIXON and POLAK-WYSS, *Mycoses*, **34**, 1 (1991).
[5] WEITZMAN et al., *Mycotaxon*, **25**, 505 (1986).

No.	**Fungus** *Synonyms*	Characteristics	Habitat Host Transmission	Associated disease
	Dermatophytes causing infections of the skin (for references, see page 95; see also text on page 89)			
284	**Epidermophyton floccosum** (HARZ) LANGERON and MILOCHEVITCH 1930 *Epidermophyton cruris* *Epidermophyton inguinale*	Slow growth of beige-colored or green-yellowish colonies, later becoming white, with cotton-like appearance and typical rounded, partly ovoid, 2- to 4-chambered macroconidia (see Fig. 19, page 98), numerous chlamydospores and, rarely, helical hyphae. No microconidia	Anthropophilic. Worldwide distribution in humid, warm climates. Infection in public baths, sportsgrounds, sauna establishments, etc., and through sexual intercourse	Main cause of tinea cruris and tinea pedis. Affects mainly the skin of the inguinal and perianal regions
285	**Microsporum amazonicum** MORAES, BORELLI and FEO 1967 Teleomorph: *Arthroderma borellii* PADHYE et al. 1986	Rapid growth of colonies at 23 to 28 °C, with woolly, later powdery surface. Unicellular microconidia. Numerous spindle-shaped, 1- to 3-chambered macroconidia with thick walls and protuberances	Infection among wild rats in the Amazonas region of Brazil reported[1]	Clinical importance not established
286	**Microsporum audouinii** GRUBY 1843 *Sabouraudites audouini* *Trichophyton decalvans*	Slow growth of white, downy colonies not forming a large mycelium. Surface light-beige to brownish, reverse side light- to dark-orange. Scanty growth on rice grains. Mycelium usually sterile, with occasional sessile microconidia and large, irregularly shaped, often bizarre fusiform macroconidia with thick, either smooth or spiky walls. Numerous chlamydospores. Seen in infected material as small, round, tightly packed spores	Anthropophilic. Worldwide distribution. Highly contagious, especially in children. Indirect transmission via communal combs, headgear, etc. Infections occasionally epidemic	Tinea capitis. Hair shafts contain branched hyphae. The fungal cuffs around affected hairs (ectothrix type) fluoresce under WOOD's light (see Fig. 33, page 99). Hair is rarely affected after puberty, only the skin below. Infected hairs break off about 1 mm above capillitium
286a	**Microsporum langeronii** ZAIAS, REBELL and TAPLIN	Considered to be a variant of *M. audouinii*	As for *M. audouinii*	Tinea capitis, tinea corporis
286b	**Microsporum rivalieri** VANBREUSEGHEM 1963	Considered to be a variant of *M. audouinii*. On glycerol-containing media, thick, woolly-flaky thallus with slight yellow color. Macroconidia – different from *M. audouinii* – are coomb-like curved, bizarre, and contain irregular chambers	As for *M. audouinii*. Rarely found in Europe, reported from Central Africa and Florida	Tinea capitis, tinea corporis
287	**Microsporum boullardii** DOMINIK and MAJCHROWICZ 1965 Teleomorph: *Arthroderma corniculatum* WEITZMAN et al. 1986	Rapid growth of colonies at 20 °C and 35 °C. Surface turns from white to ochre and carmine, reverse side red-brown or carmine. Velvety surface, later powdery. Numerous unicellular, round to ovoid or cylindric microconidia with little stems. Spindle-shaped, 3- to 9-chambered macroconidia with thin walls and protuberances when matured	Isolated from soil specimens of plants imported from West Africa[2]	Pathogenicity not known
288	**Microsporum canis** BODIN 1902 *Microsporum lanosum* *Microsporum felineum* Variants: *Microsporum obesum* *Microsporum distortum* Teleomorph: *Arthroderma otae* MCGINNIS et al. 1986	Rapid growth of white to yellow colonies, becoming beige after 2 to 4 weeks. Reverse side bright yellow, later orange-brown. Woolly aerial mycelium with irregular zones of greater proliferation; occasionally forms concentric rings with a central knob. Growth on rice grains usually good (except *M. obesum*). Numerous fusiform, 8- to 15-chambered, thick-walled macroconidia with round protuberances (see Fig. 23, page 98). In *M. distortum* the macroconidia take bizarre forms. Occasional sessile microconidia	Anthropozoophilic. Worldwide distribution. Human infections from dogs, but primarily from cats. Also affects horses, monkeys, chinchillas. Frequent transmission from man to man; occasionally epidemic	Main cause of microsporosis in the western hemisphere. Tinea corporis, tinea capitis, also tinea barbae; fairly common in adults. Lesions are of a marked inflammatory nature. Hair lesions of smallspored (2–3 µm) ectothrix type fluoresce under WOOD's light (see Fig. 33, page 99)

No.	**Fungus** *Synonyms*	Characteristics	Habitat Host Transmission	Associated disease
289	**Microsporum cookei** AJELLO et al. 1959 Teleomorph: *Arthroderma cajetanii* AJELLO et al. 1986	Rapid growth of flat colonies with powdery yellow center and thin white peripheral zone. Reverse side dark purplish-red. Hyaline septate mycelium with many 2- to 8-chambered, ellipsoidal macroconidia (12 μm by 39 μm). Thick outer walls with protuberances	Geophilic. Found in the fur of rodents	Not pathogenic in man or animals. Perforates hairs *in vitro*
290	**Microsporum ferrugineum** OTA 1921 *Trichophyton ferrugineum*	Slow growth of colonies with many radial folds and usually no aerial mycelium. Surface yellow to deep rust-colored, reverse side dark-orange. Mycelium is usually sterile with a few arthrospores. Microconidia and macroconidia have never been observed	Anthropophilic. Mainly in Africa, Asia, eastern Europe	Tinea capitis (cf. *M. audouinii, No. 286*). Hair lesions of small-spored (2–3 μm) ectothrix type fluoresce under WOOD's light (see Fig. 33, page 99)
291	**Microsporum fulvum** URIBURU 1909 Teleomorph: *Arthroderma fulvum* WEITZMAN et al. 1986	Growth of colonies similar to *M. gypseum*, but more floccose and tawny buff in color. Reverse side colorless to yellow, occasionally dark-red. Macroconidia clavate, cylindric or bullet-shaped. Few microconidia. Numerous spiral hyphae	Geophilic. Worldwide distribution	Tinea capitis, tinea corporis. Hair lesions of ectothrix type. No fluorescence under WOOD's light
292	**Microsporum gallinae** GRIGORAKIS 1929 *Trichophyton gallinae* *Epidermophyton gallinae*	Rapid growth of irregularly folded, cleft colonies. Surface white to pale-pink, reverse side strawberry-red. Pigment diffuses into medium. Pyriform or elongate microconidia along the hyphae or in clusters. Abundant cylindric or club-shaped, 2- to 10-chambered macroconidia	Zoophilic. Worldwide distribution. Mainly in poultry, occasionally transmitted to man	Favus in poultry
293	**Microsporum gypseum** (BODIN) GUIART and GRIGORAKIS 1928 *Sabouraudites gypseus* *Achorion gypseum* Teleomorphs: *Arthroderma gypseum* WEITZMAN et al. 1986 *Arthroderma incurvatum* WEITZMAN et al. 1986	Rapid growth of colonies with a powdery-granular, yellowish-brown surface. Reverse side yellow to beige, occasionally pink to red. Good growth on rice grains. Numerous fusiform, 5- to 7-chambered, ellipsoidal macroconidia with thin, spiky walls (see Fig. 22, page 98). Few microconidia	Geophilic. Affects man, also horses, dogs and cats. Occurs in Europe, Africa and America. Strains isolated from soil have only slight virulence but this is increased by passage through a host, when they may become epidemic	Tinea capitis, tinea corporis, kerion. Hair lesions of large-spored ectothrix type. No fluorescence under WOOD's light. Patients usually have only a single lesion
294	**Microsporum nanum** FUENTES 1956 Teleomorph: *Arthroderma obtusum* WEITZMAN et al. 1986	Rapid growth of flat, white to cinnamon-colored colonies with powdery or downy surface. Reverse side orange, later brownish-red. Numerous 2- to 3-chambered, ovoid or ellipsoidal macroconidia. Thin outer walls with protuberances. Sessile pyriform microconidia	Zoophilic. Pigs particularly affected. Rare in man, though it is probably transmissible from animals. Found in North and South America, Cuba, Australia, Europe, India	Occasional cause of tinea capitis and tinea corporis. Hair lesions of large-spored (5–8 μm) ectothrix type. Mycelium runs parallel inside affected hairs, with arthrospores in chains. Usually no fluorescence under WOOD's light
295	**Microsporum persicolor** (SABOURAUD) GUIART and GRIGORAKIS 1928 *Trichophyton persicolor* Teleomorph: *Arthroderma persicolor* WEITZMAN et al. 1986	Growth and macroscopic characteristics similar to *Trichophyton mentagrophytes* (*No. 307*), but large numbers of round or pointed microconidia, with or without stems. Colonies turn yellowish and take the color of peaches – probably overlooked frequently and mistaken for *Trichophyton mentagrophytes* *Remark*. No longer classified as a *Trichophyton* species owing to roughness of the macroconidial cell wall and genetic characteristics[3]	Zoophilic. Widespread in Europe in domestic animals and man	Tinea corporis

No.	Fungus *Synonyms*	Characteristics	Habitat Host Transmission	Associated disease
296	**Microsporum praecox** RIVALIER 1953	Flat, gray, granular colonies, buff or powdery with much soft folding. Elongate, 6- to 9-chambered macroconidia with thick walls. Peg-shaped microconidia occur singly	Isolated in France and the USA	Rare cause of tinea corporis with pustular lesions on the wrist
297	**Microsporum racemosum** BORELLI 1965 Teleomorph: *Arthroderma racemosum* WEITZMAN et al. 1986	Morphologically similar to *M. gypseum* (*No. 293*). Rapid growth at 23–28 °C of woolly, yellowish, later powdery and pink colonies. Abundant microconidia. Spindle-shaped, 5- to 6-chambered macroconidia with thin walls and protuberances. Early pleomorphism	Saprophyte in the fur of rats in northern Venezuela[4]	Experimentally proven cause of tinea corporis in volunteers
298	**Microsporum vanbreuseghemii** GEORG et al. 1962 Teleomorph: *Arthroderma grubyi* WEITZMAN et al. 1986	Rapid growth of flat, powdery or downy colonies with white, yellowish-beige or pink surface. Reverse side yellowish or unpigmented. Numerous cylindric or fusiform, 5- to 12-chambered macroconidia with thick, spiky walls. Many pyriform or ovoid microconidia	Geophilic. Found only in the USA and occasionally in Germany	Rare cause of tinea capitis and tinea corporis. Hair lesions of ectothrix type. No fluorescence under WOOD's light
299	**Trichophyton ajelloi** (VANBREUSEGHEM) AJELLO 1967 *Keratinomyces ajelloi* Teleomorph: *Arthroderma uncinatum* DAWSON and GENTLES 1961	Rapid growth of flat or raised, folded colonies with powdery or matt surface; cream-, beige- or orange-colored. Reverse side colorless or blue-black. Rapid development of cotton-like, pleomorphous growth zones. Numerous cylindric or fusiform, 8- to 12-chambered macroconidia with thick, smooth walls. Microconidia ovoid or pyriform, sessile	Geophilic. Worldwide distribution	Rare cause of tinea corporis in man. Mycelium inside affected hairs. Spores do not form cuffs. No fluorescence under WOOD's light
299a	**Trichophyton ajelloi** var. **nana** (KUNERT and HEJTMÁNEK) AJELLO	Granular colonies with folded center, buff colored. Ellipsoidal, 2- to 4-chambered macroconidia with thick, smooth walls	Soil (isolated in Czechoslovakia)	
300	**Trichophyton concentricum** BLANCHARD 1896 *Endodermophyton indicum*	Slow growth of cerebriform, yellow to amber colonies with short white hyphae. Numerous chlamydospores	Anthropophilic. Limited geographical distribution (South Pacific Islands, the Far East, northern South America, Central America). Direct or indirect transmission	Tinea imbricata (tokelau). Wide skin areas of the trunk and extremities are affected, but not hair
301	**Trichophyton equinum** GEDOELST 1902	Rapid growth of initially flat, later folded, colonies. Surface at first white with cotton-wool appearance and with bright-yellow margin. Older colonies flat, velvety, beige-colored. Reverse side yellow, later pink and dark brownish-red. Grows only in the presence of nicotinic acid. Varying numbers of slender, longish microconidia and a few thin-walled macroconidia with smooth walls	Zoophilic (horses). Worldwide distribution	Tinea corporis, mainly of the hair. Growth of mycelium within the hairs, with cuffs or chains of isolated spores (3–5 μm) on the surface. No fluorescence under WOOD's light
301a	**Trichophyton equinum** var. **autotrophicum** SMITH et al.	Very similar to *T. equinum*, but nicotinic acid not required for growth *in vitro*	Zoophilic (horses). Mainly in New Zealand and Australia	
302	**Trichophyton georgiae** VARSAVSKY and AJELLO 1964 Teleomorph: *Arthroderma ciferrii* VARSAVSKY and AJELLO 1964	Similar to *T. terrestre* (*No. 315*)	Soil, fur of opossum. Saprophyte on birds in Australia, Europe, the USA	Pathogenicity not known

No.	Fungus *Synonyms*	Characteristics	Habitat Host Transmission	Associated disease
303	**Trichophyton gloriae** AJELLO and CHENG 1967 Teleomorph: *Arthroderma gloriae* AJELLO 1967	Downy, slightly folded colonies with raised center, cream colored. Reverse side yellowish to brownish. Elongate, 1- to 10-chambered macroconidia in clusters on conidiophores. Conidia abundant, one-celled, singly borne	Soil (isolated in some US states)	Pathogenicity not known
304	**Trichophyton gourvilii** CATANEI 1923	Slow growth of colonies, at first glabrous with a waxy appearance, later covered by a velvety aerial mycelium. Rose-violet to deep-red pigmentation. Microconidia and macroconidia. In some respects similar to *T. violaceum* and *T. soudanense*. L-Histidine or thiamine not required for growth	Anthropophilic. Mainly in North, West and Central Africa	Tinea capitis, onychomycosis. Endothrix type of hair lesions (see Fig. 34, page 99)
305	**Trichophyton longifusum** (FLORIAN and GALGOCZY) AJELLO 1964	Cottony or powdery colonies with central knob, white to pale yellow. Cylindric, 4- to 15-chambered macroconidia with thin walls, distal ends club-shaped; with age they germinate to form new macroconidia	Soil (isolated in Hungary)	Tinea capitis in association with *Microsporum gypseum*
306	**Trichophyton megninii** BLANCHARD 1896 *Trichophyton rosaceum* *Aleurosporium rosaceum* *Trichophyton kuryangei*	Slow growth of flat colonies with deep radial folds. Velvety surface, white at first, later light or dark pink. Pigment intracellular. Reverse side deep-red. Many small pyriform microconidia, less numerous, slightly club-shaped, 2- to 8-chambered macroconidia. Requires L-histidine for growth. Urease-positive	Anthropophilic. Mainly in Europe (Sardinia, Portugal) and Africa	Tinea barbae, tinea corporis. Ectothrix type of hair lesions
307	**Trichophyton mentagrophytes** (ROBIN) BLANCHARD 1896 *Trichophyton granulosum* *Trichophyton quinckeanum* *Trichophyton interdigitale* *Trichophyton erinacei* Teleomorphs: *Arthroderma benhamiae* AJELLO and CHENG 1967 *Arthroderma vanbreuseghemii* TAKASHIO 1973	Var. *mentagrophytes*. Rapid growth of flat, granular colonies. Mycelium is usually sparce. Colonies variable in color from greyish-white, yellow, buff to tan or reddish-brown. Reverse side rosy-brown, yellow-orange or dark-red. Masses of round or slender microconidia growing singly along hyphae or in pine-needle-like clusters (see Fig. 10, page 97). Some cigar-shaped, 3- to 5-chambered macroconidia with thin walls (see Fig. 20, page 98). Spiral hyphae	Zoophilic. Worldwide distribution. Often affects domestic animals with transmission to man	Tinea pedis, tinea corporis, tinea capitis, tinea barbae, tinea cruris. Ectothrix type of hair lesions. No fluorescence under WOOD's light
		Var. *interdigitale*. Growth similar to that of var. *mentagrophytes*, but surface of colonies downy. Microconidia less abundant	Anthropophilic. Worldwide distribution. Transmission from man to man in swimming-pools, schools, etc.	Common cause of tinea pedis ('athlete's foot'), also onychomycosis (tinea unguium), tinea cruris, tinea barbae. Ectothrix type of hair lesions. No fluorescence under WOOD's light
		Var. *quinckeanum*. Growth similar to that of var. *mentagrophytes*, but colonies have prominent radial folds	Zoophilic (mice, rabbits, fowl, guinea pigs). Worldwide distribution. Transmission by mice	Tinea corporis, tinea capitis. May produce endothrix type of hair lesions
		Var. *erinacei*. Growth similar to that of var. *mentagrophytes*. Urease-negative	Zoophilic (hedgehogs, dogs). Mainly in Europe and New Zealand	Tinea corporis. Ectothrix type of hair lesions. No fluorescence under WOOD's light
308	**Trichophyton proliferans** ENGLISH and STOCKDALE Teleomorph: *Arthroderma benhamiae* var. *erinacei*	Very similar to *T. mentagrophytes* var. *erinacei*. Pleomorphic macroconidia and chlamydospore-like structures near the surface of and within the culture medium. Urease-negative		Tinea corporis in children reported from England and New Zealand[5]

No.	**Fungus** *Synonyms*	Characteristics	Habitat Host Transmission	Associated disease
309	**Trichophyton phaseoliforme** BORELLI and FEO 1966	White cotton-like colonies becoming granular and ochrous in color. Abundant microconidia, characteristically bean-shaped, inserted laterally along the hyphae. Clavate, cylindric macroconidia consisting of several chambers	Soil (isolated in Poland, Switzerland, Venezuela)	Not pathogenic in man or animals
310	**Trichophyton raubitschekii** KANE et al. 1981	Growth in granular to velutinous colonies with deep-red surface, abundant macroconidia in primary isolate, subglobose, pyriform and clavate microconidia (similar to *T. rubrum*). Urease-positive	Anthropophilic. Mainly in Asia and southern Europe	Tinea corporis, tinea cruris, tinea pedis[6]
311	**Trichophyton rubrum** (CASTELLANI) SABOURAUD 1912 *Epidermophyton rubrum* *Trichophyton purpureum*	Slow growth of white, later reddish colonies, partly flat, partly elevated; surface woolly, sometimes with radial folds. Reverse side red to purple. According to surface structure, pigmentation, etc. five growth forms have been distinguished. Microconidia and macroconidia in varying numbers, the latter usually pencil-shaped, 3- to 8-chambered with rounded ends, sessile (see Fig. 21, page 98)	Anthropophilic. Worldwide distribution. Direct or indirect transmission	Common cause of tinea cruris[7], tinea pedis, tinea manuum; also onychomycosis. Hair hardly ever affected
312	**Trichophyton schoenleinii** (LEBERT) LANGERON and MILOCHEVITCH 1930 *Achorion schoenleinii*	Snow-white, star-shaped colonies on gelatin. On SABOURAUD glucose agar slow growth of (at 22°C and 37°C) irregularly folded, tough, leathery colonies that often split the agar surface. Surface white to beige-colored, wax-like, powdery or downy. Chlamydospores. Few microconidia. Terminal hyphae with club-like swellings ('chandeliers') (see Fig. 3, page 97)	Anthropophilic. Worldwide distribution. Transmission mainly under poor hygienic conditions, especially among children	Favus, a distinct type of tinea capitis with characteristic golden-yellow scutula around the hairs. Infected hairs contain branched mycelium and cavities, also fat droplets, and have a dull gray color
313	**Trichophyton simii** (PINOY) STOCKDALE et al. 1965 *Epidermophyton simii* Teleomorph: *Arthroderma simii* STOCKDALE et al. 1965	Similar to *T. mentagrophytes* except that colonies are thinner and have a finer granulation; abundant macroconidia with several chambers and characteristic endochlamydospores	Zoophilic. Mainly in monkeys, also in poultry, dogs and man in India	Tinea capitis, tinea corporis. Hair lesions of endoectothrix type fluoresce under WOOD's light[8]
314	**Trichophyton soudanense** JOYEUX 1912 *Langeronia soudanensis*	Slow growth of flat colonies with an elevated, sometimes wrinkled center. Surface glabrous, dry or powdery, dark-apricot in color. Reverse side yellow or orange. Microconidia in varying numbers. Mycelium disintegrates to form arthrospores	Anthropophilic. Mainly in Central and West Africa	Tinea capitis. Endothrix type of hair lesions
315	**Trichophyton terrestre** DURIE and FREY 1957 Teleomorphs: *Arthroderma quadrifidum* DAWSON and GENTLES 1961 *Arthroderma lenticulorum* PORE et al. 1965 *Arthroderma insingulare* PADHYE and CARMICHAEL 1972	Rapid growth of flat, white, cream-colored or sulfur-yellow colonies with powdery, granular or velvety surface. Reverse side yellowish-brown or reddish. Abundant elongate, pyriform or ellipsoidal microconidia on aerial hyphae. Microconidia sit on short conidiophores or on a wide upright base. Few thin-walled, cigar-shaped macroconidia containing several chambers	Geophilic. Worldwide distribution	Not pathogenic in man or animals

No.	Fungus *Synonyms*	Characteristics	Habitat Host Transmission	Associated disease
316	**Trichophyton tonsurans** MALMSTEN 1845 *Trichophyton crateriforme* *Trichophyton acuminatum* *Trichophyton sulfureum*	Slow growth of cream- or beige-colored, flat colonies with a yellow or rose tint and central crater or central knob. Surface at first powdery, later velvety; older colonies have deep folds. Abundant delicate, oblong or oval microconidia; old cultures have many chlamydospores. Rarely there are club-shaped, irregular macroconidia with thin, smooth walls. Requires thiamine for growth	Anthropophilic. Worldwide distribution, mainly in northern South America, Central America, the USA. Direct and indirect transmission	Tinea capitis, tinea corporis. Usually superficial, with moderate alopecia, but often chronic and protracted. In adult males primarily cause of tinea barbae. Endothrix type of hair lesions, with spores 4–7.5 µm in diameter. No fluorescence under WOOD's light
317	**Trichophyton vanbreuseghemii** RIOUX, JARRY and JUMINER 1964 Teleomorph: *Arthroderma gertleri* BÖHME 1967	Initially flat white colonies turning granular and folded. Buff-ochrous in color. Pyriform microconidia along the hyphae and many cylindric or club-shaped macroconidia with rounded ends and smooth walls *Remark.* Not to be confused with *Microsporum vanbreuseghemii*	Geophilic. Mainly in Africa, Europe and North America	Not pathogenic in man or animals
318	**Trichophyton verrucosum** BODIN 1902 *Trichophyton discoides* *Trichophyton album* *Trichophyton faviforme* *Trichophyton ochraceum*	Very slow growth at 22 °C, better at 37 °C (10–14 days) in form of small, elevated, folded colonies, sometimes disk-shaped; appearance at first leathery or waxy, sometimes with a white or yellow, powdery or downy surface. Thiamine and inositol necessary for growth. Forms a thin mycelium with chlamydospores on SABOURAUD glucose agar; on vitamin-enriched media forms small, fine microconidia along the hyphae, very rarely 3- to 5-chambered macroconidia of varying size with thin, smooth walls. Three variants are distinguished according to colonial appearance: var. *album*, var. *discoides*, var. *ochraceum*	Zoophilic. Worldwide distribution. Human infections originate from animals (cattle, etc.)	Tinea corporis, tinea capitis. Ectothrix type of hair lesions with cuffs of spores 5–10 µm in diameter. No fluorescence under WOOD's light
319	**Trichophyton violaceum** SABOURAUD and BODIN 1902 *Achorion violaceum*	Slow growth of glabrous colonies, initially cream-colored, later violet, occasionally with greyish-white patches. Old cultures often colorless (var. *glabrum*). Scanty aerial mycelium, usually with warty elevations. Thin, irregular mycelium with chlamydospores. No macroconidia. Requires thiamine for growth	Anthropophilic. Worldwide distribution, mainly in India, the Middle East and some parts of Africa. Direct or indirect transmission	Tinea capitis, tinea corporis. Endothrix type of hair lesions, with spores 4–7.5 µm in diameter (see Fig. 34, page 99). No fluorescence under WOOD's light
320	**Trichophyton yaoundei** COCHET and DOBY-DUBOIS 1957	Slow growth of glabrous colonies with an elevated, wrinkled surface. Color at first white to cream, later deep chocolate-brown. Irregularly formed mycelium with many chlamydospores. Pyriform microconidia, no macroconidia	Anthropophilic. Mainly in children in Central Africa	Tinea capitis. Endothrix type of hair lesions

[1] MORAES et al., *Med. cutanea*, **2**, 201 (1967).
[2] DOMINIK and MAJCHROWICZ, *Mycopathologia (Den Haag)*, **28**, 202 (1966).
[3] STOCKDALE, P. M., *Sabouraudia*, **5**, 33 (1967).
[4] BORELLI, D., *Acta med. venez.*, **12**, 148 (1965).
[5] RUSH-MUNRO, F. M., *Rev. Méd.*, **19**, 639 (1978).
[6] KANE et al., *Mycoses*, **33**, 499 (1990).
[7] PUISSANT and BADILLET, *Rev. Méd.*, **19**, 633 (1978).
[8] RIPPON and MALKINSON, *Arch. Derm.*, **98**, 615 (1968).

No.	**Fungus** *Synonyms*	Characteristics	Habitat Host Transmission	Associated disease
	Other fungi, including algae, implicated in disease			
321	**Arnium leporinum** (CAIN) LUNDQVIST and KRUG	Colonies 6–8 cm after 2 months at 22 °C on cornmeal agar, dotted irregularly with black pyriform ascomata. Reverse side grayish-black. Hyphal appendages on asci. Ovoid ascospores with or without gelatinous appendages	Coprophilic. Found in northern Europe, Canada, the USA, Colombia	A case of endocarditis reported from Colombia[1]
322	**Cercospora apii** FRESENIUS 1863	Compact, dome-shaped colonies with short aerial hyphae, olive colored. Brown conidia terminally or laterally on brown conidiophores, becoming rather long and multicellular with truncate base	Infects leaves of crop plants	A case of human infection reported from Indonesia[2]
323	**Chrysosporium parvum** (EMMONS and ASHBURN) CARMICHAEL 1962 *Haplosporangium parvum* *Emmonsia parva* *Emmonsia crescens*	White, felty to floccose colonies of tough consistency, occasional zoning and coremia. Septate hyphae with short, slender microconidia on erect conidiophores. On media containing blood, development of adiaspores at 35 to 40 °C with thick walls, 10–25 µm in diameter. These adiaspores may contain one nucleus (var. *parva*) or several (var. *crescens*). They are exclusively present in tissue sections from adiaspiromycosis	Saprophyte in soil. Worldwide distribution. Rodents, occasionally man	Adiaspiromycosis[3]. Asymptomatic pulmonary infection
324	**Piedraia hortae** (BRUMPT) FONSECA and AREÂ LEÃO 1928 *Trichosporon hortai* *Piedraia javanica*	Slow growth of small, smooth, greenish-black colonies with dark septate mycelium. Gelatine not liquefied. Affected hairs show black nodules containing oval asci with 2–8 spindle-shaped, slightly curved ascospores	Mainly in warm and humid areas (South America, the Far East, Pacific Islands)	Black piedra (black hair-nodule disease)[4]
325	**Prototheca wickerhamii** TUBAKI and SONEDA 1959	Achlorophyllous algae. Moist, cream-colored, yeast-like colonies at 25 °C and 30 °C on SABOURAUD glucose agar. Ovoid cells, 8–13 µm by 11–16 µm. Numerous autospores (4–5 µm in diameter). Utilizes trehalose	Soil, sewage, water. Widely distributed	Protothecosis in man[5]. Skin involvement, olecranal bursitis, disseminated disease[6]
326	**Pythium insidiosum** DE COCK 1987	Glabrous, white or yellowish-white colonies on SABOURAUD glucose agar. Nonseptate hyphae. Biflagellate zoospore formation	Plants, fish, mammals such as horses, cattle, dogs[7]. Human infections reported from Thailand[8]	Pythiosis in man. Cutaneous lesions, arteritis in association with thalassemia[8]
327	**Rhinosporidium seeberi** (WERNICKE) SEEBER 1912	Not yet cultivated. Seen in affected tissues as spherical sporangia of varying size (up to 350 µm) filled with endospores (7–9 µm)	Man and animals. Endemic in India, Sri Lanka, South America and the CIS. Mode of transmission not known for certain; not transmissible from man to man	Rhinosporidiosis[9], especially of the nasal mucosa, with formation of polypoid tumors in affected tissues, including the conjunctiva. Recurrence of infection is characteristic

[1] RESTREPO et al., *Sabouraudia*, **22**, 225 (1984).
[2] EMMONS et al., *Mycologia*, **49**, 1 (1957); LIE-KIAN-JOE et al., *Arch. Derm.*, **75**, 864 (1957).
[3] RIPPON, J.W., *Medical Mycology*, 3rd ed., Saunders, Philadelphia, 1988, page 718.
[4] RIPPON, J.W., *Medical Mycology*, 3rd ed., Saunders, Philadelphia, 1988, page 163.
[5] RIPPON, J.W., *Medical Mycology*, 3rd ed., Saunders, Philadelphia, 1988, page 723.
[6] SANDS et al., *Rev. infect. Dis.*, **13**, 376 (1991).
[7] DE COCK et al., *J. clin. Microbiol.*, **25**, 344 (1987).
[8] SATHAPATAYAVONGS et al., *J. infect. Dis.*, **159**, 274 (1989).
[9] RIPPON, J.W., *Medical Mycology*, 3rd ed., Saunders, Philadelphia, 1988, page 362.

Forms of mycelium

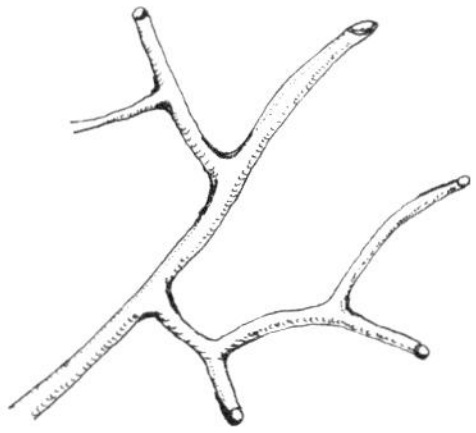

Fig. 1 Mycelium, nonseptate

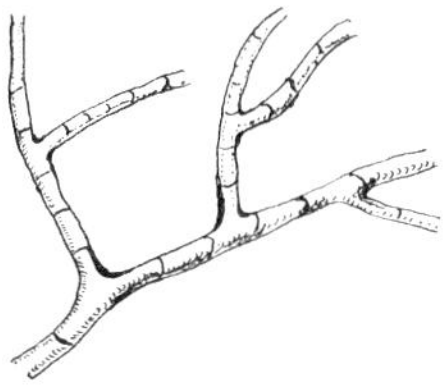

Fig. 2 Mycelium, septate

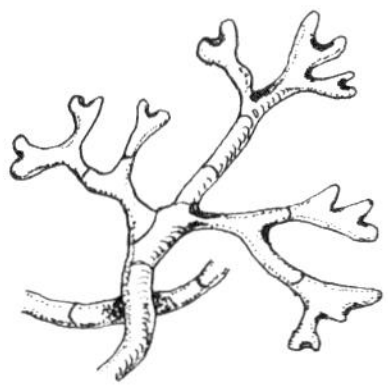

Fig. 3 Mycelium, septate, terminal dichotomous branching

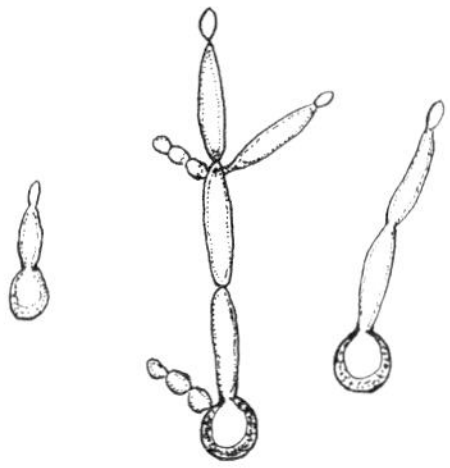

Fig. 4 Pseudomycelium (blastospores)

Vegetative forms of spores

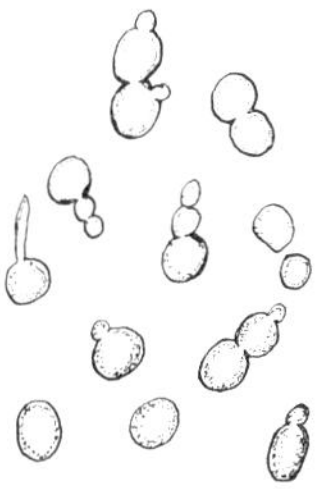

Fig. 5 Budding forms with blastospores (yeast cells of *Candida*)

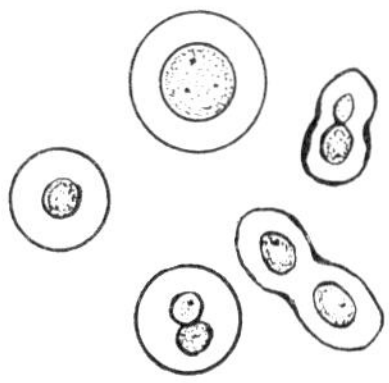

Fig. 6 Blastospores with capsule (*Cryptococcus neoformans*)

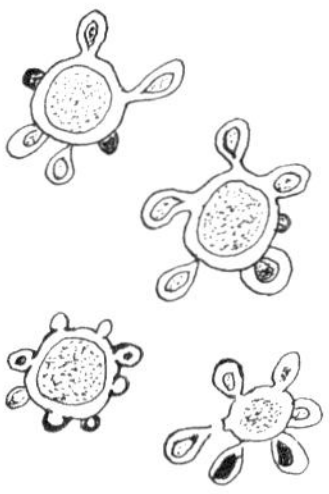

Fig. 7 Multilocular budding (*Paracoccidioides brasiliensis*)

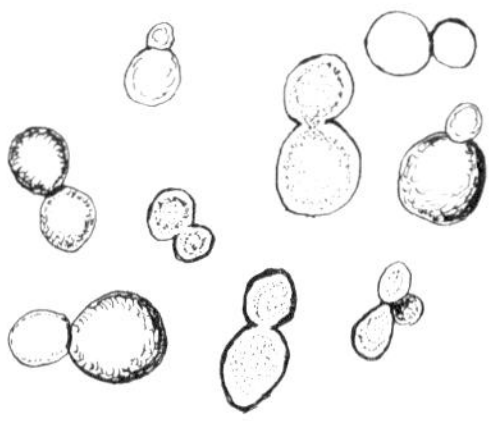

Fig. 8 Unilocular budding (yeast phase of *Blastomyces dermatitidis*)

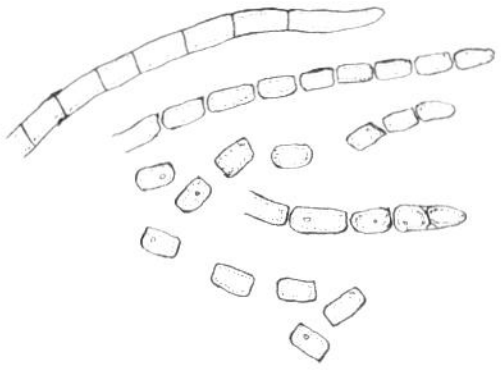

Fig. 9 Arthrospores produced by division and fragmentation of a hypha (*Geotrichum candidum*)

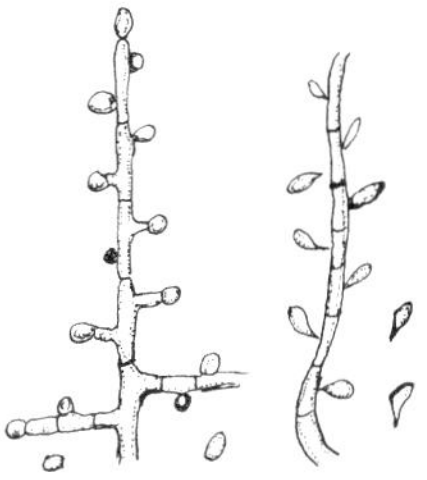

Fig. 10 Microconidia produced along mycelium (left *Trichophyton mentagrophytes*, right *Trichophyton rubrum*)

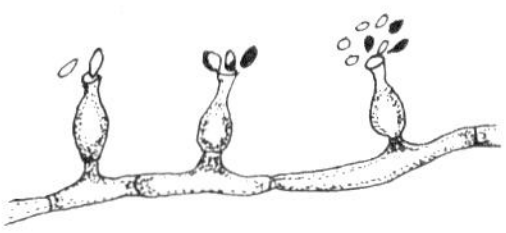

Fig. 11 Spores produced by expulsion out of a 'container' (*Phialophora* spp.)

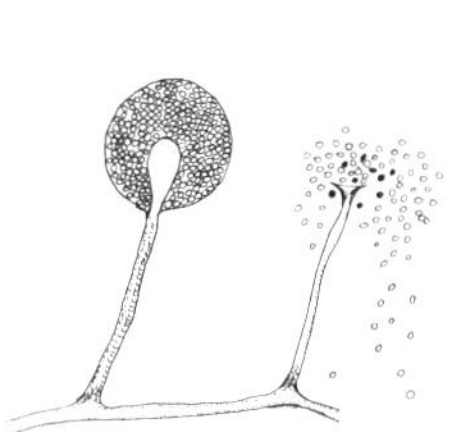

Fig. 12 Endospores produced in a sporangium (*Mucor* spp.)

Vegetative forms of spores (conidiophores with genus specific appearance)

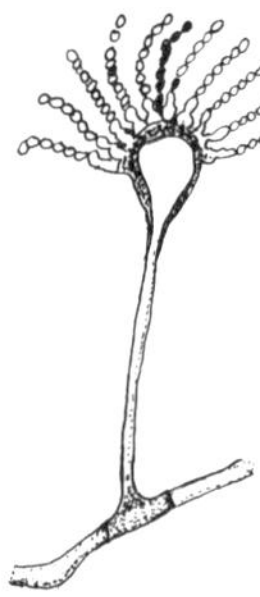

Fig. 13 *Aspergillus*-type of conidial formation

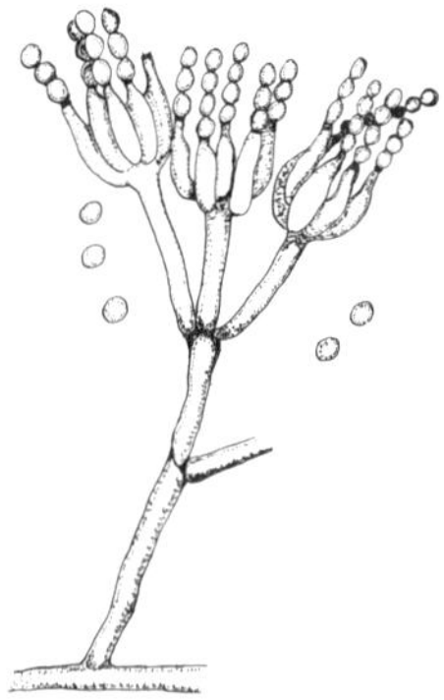

Fig. 14 *Penicillium*-type of conidial formation

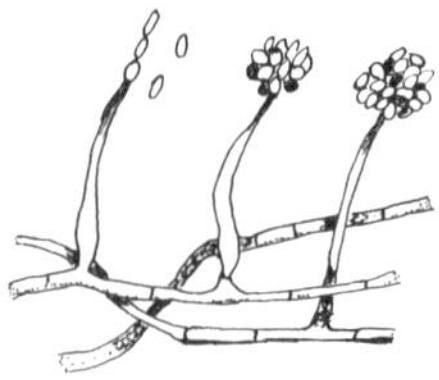

Fig. 15 *Cephalosporium*-type of conidial formation

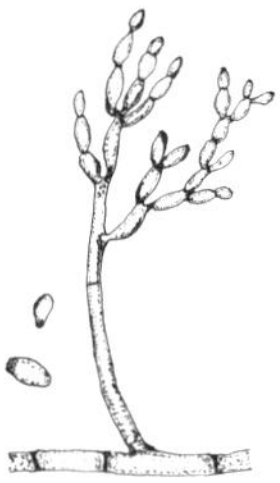

Fig. 16 *Cladosporium*-type of conidial formation

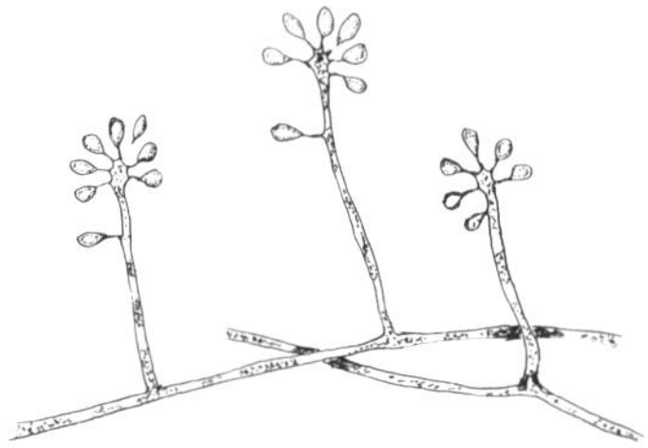

Fig. 17 *Sporothrix*-type of conidial formation

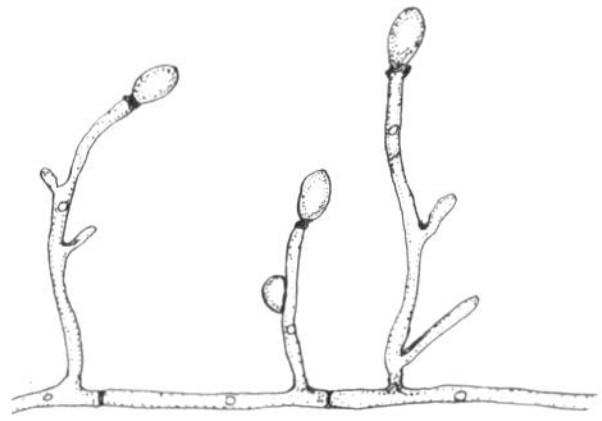

Fig. 18 'Monosporium-type' of conidial formation. Terminal single conidium on conidiophore (*Pseudoallescheria sheari*)

Macroconidia of dermatophytes

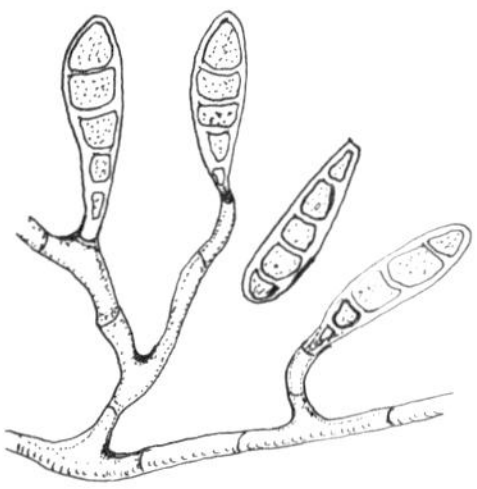

Fig. 19 Epidermophyton floccosum

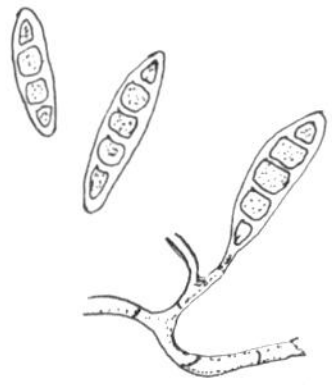

Fig. 20 Trichophyton mentagrophytes

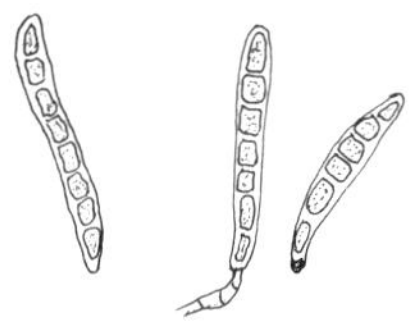

Fig. 21 Trichophyton rubrum

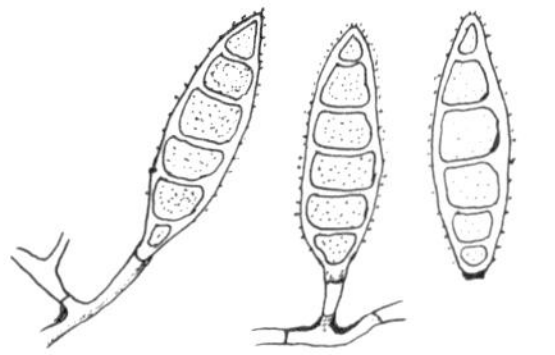

Fig. 22 Microsporum gypseum

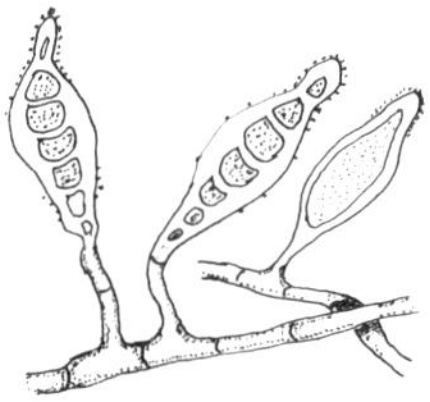

Fig. 23 Microsporum canis

Generative sporulation after nuclear fusion

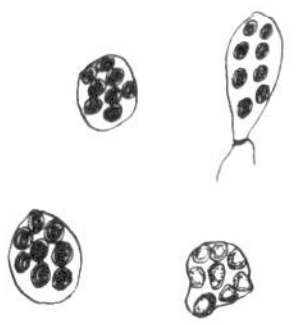

Fig. 24 Asci containing ascospores

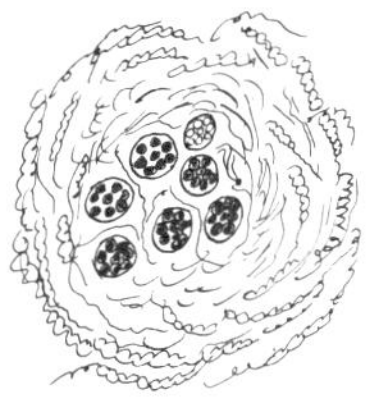

Fig. 25 Cleistothecium with asci containing ascospores

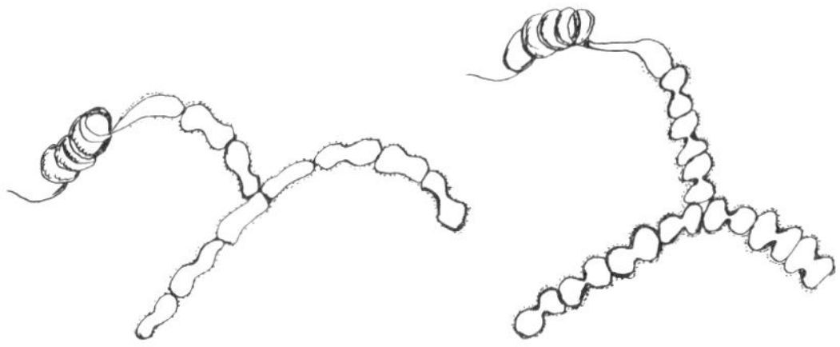

Fig. 26 Peridial hyphae at the outside of cleistothecia (*Arthroderma*)

Tissue-form elements of dimorphic fungi

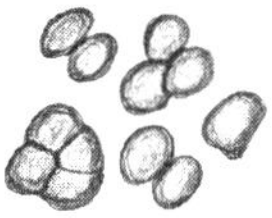

Fig. 27 Chromoblastomycosis. Sclerotial cells in tissue sections and pus (homogenously dark-brown)

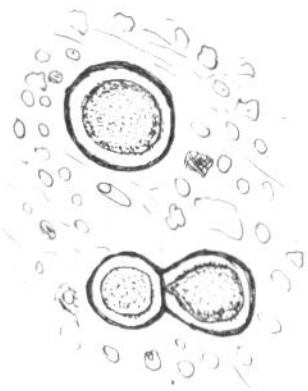

Fig. 28 North American blastomycosis. Thick-walled, double-refractory yeast phase cell and budding cell with broad basis of *Blastomyces dermatitidis* in tissue sections and pus

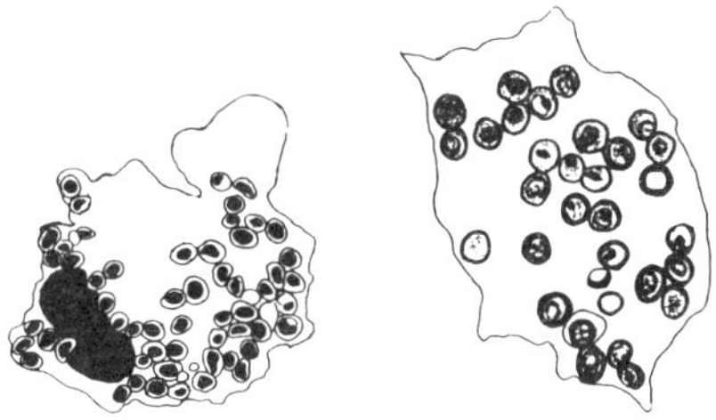

Fig. 29 Histoplasmosis. (a) Small cell type (*Histoplasma capsulatum*), (b) large cell type (*Histoplasma duboisii*)

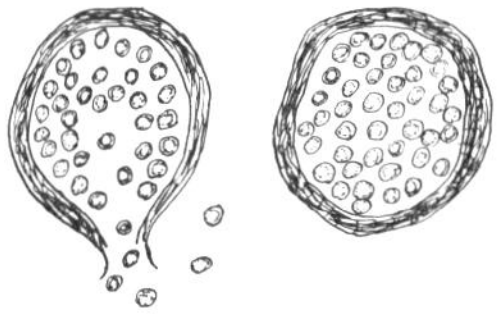

Fig. 30 Coccidioidomycosis. Ripening stages of spherules containing endospores of *Coccidioides immitis*

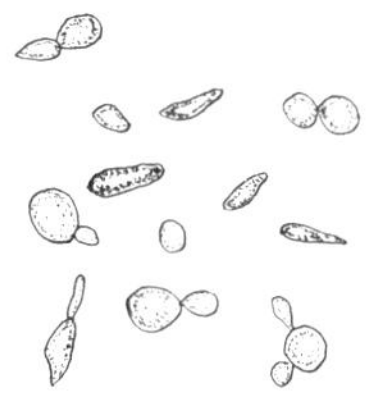

Fig. 31 Sporotrichosis. Yeast-like and cigar-shaped cells of *Sporothrix schenckii* in tissue sections and pus

Hair lesions

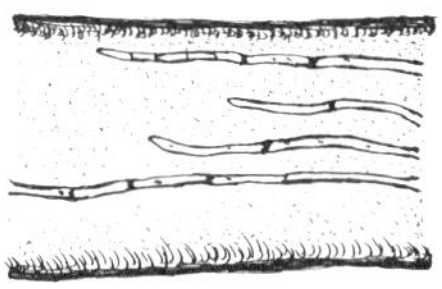

Fig. 32 Early stage of hair lesion with septate mycelium. No sporulation (hyphae and occasionally vacuoles)

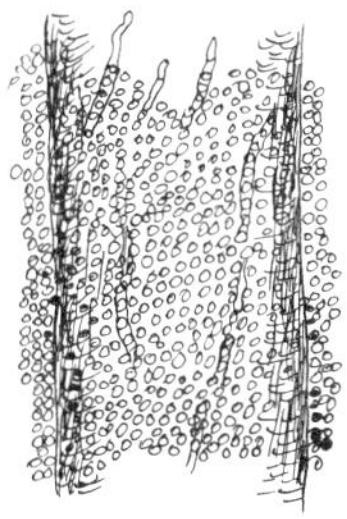

Fig. 33 Ectothrix type of hair lesion. Fragmentation of mycelium outside the hair

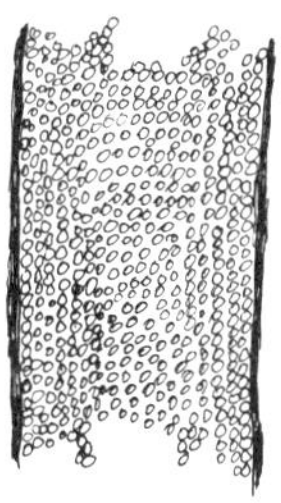

Fig. 34 Endothrix type of hair lesion. Fragmentation of mycelium within the hair

Introduction

Protozoa contain within a single cell all the organelles essential for adaptation to either a free living or parasitic existence. Their life cycles may be simple and direct with a single life cycle stage (for example *Entamoeba gingivalis*, which spreads from mouth to mouth with no external development) or extremely complex with distinct definitive and intermediate hosts and a great variety of different development stages (for example malaria in man and mosquitoes). Many species of protozoa have had a long and intimate evolutionary relationship with man and may be completely nonpathogenic, as for example *Entamoeba coli*. Other species can produce devastating epidemics, such as *Trypanosoma brucei rhodesiense*, primarily a parasite of wild animals which has been acquired by man relatively recently. This type of sleeping sickness is a zoonosis which was defined by a Joint WHO/FAO Expert Committee as 'those diseases and infections which are naturally transmitted between vertebrate animals and man'. Many of the protozoal infections of man, including toxoplasmosis, leishmaniasis, trypanosomiasis and balantidiasis, have long been recognized as zoonoses, but more recent epidemiological studies have revealed that there are animal hosts of most of the other protozoa infecting man.

The protozoa of medical importance are not uniform species, and both pathogenic and nonpathogenic strains occur which are morphologically identical but can be distinguished on the basis of their biological properties, their isoenzyme profiles (zymodemes) or on their genetic material. This has been most clearly demonstrated with the leishmanias and trypanosomes, but similar variations are now known to account for the existence of both pathogenic and nonpathogenic strains of *Entamoeba histolytica*. Antigenic variation is a characteristic of trypanosomes and malaria parasites, and this has become a major problem in developing antiprotozoal vaccines. Variations in susceptibility to drugs have also become a major public health problem, particularly since the spread of drug-resistant strains of *Plasmodium falciparum* to many parts of the world.

Some protozoal infections which were thought to be rare are now known to be extremely common and widespread. This is the result of improved methods of diagnosis and new knowledge of the life cycles and diversity of natural hosts, for example of *Toxoplasma* and *Cryptosporidium*. There is also an increasing awareness of opportunistic protozoal infections such as *Pneumocystis**, *Enterocytozoon* and *Isospora* in immunocompromised hosts including individuals with the acquired immunodeficiency syndrome.

The diagnosis of protozoal infections usually depends on recognizing the organisms in blood, tissues or excreta, but there have been many important advances in the development of immunodiagnostic techniques which are particularly valuable in epidemiological surveys and for detecting cryptic infections such as ocular toxoplasmosis or hepatic amebiasis. There have been relatively few advances in the chemotherapy of protozoal infection in the past 20 years, but many advances in knowledge of the epidemiology, immunology and pathogenicity of protozoal infections, mainly as a result of the stimulus provided by the World Health Organization's Special Programme for Research and Training in Tropical Diseases.

The tables on pages 101–116 list the most important species of protozoa pathogenic in man together with nonpathogenic species which may cause confusion in diagnosis. The species are ordered on the basis of the following classification.

For a detailed description of the protozoa and the diseases caused by them the reader is referred to more extensive publications on parasitology and tropical diseases (see General References).

General References

ASH and ORIHEL, *Atlas of Human Parasitology*, 3rd ed., Raven, New York, 1990.

TAYLOR and MULLER (Eds.), *Problems in the Identification of Parasites and Their Vectors*, Blackwell, Oxford, 1979.

COHEN and WARREN (Eds.), *Immunology of Parasitic Infections*, 2nd ed., Blackwell, Oxford, 1982.

BINFORD and CONNOR (Eds.), *Pathology of Tropical and Extraordinary Diseases*, 2 vols, US Armed Forces Institute of Pathology, Washington, 1976.

DONALDSON, R. J. (Ed.), *Parasites and Western Man*, MPT Press, Lancaster, 1979.

PETERS and GILLES, *A Colour Atlas of Tropical Medicine and Parasitology*, 3rd ed., Wolfe, London, 1989.

World Health Organization, *The 'In Vitro' Culture of Pathogens of Tropical Diseases*, Tropical Diseases Research Series, No. 3, Schwabe, Basel, 1980.

World Health Organization, *New Approaches to the Identification of Parasites and Their Vectors*, Tropical Diseases Research Series, No. 5, Schwabe, Basel, 1984.

BEAVER et al., *Clinical Parasitology*, 9th ed., Lea & Febiger, Philadelphia, 1984.

STRICKLAND, G. T. (Ed.), *Hunter's Tropical Diseases*, 7th ed., Saunders, Philadelphia, 1991.

Classification of the protozoa
(abridged from LEVINE et al., *J. Protozool.*, **27**, 37 [1980].)

The italic numbers are the serial numbers appearing in column 1 of the tables.

KINGDOM	Animalia	
SUBKINGDOM	Protozoa	
Phylum	Sarcomastigophora HONIGBERG and BALAMUTH	
Subphylum	Mastigophora DIESING	
Class	Zoomastigophorea CALKINS	
Order	Kinetoplastida HONIGBERG emend. VICKERMAN	
Suborder	Trypanosomatina KENT *Leishmania, Trypanosoma*	*328–336*
Order	Retortamonadida GRASSÉ *Retortamonas, Chilomastix*	*337–338*
Order	Diplomonadida WENYON	
Suborder	Enteromonadina BRUGEROLLE emend. KULDA and NOHÝNKOVÁ *Enteromonas*	*339*
Suborder	Diplomonadina WENYON *Giardia*	*340*
Superorder	Parabasalidea HONIGBERG	
Order	Trichomonadida KIRBY *Trichomonas, Dientamoeba*	*341–344*
Subphylum	Sarcodina SCHMARDA	
Superclass	Rhizopoda VON SIEBOLD	
Class	Lobosea CARPENTER	
Subclass	Gymnamoebia HAECKEL	
Order	Amoebida EHRENBERG	
Suborder	Tubulina BOVEE and JAHN *Entamoeba, Endolimax, Iodamoeba*	*345–350*
Suborder	Acanthopodina PAGE *Acanthamoeba*	*351, 352*
Order	Schizopyrenida SINGH *Naegleria*	*353*
Phylum	Apicomplexa LEVINE	
Class	Sporozoea LEUCKART	
Subclass	Coccidia LEUCKART	
Order	Eucoccidiida LÉGER and DUBOSCQ	
Suborder	Eimeriina LÉGER *Cryptosporidium, Isospora, Pneumocystis*, Sarcocystis, Toxoplasma*	*354–359*
Suborder	Haemosporina DANILEWSKY *Plasmodium*	*360–363*
Subclass	Piroplasmia LEVINE	
Order	Piroplasmida WENYON *Babesia*	*364*
Phylum	Microspora SPRAGUE	
Class	Microsporea DELPHY	
Order	Microsporidia BALBIANI	
Suborder	Apansporoblastina TUZET et al. *Enterocytozoon*	*365*
Phylum	Ciliophora DOFLEIN	
Class	Kinetofragminophorea DE PUYTORAC et al.	
Subclass	Vestibuliferia DE PUYTORAC et al.	
Order	Trichostomatida BÜTSCHLI	
Suborder	Trichostomatina BÜTSCHLI *Balantidium*	*366*

* Although there is some evidence suggesting that *Pneumocystis* should be reclassified as a fungus, it is retained in this section because it has been studied mainly by parasitologists.

No.	**Protozoa** *Synonyms*	Characteristics	Habitat Host Transmission	Associated disease
328	**Leishmania donovani** (LAVERAN and MESNIL) ROSS *Leishmania canis* *Leishmania chagasi* *Leishmania infantum*	Length 2–3 µm. The different species and subspecies of *Leishmania* are morphologically indistinguishable, and it is necessary to culture the organisms so that they can be characterized either biochemically by examining isoenzyme profiles[1] or by use of DNA probes[2,3]. Material should be sent to one of the WHO Reference Centers[4]	Transmitted by *Phlebotomus* (sandflies). Reservoir hosts: dogs, wild carnivores, rodents (Africa), but epidemics are due to interhuman transmission[5-8]	Visceral leishmaniasis (kala azar). Involves the reticuloendothelial system with splenomegaly, hepatomegaly, lymphadenopathy, bone marrow dyshematopoiesis, pancytopenia, fever and wasting. Mucous membranes may be affected, and generalized skin lesions occur as 'post-kala azar' dermal leishmaniasis Epidemics occur in India, East Africa and Brazil, but also endemic in many other countries (see map on page 117). Leishmaniasis infantum is especially common in children in the Mediterranean area, but adult cases do occur: they may appear as opportunistic infection in patients with AIDS[9] with unusual gastrointestinal features[10] Diagnosis: demonstration of amastigotes from bone marrow or spleen biopsy; serology including formol gel test for high-level immunoglobulins useful in surveys[11] *Remarks.* For treatment, a pentavalent antimony compound (e.g. sodium stibogluconate, meglumine antimoniate) is the drug of choice[4,12,13]. Treatment with pentamidine, amphotericin B or allopurinol should be limited to persons unresponsive to antimony compounds[4,12]. Paromomycin may be effective[14]. For review of *Leishmania* biochemistry relevant to chemotherapy, see BERMAN[15]

[1] KREUTZER et al., *Amer. J. trop. Med. Hyg.*, N.S. **32**, 703 (1983).
[2] BARKER and BUTCHER, *Trans. roy. Soc. trop. Med. Hyg.*, **77**, 285 (1983).
[3] SPITHILL and GRUMONT, *Molec. biochem. Parasit.*, **12**, 217 (1984).
[4] WHO Expert Committee on Control of the Leishmaniases, *Wld Hlth Org. techn. Rep. Ser.*, No. 793 (1990).
[5] MOLYNEUX and ASHFORD, *The Biology of Trypanosoma and Leishmania; Parasites of Man and Animals*, Taylor & Francis, London, 1983.
[6] KILLICK-KENDRICK, R., *Med. vet. Entom.*, **4**, 1 (1990).
[7] *Proceedings Indo-UK Workshop on Leishmaniasis*, Indian Council of Medical Research, New Delhi, 1983.
[8] HART, D. T. (Ed.), *Leishmaniasis; the Current Status and New Strategies for Control*, NATO ASI Series, Ser. A, Life Sciences, Vol. 163, Plenum, New York, 1989.
[9] ALVAR et al., *J. infect. Dis.*, **160**, 560 (1989).
[10] DATRY et al., *Trans. roy. Soc. trop. Med. Hyg.*, **84**, 239 (1990).
[11] HO et al., *Amer. J. trop. Med. Hyg.*, N.S. **32**, 943 (1983).
[12] WHO Model Prescribing Information, *Drugs Used in Parasitic Diseases*, World Health Organization, Geneva, 1990.
[13] *Med. Lett. Drug. Ther.*, **34**, No. 865 (1992).
[14] CHUNGE, C. N., *Trans. roy. Soc. trop. Med. Hyg.*, **84**, 221 (1990).
[15] BERMAN, J. D., *Rev. infect. Dis.*, **10**, 560 (1988).

General References (Continued)

MANSON-BAHR and BELL, *Manson's Tropical Diseases*, 19th ed., Baillière Tindall, London, 1987.

WARREN and MAHMOUD (Eds.), *Tropical and Geographical Medicine*, 2nd ed., McGraw-Hill, New York, 1990.

ZAMAN, V., *Atlas of Medical Parasitology*, 2nd ed., ADIS Health Science Press, Sydney, 1985.

HUBBERT et al. (Eds.), *Diseases Transmitted from Animals to Man*, 6th ed., Thomas, Springfield, 1975.

BAER, J. G., *Ecology of Animal Parasites*, University of Illinois Press, Urbana, 1951.

JENSEN, J. B., *'In Vitro' Cultivation of Protozoan Parasites*, CRC Press, Boca Raton, FL, 1983.

MANSFIELD, J. M., *Parasitic Disease, The Chemotherapy*, Vol. 2, Dekker, New York, 1984.

WERY, M., *Notes de protozoologie médicale*, Institut de Médecine Tropicale Prince Léopold, Brussels, 1983.

MARCIAL-ROJAS, R. A., *Pathology of Protozoal and Helminthic Disease*, Williams & Wilkins, Baltimore, 1971.

BELL, D. R., *Lecture Notes on Tropical Medicine*, Blackwell, Oxford, 1981.

LUMSDEN and EVANS (Eds.), *Biology of Kinetoplastida*, 2 vols, Academic Press, London, 1976.

GILLES, H. M. (Ed.), *Recent Advances in Tropical Medicine*, Churchill Livingstone, London, 1984.

TAYLOR and BAKER, *The Cultivation of Parasites 'In Vitro'*, Blackwell, Oxford, 1968.

GENTILINI et al., *Médecine tropicale*, 2nd ed., Flammarion, Paris, 1977.

KEAN et al. (Eds.), *Tropical Medicine and Parasitology; Classic Investigation*, 2 vols, Cornell University Press, Ithaca, 1978.

GEIGY and HERBIG, *Erreger und Überträger tropischer Krankheiten*, Verlag für Recht und Gesellschaft, Basel, 1955.

PIERKARSKI, G., *Medizinische Parasitologie in Tafeln*, 3rd ed., Springer, Berlin, 1987.

GARNHAM, P. C. C., *Malaria Parasites and other Haemosporidia*, Blackwell, Oxford, 1966.

KREIER and BAKER (Eds.), *Parasitic Protozoa*, Allen & Unwin, Boston, 1987.

LIEW, F. Y., *Vaccination Strategies of Tropical Diseases*, CRC Press, Boca Raton, FL, 1989.

Parasitic and Other Infections in AIDS, *Trans. roy. Soc. trop. Med. Hyg.*, **84**, Suppl. 1, 1–39 (1990).

No.	**Protozoa** *Synonyms*	Characteristics	Habitat Host Transmission	Associated disease
329	**Leishmania tropica** (Wright) Lühe *Leishmania tropica minor*	As for *L. donovani*	Transmitted by *Phlebotomus* (sandflies). Main reservoir host: man[1]	Anthroponotic or urban cutaneous leishmaniasis (Aleppo boil, bouton d'Orient, Delhi boil, Jericho boil, oriental sore). Painless ulceration of skin leading to disfiguring scars; usually heals spontaneously within a year Endemic in the Middle East and India. See map on page 118 Diagnosis: demonstration of amastigotes from edge of lesion; intradermal test (Montenegro test) supporting evidence *Remarks.* Antimony compounds used for *L. donovani* – either given systemically or by local infiltration – are effective[1,2]. Local heat application may accelerate healing[1]. A vaccine has been tested in Israel[3]
330	**Leishmania major** Yakimov and Schockov *Leishmania tropica major*	Length 3–5 µm	Transmitted by *Phlebotomus* (sandflies). Reservoir host: rodents	Zoonotic or rural cutaneous leishmaniasis. Painless but often multiple ulcers in the skin may become confluent leaving large disfiguring scars Endemic in the Middle East, North Africa, the CIS, Afghanistan; sporadic cases in East and West Africa[1] Diagnosis and treatment as for *L. tropica*
331	**Leishmania aethiopica** Bray, Ashford and Bray	As for *L. donovani*	Transmitted by *Phlebotomus* (sandflies). Confined to East Africa highlands where the cave dwelling hyrax is the reservoir. Probably no interhuman transmission[4]	Cutaneous leishmaniasis as for *L. tropica*, but with some diffuse nodular cutaneous lesions (pseudolepromatous)[5,6] Diagnosis and treatment as for *L. tropica*, but *L. aethiopica* is much less responsive to antimony compounds[2]
332	**Leishmania brasiliensis** Vianna Subspecies: *Leishmania braziliensis braziliensis* *L. b. guyanensis* *L. b. panamensis*	As for *L. donovani*	Transmitted by *Lutzomyia* (sandflies). All forms are zoonoses with numerous reservoir hosts including forest rodents, marsupials in Brazil and sloths and monkeys in Panama. No interhuman transmission[7,8]	Cutaneous and mucocutaneous leishmaniasis with ulceration and lymphatic spread; often multiple lesions which fail to heal spontaneously. The Brazilian form (espundia) produces destructive lesions of the oronasopharyngeal mucosa which may lead to death due to secondary infection and pneumonia. *L. b. guyanensis* produces forest yaws or 'pian bois', often with multiple lesions. *L. b. panamensis* is the least pathogenic member of this group[1] Diagnosis as for *L. tropica* *Remark.* Treatment as for *L. donovani*; patients with mucocutaneous lesion may not respond, and plastic surgery is often necessary[9]. In treatment of *L. b. panamensis* infections, a combination of allopurinol with meglumine antimoniate was more effective than meglumine antimoniate alone[10]

[1] WHO Expert Committee on Control of the Leishmaniases, *Wld Hlth Org. techn. Rep. Ser.*, No. 793 (1990).
[2] WHO Model Prescribing Information, *Drugs Used in Parasitic Diseases*, World Health Organization, Geneva, 1990.
[3] Green et al., *Trans. roy. Soc. trop. Med. Hyg.*, **77**, 152 (1983).
[4] Molyneux and Ashford, *The Biology of Trypanosoma and Leishmania; Parasites of Man and Animals*, Taylor & Francis, London, 1983.
[5] Bryceson, A. D., *Trans. roy. Soc. trop. Med. Hyg.*, **63**, 708 (1969).
[6] Bryceson, A. D., *Trans. roy. Soc. trop. Med. Hyg.*, **64**, 369, 380 (1970).
[7] Lainson, R., *Trans. roy. Soc. trop. Med. Hyg.*, **77**, 569 (1983).
[8] Christensen et al., *J. med. Entom.*, **20**, 463 (1983).
[9] Marsden and Monata, *Rev. Soc. brasil. Med. trop.*, **9**, 297 (1975).
[10] Martinez and Marr, *New Engl. J. Med.*, **326**, 741 (1992).

No.	**Protozoa** *Synonyms*	Characteristics	Habitat Host Transmission	Associated disease
333	**Leishmania mexicana** Subspecies: *Leishmania mexicana mexicana* *L.m. amazonensis* *L.m. venezuelensis* *L.m. garnhami*	As for *L. donovani*	Transmitted by *Lutzomyia* (sandflies). As with *L. braziliensis*, all forms of *L. mexicana* are zoonoses with forest animals as reservoir hosts. No interhuman transmission[1,2]	Mainly cutaneous indolent nodular or ulcerating lesions. *L.m. mexicana* cause 'chiclero's ulcer', an affection of gum collectors causing severe destruction of the ear[3]. The relatively mild condition known as 'uta' which affects children in the Andes is caused by *L. peruviana*[3] Diagnosis and treatment as for *L. braziliensis*
334	**Trypanosoma brucei gambiense** DUTTON	Flagellate, 15–30 µm in length, with an undulating membrane and characteristic internal organelles including the kinetoplast which contains DNA. Members of the *T. brucei* group are polymorphic with short, intermediate and long forms. The two subspecies infecting man are indistinguishable morphologically from the animal parasite *T.b. brucei*, but can be separated on the basis of host infectivity and pathogenicity and by biochemical techniques to characterize their isoenzymes or DNA[4,5]	Transmitted by tsetse flies (*Glossina palpalis*, *G. fuscipes* and *G. tachinoides*) which are mainly confined to riverine and lacustrine habitats[6]. Although pigs, dogs and some antelopes have been found infected, man is the main reservoir host. Transmission predominantly interhuman[7,8]	African trypanosomiasis (sleeping sickness) is of the chronic type[9-11]. Following the initial trypanosome chancre in the skin there is involvement of the lymph nodes, especially in the neck, associated with irregular pyrexia and headache with the eventual involvement of the central nervous system: meningoencephalitis characterized by mental and speech disturbances, ataxia, somnolence and, after many months of illness, coma and death Occurs mainly in the tropical region of West and Central Africa extending into the southern Sudan and Uganda and Kenya[11,12]. See map on page 120 Diagnosis: finding of trypanosomes in the blood, lymph node juice, or CSF. There are usually very few parasites in the peripheral circulation, and it is necessary to use a concentration method such as the anion exchange centrifugation technique[13]. A card agglutination test is available for epidemiological studies[14] *Remarks*. For treatment of early hematolymphopathic stage, suramin or eflornithine are the drugs of choice, pentamidine an effective alternative[15,16]. In the late stage with central nervous system involvement, drugs which cross the blood–brain barrier, such as melarsoprol[15,16], nifurtimox[17], or preferentially eflornithine[16,18], should be used

[1] LAINSON, R., *Trans. roy. Soc. trop. Med. Hyg.*, **77**, 569 (1983).
[2] CHRISTENSEN et al., *J. med. Entom.*, **20**, 463 (1983).
[3] WHO Expert Committee on Control of the Leishmaniases, *Wld Hlth Org. techn. Rep. Ser.*, No. 793 (1990).
[4] GODFREY et al., *Advanc. Parasit.*, **29**, 1 (1990).
[5] GIBSON et al., *Advanc. Parasit.*, **18**, 175 (1980).
[6] MULLIGAN and POTTS, *African Trypanosomiases*, Allen & Unwin, London, 1970.
[7] MOLYNEUX and ASHFORD, *The Biology of Trypanosoma and Leishmania: Parasites of Man and Domestic Animals*, Taylor & Francis, London, 1983.
[8] NELSON, G. S., in DUNSMORE, J. D. (Ed.), *Tropical Parasitoses and Parasitic Zoonoses*, World Association for the Advancement of Veterinary Parasitology, Perth, 1983, page 59.
[9] MANSON-BAHR and BELL, *Manson's Tropical Diseases*, 19th ed., Baillière Tindall, London, 1987.
[10] HAJDUK et al., in WARREN and MAHMOUD (Eds.), *Tropical and Geographical Medicine*, 2nd ed., McGraw-Hill, New York, 1990, page 268.
[11] WHO Expert Committee on Epidemiology and Control of African Trypanosomiasis, *Wld Hlth Org. techn. Rep. Ser.*, No. 739 (1986).
[12] FREZIL, J. L., *La trypanosomiase humaine en république populaire du Congo*, Travaux et documents de l'ORSTOM, No. 155, 1983.
[13] LUMSDEN et al., *Trans. roy. Soc. trop. Med. Hyg.*, **74**, 41 (1980).
[14] VICKERMAN and BARRY, in COHEN and WARREN (Eds.), *Immunology of Parasitic Infections*, 2nd ed., Blackwell, Oxford, 1982, page 204.
[15] WHO Model Prescribing Information, *Drugs Used in Parasitic Diseases*, World Health Organization, Geneva, 1990.
[16] *Med. Lett. Drug. Ther.*, **34**, No. 865 (1992).
[17] PEPIN et al., *Trans. roy. Soc. trop. Med. Hyg.*, **83**, 514 (1989).
[18] EOZENOU et al., *Méd. trop.*, **49**, 149 (1989).

No.	Protozoa *Synonyms*	Characteristics	Habitat Host Transmission	Associated disease
335	**Trypanosoma brucei rhodesiense** STEPHENS and FANTHAM	Morphologically identical with *T.b.gambiense* and *T.b.brucei*	Zoonosis, maintained in nature in wild antelopes. Transmitted by the savanna tsetse flies *Glossina morsitans*, *G.pallidipes* and *G.swynnertoni* from wild animals to man, cattle and dogs[1,2]. Epidemics have occurred with interhuman transmission by *G.fuscipes* in Kenya and Uganda and by *G.tachinoides* in Ethiopia[3]	African trypanosomiasis (sleeping sickness) of the more acute type[4-6]. Usually severe pyrexial illness with lymphadenopathy and involvement of the CNS with a fatal outcome within a few weeks of onset. A few individuals may harbor the parasites for long periods with no ill effects Occurs mainly in East Africa from Ethiopia as far south as Zimbabwe. See map on page 120 Diagnosis: as for *T.b.gambiense*, but trypanosomes are more easily found in the peripheral blood, and the parasite is much more virulent in laboratory animals. A test for circulating antigen has been developed[7] *Remark*. Treatment as for *T.b. gambiense*, but with less response to eflornithine[8]
336	**Trypanosoma cruzi** CHAGAS *Schizotrypanum cruzi*	Blood forms: crescent-shaped trypanosomes with an undulating membrane, free flagellum and large, round kinetoplast; length 20 µm. Leishmanial tissue forms: 1.5–4.5 µm in length. Isoenzyme techniques have shown that there are several distinct zymodemes of *T.cruzi* with differences in host infectivity, pathogenicity and epidemiology[9,10]. *T.cruzi* must be distinguished from *T.rangeli*, a nonpathogenic trypanosome which is transmitted to man by bugs in Central and South America[11]	Zoonosis, maintained in nature in a wide range of South American wild and domestic animals including rodents, bats, marsupials, dogs and edentates. Transmitted by the feces of bugs of the family Reduviidae (*Triatoma*, *Rhodnius*, *Panstrongylus*, etc.)[12]. Man can be infected by bugs from a reservoir host or by interhuman transmission. Transmission can occur by blood transfusion or congenitally[12]	American trypanosomiasis (CHAGAS' disease)[12-14]. 3 stages are recognized: – Acute stage: swelling of the eyelids and edema of the face (ROMAÑA's sign). Often mild and atypical symptoms (fever, hepatomegaly, splenomegaly, generalized edema, lymphadenopathy) – Indeterminate stage: begins 8–10 weeks after the acute stage, may last for years or persist indefinitely. No clinical symptoms – Chronic stage: 10–20 years after contamination up to 30% of persons with the indeterminate form will suffer from cardiomyopathy, digestive tract damage (megaviscera), or neurological symptoms Widespread in Central and South America with the highest prevalence in Venezuela, Brazil and Argentina, especially in rural areas Diagnosis: finding of *T.cruzi* in the blood – either by direct examination or by xenodiagnosis[15] using clean bugs fed on the patient. Serology[12,16] and DNA probes[17] may be helpful *Remarks*. For treatment of the acute stage, nifurtimox is the drug of choice, benznidazole an effective alternative[12,18]. Symptomatic treatment during the chronic stage[12]

1 MULLIGAN and POTTS, *African Trypanosomiases*, Allen & Unwin, London, 1970.
2 MOLYNEUX and ASHFORD, *The Biology of Trypanosoma and Leishmania; Parasites of Man and Domestic Animals*, Taylor & Francis, London, 1983.
3 BAKER, J. R., in *Trypanosomiasis and Leishmaniasis*, Ciba Foundation Symposium 20 (new series), Elsevier, Amsterdam, 1974, page 29.
4 MANSON-BAHR and BELL, *Manson's Tropical Diseases*, 19th ed., Baillière Tindall, London, 1987.
5 HAJDUK et al., in WARREN and MAHMOUD (Eds.), *Tropical and Geographical Medicine*, 2nd ed., McGraw-Hill, New York, 1990, page 268.
6 WHO Expert Committee on Epidemiology and Control of African Trypanosomiasis, *Wld Hlth Org. techn. Rep. Ser.*, No. 739 (1986).
7 NANTULYA, V. M., *Parasite Immun.*, **11**, 69 (1989).
8 *TDR News*, **34**, 1 (1990).
9 MILES et al., *Nature (Lond.)*, **272**, 819 (1978).
10 BARRETT et al., *Trans. roy. Soc. trop. Med. Hyg.*, **74**, 84 (1980).
11 AÑEZ, N., *Mem. Inst. Oswaldo Cruz*, **77**, 405 (1982).
12 WHO Expert Committee on Control of Chagas disease, *Wld Hlth Org. techn. Rep. Ser.*, No. 811 (1991).
13 MANSON-BAHR and BELL, *Manson's Tropical Diseases*, 19th ed., Baillière Tindall, London, 1987.
14 NOGUEIRA and COURA, in WARREN and MAHMOUD (Eds.), *Tropical and Geographical Medicine*, 2nd ed., McGraw-Hill, New York, 1990, page 281.
15 MARSDEN, P. D., *Int. Rev. trop. Med.*, **4**, 97 (1971).
16 SCOTT and SNARY, in COHEN and WARREN (Eds.), *Immunology of Parasitic Diseases*, 2nd ed., Blackwell, Oxford, 1982, page 261.
17 MOSER et al., *J. clin. Microbiol.*, **27**, 1477 (1989).
18 *Med. Lett. Drug. Ther.*, **34**, No. 865 (1992).

No.	Protozoa *Synonyms*	Characteristics	Habitat Host Transmission	Associated disease
337	**Retortamonas intestinalis** (WENYON and O'CONNOR) WENRICH *Embadomonas intestinalis*	Length 4–9 µm; 2 flagella. Cysts, 4–6 µm in length	Probably zoonosis. Colon; rare in man	Probably nonpathogenic
338	**Chilomastix mesnili** (WENYON) ALEXEIEFF	Length 6–20 µm; 3 flagella. Lemon-shaped cysts, 7–10 µm in length	Cecum. Worldwide distribution; 1–10% infection rate	Probably nonpathogenic
339	**Enteromonas hominis** DA FONESCA	Length 4–10 µm; 4 flagella. Ovoid cysts, 6–8 µm in length	Cecum. Worldwide distribution	Probably nonpathogenic
340	**Giardia intestinalis** (LAMBL) *Giardia lamblia*	Length 10–20 µm; pear-shaped with 2 sucking discs, 2 nuclei, 8 flagella. Ovoid cysts, 8–12 µm in length	Duodenum, jejunum. Worldwide distribution. Most infections from food and water contaminated by cysts from human feces, but beavers and dogs suspected reservoir hosts. *Giardia* is not a uniform species and not all strains are infective to man[1]	Giardiasis[2,3]. May be commensal, but is a common cause of diarrhea in children[4] and travellers[5], promiscuous male homosexuals and immunocompromised persons[6,7]. Chronic disease with malabsorption resembling celiac disease (sprue). Incubation period usually 1–3 weeks. Infection may last, if untreated, 4–6 weeks. Symptoms occur in as few as 20% of infections[12] About 200 million infections occur annually in Africa, Asia and Latin America[8] Diagnosis: usually by finding cysts in feces, but sometimes by jejunal aspirations, by string test, or by serology[9–11] *Remark*. Treatment with a 5-nitroimidazole (e.g. metronidazole, tinidazole) is highly effective[8]
341	**Trichomonas hominis** (DAVAINE) LEUCKART	Length 5–14 µm, 4 free flagella, 1 on undulating membrane. No cyst	Colon; commonest intestinal flagellate. Worldwide distribution	Probably nonpathogenic, but associated with diarrhea *Remark*. Treatment usually unnecessary, but metronidazole is effective
342	**Trichomonas vaginalis** (DONNÉ)	Length up to 23 µm; 4 free flagella, 1 on undulating membrane. No cyst	Vagina, prostate. Worldwide distribution. Transmitted by sexual intercourse. In the USA, infection rates about 5% in adult women consulting family planning clinics, 13–25% in women attending gynecology clinics[1]; in tropical countries, 15–40% in healthy women in child-bearing age[2]	Trichomoniasis[13–16]. Most prevalent venereal disease. Lesions usually confined to lower urogenital tract causing vaginitis and urethritis Diagnosis: direct demonstration of the organisms in genital exudates or urine, especially in men after prostatic massage *Remarks*. Oral treatment with a 5-nitroimidazole (e.g. metronidazole, tinidazole) is highly effective[8,16,17]. Intravaginal treatment with acidifying jellies or clotrimazole in pregnancy, when 5-nitroimidazoles are contraindicated, or in women when drug resistance occurs, may be effective[8,16]. Sexual partners should be treated

1 THOMPSON et al., *Protozool. Abstr.*, **14**, 1 (1990).
2 MANSON-BAHR and BELL, *Manson's Tropical Diseases*, 19th ed., Baillière Tindall, London, 1987.
3 STEVENS and GILLIN, in WARREN and MAHMOUD (Eds.), *Tropical and Geographical Medicine*, 2nd ed., McGraw-Hill, New York, 1990, page 344.
4 KEYSTONE et al., *Canad. med. Ass. J.*, **119**, 241 (1978).
5 BRANDBORG, L. L., *Gastroenterology*, **78**, 1602 (1980).
6 STEVENS, D. P., in COHEN and WARREN (Eds.), *Immunology of Parasitic Infections*, 2nd ed., Blackwell, Oxford, 1982, page 192.
7 FARTHING, M. J., *Quart. J. Med.*, N.S. **70**, 191 (1989).
8 WHO Model Prescribing Information, *Drugs Used in Parasitic Diseases*, World Health Organization, Geneva, 1990.
9 JOKIPII and JOKIPII, *Ann. trop. Med. Parasit.*, **74**, 93 (1980).
10 CRAFT and NELSON, *J. infect. Dis.*, **145**, 499 (1982).
11 WIENECKA et al., *Scand. J. infect. Dis.*, **21**, 443 (1989).
12 CASEMORE, D. P., *Lancet*, **336**, 1427 (1990).
13 SOBEL, J. D., *Med. Clin. N. Amer.*, **74**, 1573 (1990).
14 WHO Scientific Group on Nongonococcal Urethritis and Other Selected Sexually Transmitted Diseases of Public Health Importance, *Wld Hlth Org. techn. Rep. Ser.*, No. 660 (1981).
15 REIN and MÜLLER, in HOLMES et al. (Eds.), *Sexually Transmitted Diseases*, 2nd ed., McGraw-Hill, New York, 1990, page 481.
16 QUINN and KRIEGER, in WARREN and MAHMOUD (Eds.), *Tropical and Geographical Medicine*, 2nd ed., McGraw-Hill, New York, 1990, page 358.
17 *Med. Lett. Drug. Ther.*, **34**, No. 865 (1992).

No.	**Protozoa** *Synonyms*	Characteristics	Habitat Host Transmission	Associated disease
343	**Trichomonas tenax** (MÜLLER) DOBELL *Tetratrichomonas buccalis*	Length 6–10 μm; similar to other *Trichomonas* species	Oral cavity, possibly also respiratory tract. Worldwide distribution. Transmitted by kissing and probably droplets	Probably nonpathogenic, but may be associated with other oral diseases *Remark*. Treatment not usually necessary, but metronidazole can be used
344	**Dientamoeba fragilis** (JEPPS and DOBELL)	Length 5–12 μm; 2 nuclei. No cyst	Colon. Widespread. Prevalence underestimated because rarely seen with standard fecal examination methods. May be transmitted through the egg of *Enterobius vermicularis*	Probably nonpathogenic[1], abdominal discomfort possible *Remark*. Treatment not usually necessary, but metronidazole can be used
345	**Entamoeba histolytica** (SCHAUDINN) *Entamoeba dysenteriae* *Entamoeba dispar*	Trophozoite diameter 20–60 μm; clear ectoplasm, granular endoplasm; single nucleus. Pathogenic strains contain ingested erythrocytes. Cysts (10–20 μm, 'large race') with 4 nuclei when mature. Isoenzyme characterization helps to distinguish pathogenic from nonpathogenic strains of *E. histolytica*. It is essential to distinguish *E. histolytica* from nonpathogenic intestinal amebae	Cecum and colon. Worldwide distribution, but pathogenic strains mainly tropical. Transmission by ingestion of cysts by fecal–oral route or by homosexual activities. No animal reservoir	Amebiasis. See text on next page
346	**Entamoeba hartmanni** (VON PROWAZEK)	Trophozoite diameter 4–12 μm; cysts 5–10 μm ('small race'). Easily mistaken for *E. histolytica*	Host and transmission as for *E. histolytica*	Nonpathogenic
347	**Entamoeba coli** (GRASSI)	Trophozoite diameter 15–50 μm; cysts (10–30 μm) with 8 nuclei when mature	Host and transmission as for *E. histolytica*. Worldwide distribution; up to 50% infection rate in the tropics	Nonpathogenic
347a	**Entamoeba polecki** VON PROWAZEK	Similar to *E. histolytica*; uninucleated cysts	Common pathogen of pigs and monkeys, occasionally infects man	Nonpathogenic
348	**Entamoeba gingivalis** (GROS) BRUMPT	Diameter 10–20 μm; similar to *E. histolytica*, but very rarely ingests erythrocytes. No cysts	Worldwide distribution. In healthy and unhygienic mouths. Lives in gingival tissue around teeth; also reported from vagina when intrauterine devices are used. Direct spread. Similar if not identical species in many animals	Probably never pathogenic
349	**Endolimax nana** (WENYON and O'CONNOR)	Diameter 6–15 μm. Ovoid cysts with up to 4 nuclei	Worldwide distribution. Transmission as for *E. histolytica*. Also a common parasite of monkeys	Nonpathogenic
350	**Iodamoeba bütschii** (VON PROWAZEK) DOBELL	Diameter 6–25 μm. Ovoid cysts (6–15 μm) with single nucleus and large vacuole	Worldwide distribution. Transmission as for *E. histolytica*	Nonpathogenic

[1] YANG and SCHOLTEN, *Amer. J. trop. Med. Hyg.*, N.S. **26**, 16 (1977).

Amebiasis

Over 90% of individuals passing cysts of *Entamoeba histolytica* show no evidence of disease. *E. histolytica* has been reported from almost every country in the world including the Arctic regions, but the parasite is most prevalent in areas with poor hygiene in the tropics and subtropics, where infection rates may exceed 50%[1]. It has been estimated that 480 million people are infected with *E. histolytica* and 36–48 million suffer from invasive amebiasis. The latter, in the intestinal and extraintestinal forms, accounts for 40000 to 110000 deaths annually[2].

Most of the strains of *E. histolytica* are nonpathogenic, and they can be distinguished from pathogenic or invasive strains by their isoenzyme pattern[3,4], their genomic DNA[5] and by the use of monoclonal antibodies[6]. It is not known why some strains (or zymodemes) are invasive and become disseminated whereas other strains remain as commensals[7]. Both parasite and host factors, such as nutritional status, are involved, and immunosuppression can result in the activation of silent infections.

The normal habitat of *E. histolytica* is the large intestine, especially the cecum and rectosigmoid colon. The life cycle consists of 3 consecutive stages: trophozoite, cyst, metacyst. The trophozoites multiply by binary fission and invade the wall of the colon, where they can cause ulceration with dysentery and some may be disseminated and produce abscesses in the liver, lungs or brain. Most of the infections in the bowel are harmless, the trophozoites encyst and are passed out in the feces to complete the life cycle when the cysts are ingested, usually from contaminated water or food. *E. histolytica* has become increasingly prevalent among male homosexuals, probably as a result of colonic irrigation or direct transfer of trophozoites or cysts into the lower bowel[8], but there is no evidence that AIDS precipitates invasive amebiasis[9].

Clinical manifestations

The manifestations of intestinal amebiasis are acute and chronic amebic dysentery. Rare complications of intestinal amebiasis include perforation, peritonitis, ameboma, intussusception, amebic appendicitis, postdysenteric colitis, stricture and cutaneous amebiasis around the anus. The commonest form of extra-intestinal amebiasis, which may or may not be associated with or preceded by amebic dysentery, is amebic liver abscess, commonly involving the right lobe of the liver. The cysts may be single or multiple, and rupture of the cysts may occur into the pleura, pericardium or peritoneal cavity. Other extra-intestinal complications include amebic abscess of the brain and lung. In more than half the patients with extra-intestinal amebiasis, *E. histolytica* cannot be isolated from the feces.

Diagnosis

In amebic dysentery active trophozoites with ingested erythrocytes can be seen in fresh fecal specimens, and in noninvasive infections *E. histolytica* cysts can be found in the feces especially if concentration techniques are used. *In vitro* culture of the trophozoites is of value for diagnosis and essential for obtaining material for isoenzyme characterization of the organisms[10]. In disseminated or invasive amebiasis immunodiagnosis is invaluable for diagnosis and for monitoring the effect of treatment[11]. Where serological tests are not available the probable diagnosis is suggested following successful specific chemotherapy. Radiological and scanning techniques are often diagnostic.

Treatment

Intestinal amebiasis. Where the only evidence of infection is the discovery of *E. histolytica* cysts in the feces, treatment is usually not necessary, but the cysts can be eliminated with diloxanide furoate, iodoquinol or paromomycin[12,13]. Treatment of cyst carriers is essential with food handlers[14]. In amebic dysentery and other forms of active intestinal amebiasis, the infection can be treated with a 5-nitroimidazole (e.g. metronidazole, tinidazole, ornidazole) either alone or combined with a tetracycline, paromomycin, iodoquinol or diloxanide furoate[12,13]. Corticosteroids may cause fulminating amebiasis, so it is essential to differentiate acute amebiasis from ulcerative colitis.

Extra-intestinal amebiasis (liver and other amebic abscesses). In most cases a 5-nitroimidazole (e.g. metronidazole, tinidazole, ornidazole) either alone or combined with paromomycin, iodoquinol or diloxanide furoate is effective[12,13]. Surgical drainage may be necessary for large abscesses. Other drugs which have proved effective, but which are now rarely used, include emetine or dehydroemetine in combination with chloroquine or diloxanide furoate.

Control

Amebiasis is a problem of poverty and insanitary conditions where human feces contaminate the environment. A decrease in incidence can be expected with the general improvement of the economic well-being of the community. In the past specific measures have been impossible to implement because of the inability to distinguish pathogenic from nonpathogenic strains of *E. histolytica*.

Recent advances hold out hope of a much better understanding of the epidemiology, pathogenesis, treatment and control of amebiasis[15–17].

References

1 Elsdon-Dew, R., *Advanc. Parasit.*, **6**, 1 (1968).
2 Ahmed et al., *Rev. infect. Dis.*, **12**, 330 (1990).
3 Sargeaunt and Williams, *Trans. roy. Soc. trop. Med. Hyg.*, **73**, 225 (1979).
4 Sargeaunt, P. G., *Trans. roy. Soc. trop. Med.*, **79**, 86 (1985).
5 Tannich et al., *Proc. Nat. Acad. Sci. (USA)*, **86**, 5118 (1989).
6 Strachan et al., *Lancet*, **1**, 561 (1988).
7 Gathiram and Jackson, *Trans. roy. Soc. trop. Med. Hyg.*, **84**, 806 (1990).
8 Istre et al., *New Engl. J. Med.*, **307**, 339 (1982).
9 Lukas, S. B., *Trans. roy. Soc. trop. Med. Hyg.*, **84**, Suppl. 1, 34 (1990).
10 Gathiram and Jackson, *Lancet*, **2**, 719 (1985).
11 Patterson et al., *Gastroenterology*, **78**, 136 (1980).
12 WHO Model Prescribing Information, *Drugs Used in Parasitic Diseases*, World Health Organization, Geneva, 1990.
13 *Med. Lett. Drug. Ther.*, **34**, No. 865 (1992).
14 Keystone et al., *Trans. roy. Soc. trop. Med. Hyg.*, **77**, 84 (1983).
15 WHO Expert Committee on Amoebiasis, *Wld Hlth Org. techn. Rep. Ser.*, No. 421 (1969).
16 Martinez-Palomo, A. (Ed.), *Amebiasis*, Elsevier, Amsterdam, 1986.
17 Ravdin, J. I. (Ed.), *Amebiasis: Human Infection by Entamoeba histolytica*, Churchill Livingstone, New York, 1988.

No.	**Protozoa** *Synonyms*	Characteristics	Habitat Host Transmission	Associated disease
351	**Acanthamoeba culbertsoni** (SINGH and DAS) SAWYER and GRIFFIN *Hartmanella culbertsoni*	Diameter 10–40 µm. Ameboid form with spiral-like pseudopodia. Double-walled irregular cysts (15–30 µm)	Worldwide distribution. Free-living organism, e.g. in soil, water, dust. Infection by inhalation of dust, aspiration of water, penetration of skin. Invasion through the olfactory neuroepithelium[1]. Direct infection of the cornea, e.g. after contact lens wear, possible[1]	Rare cause of granulomatous amebic encephalitis, uveitis, keratitis, chronic granuloma of the skin and internal organs[1–4]. Debilitated and immunocompromised persons are at risk[1–3]. Incubation period: several weeks or months are necessary to establish granulomatous amebic encephalitis[1] Diagnosis: culture and immunodifferentiation to detect parasites from tissues *Remarks. Acanthamoeba* infections are highly resistant to chemotherapeutic agents, especially in the encysted stage. For local lesions of eye and skin, topical use of propamidine plus neosporin, or oral itraconazole plus topical miconazole[5,6]
352	Other *Acanthamoeba* species of clinical importance: **Acanthamoeba castellanii** **Acanthamoeba astronyxis** **Acanthamoeba hatchetti** **Acanthamoeba palestinensis** **Acanthamoeba polyphaga** **Acanthamoeba rhysodes**	Morphologically similar to *A. culbertsoni*	As for *A. culbertsoni*	As for *A. culbertsoni*
353	**Naegleria fowleri** (CARTER) *Naegleria aerobia* *Naegleria invadens*	Ameboid form, diameter 7 to 20 µm, some transform to flagellate forms with 2 flagella, 20 to 30 µm in length. Uninucleated cysts (7–10 µm)	Worldwide distribution. Free-living organism, e.g. in soil, dust, water, including swimming pools which are the main source of infection in man due to aspiration. Invasion through the olfactory neuroepithelium[1]	Naegleriasis (primary amebic meningoencephalitis) in children and young adults[1–4]. Incubation period varies from 2–3 days to as long as 7–15 days[1]. Disease usually fatal after 3–7 days[1–3] More than 140 cases reported from many parts of the world including Europe and the USA[1] Diagnosis: recognition of the organism in CSF or brain tissue with the finding of trophozoites. For confirmation culture and/or special staining, e.g. indirect antibody tests *Remark.* Treatment with amphotericin B[7]
354	**Cryptosporidium spp.** LÉGER	Trophozoites and schizonts 2 to 5 µm in diameter. Oocysts 4 to 5 µm in diameter when mature	Worldwide distribution. In man and many species of wild and domestic animals. All stages develop in the mucosal epithelium of the intestine. Transmission by the fecal–oral route with large waterborne epidemics[8,9]	Cryptosporidiosis[10], a common cause of acute diarrhea in man and animals, but *Cryptosporidium* may occur as a commensal. Chronic diarrhea in immunocompromised persons, e.g. in patients with AIDS[10–12] Diagnosis: usually by finding of oocysts in feces using acid-fast staining[10] *Remarks.* No satisfactory chemotherapy known. Recovery spontaneous except in immunocompromised persons where octreotide may control diarrhea but not the infection[13]

[1] MA et al., *Rev. infect. Dis.*, **12**, 490 (1990).
[2] BEAVER et al., *Clinical Parasitology*, 9th ed., Lea & Febiger, Philadelphia, 1984.
[3] DUMA, R. J., in WARREN and MAHMOUD (Eds.), *Tropical and Geographical Medicine*, 2nd ed., McGraw-Hill, New York, 1990, page 321.
[4] SEIDEL, J., *Pediat. Clin. N. Amer.*, **32**, 881 (1985).
[5] MOORE and MCCULLEY, *Brit. J. Ophthal.*, **73**, 271 (1989).
[6] ISHIBASHI et al., *Amer. J. Ophthal.*, **109**, 121 (1990).
[7] *Med. Lett. Drug. Ther.*, **34**, No. 865 (1992).
[8] SMITH et al., *Lancet*, **2**, 1484 (1988).
[9] HAYES et al., *New Engl. J. Med.*, **320**, 1372 (1989).
[10] CURRENT and GARCIA, *Clin. Microbiol. Rev.*, **4**, 325 (1991).
[11] CURRENT, W. L., in WALZER and GENTA (Eds.), *Parasitic Infections in the Compromised Host*, Dekker, New York, 1989, page 281.
[12] CANNING, E. U., *Trans. roy. Soc. trop. Med. Hyg.*, **84**, Suppl. 1, 19 (1990).
[13] COOK et al., *Ann. intern. Med.*, **108**, 708 (1988).

No.	Protozoa *Synonyms*	Characteristics	Habitat Host Transmission	Associated disease
355	**Isospora belli** WENYON	Trophozoites and schizonts 12 to 15 µm in diameter. Ovoid oocysts (10–15 µm by 22–33 µm)	Worldwide distribution. Probably a zoonosis. Typical coccidial life cycle with all stages developing in the mucosal epithelium of the intestine. Transmission by ingestion of oocysts	Isosporiasis (human coccidiosis), a rare cause of chronic diarrhea with possible malabsorption which may be accelerated in patients with AIDS[1] Diagnosis: finding of oocysts in feces *Remark.* Treatment with trimethoprim–sulfamethoxazole or pyrimethamine may be effective[2,3]
356	**Pneumocystis carinii** DELANOË and DELANOË	Trophozoites, 1–4 µm in diameter, pleomorphic, commonly in clusters. Thick-walled cysts (5 to 8 µm) contain up to 8 intracystic bodies (sporozoites) 1–2 µm in diameter. The precyst (4–6 µm) is an intermediate stage	Widespread saprophyte in lungs of man and animals. Probably transmitted by respiratory droplets[4,5]	*Pneumocystis carinii* pneumonia[6–8]. Often fatal in debilitated and malnourished infants (e.g. marasmus, kwashiorkor). Common in immunocompromised persons, e.g. in patients with AIDS, especially in Europe and North America[8,9]. Rarely extrapulmonary pneumocystosis in AIDS patients, involving lymph nodes, spleen, liver and bone marrow[10] Diagnosis: demonstration of the parasite in material from the lungs strained by either the silver nitrate GOMORI method or with toluidine blue or GIEMSA[11,12]. DNA probes appear promising as diagnostic test[13] *Remarks.* For treatment, trimethoprim–sulfamethoxazole or pentamidine are the drugs of choice[3,14], trimethoprim combined with dapsone or primaquine combined with clindamycin are alternatives[3]. Relapses are common and it may be necessary to give trimetrexate combined with folinic acid[3]. For prophylaxis in patients with AIDS, aerosol pentamidine is suggested[3,15]
357	**Sarcocystis hominis** (RAILLIET and LUCET) LEVINE	Sporocysts, 8–16 µm in diameter, containing 4 sporozoites. Sarcocysts in the muscles of cattle	Worldwide distribution. Zoonosis with cattle as intermediate hosts. Transmission to man by eating inadequately cooked meat and transmission to cattle by sporocysts from human feces[16]	Usually nonpathogenic in man[17], but enteritis has been reported from Thailand[18]
358	**Sarcocystis suihominis** (HEYDORN)	Sporocysts, 10–13 µm in diameter. Other stages similar to *S. hominis*	Worldwide distribution. Zoonosis with pigs as main intermediate hosts[19]. Life cycle similar to *S. hominis* with transmission of sporocysts to pigs from human feces. Occasional reports of sarcocysts in human muscle including heart muscle (*S. 'lindemanni'*) represent the reverse situation with man as an incidental intermediate host[20]	Probably nonpathogenic in man

1 SMITH et al., *Ann. intern. Med.*, **108**, 328 (1988).
2 PAPE et al., *New Engl. J. Med.*, **320**, 1044 (1989).
3 *Med. Lett. Drug. Ther.*, **34**, No. 865 (1992).
4 HUGHES, W. T., *J. infect. Dis.*, **145**, 842 (1982).
5 MATSUMOTO and YOSHIDA, *Parasit. Today*, **2**, 137 (1986).
6 WALZER et al., in WALZER and GENTA (Eds.), *Parasitic Infections in the Compromised Host*, Dekker, New York, 1989, page 83; WALZER, P. D., in MANDELL et al. (Eds.), *Principles and Practice of Infectious Diseases*, 3rd ed., Churchill Livingstone, New York, 1990, page 2103.
7 GLATT and CHIRGWIN, *Arch. intern. Med.*, **150**, 271 (1990).
8 BARTLETT and SMITH, *Clin. Microbiol. Rev.*, **4**, 137 (1991).
9 BLASER and COHN, *Rev. infect. Dis.*, **8**, 21 (1986).
10 RAVIGLIONE, M. C., *Rev. infect. Dis.*, **12**, 1127 (1990).
11 YOSHIDA and IKAI, *Zbl. Bakt.*, **244**, 405 (1979).
12 PINTOZZI et al., *Acta cytol. (Baltimore)*, **23**, 35 (1979).
13 WAKEFIELD et al., *Trans. roy. Soc. trop. Med. Hyg.*, **84**, Suppl. 1, 17 (1990).
14 WHO Model Prescribing Information, *Drugs Used in Parasitic Diseases*, World Health Organization, Geneva, 1990.
15 FALLOON and MASUR, *Amer. J. Med.*, **90**, 415 (1991).
16 ROMMEL et al., *Berl. Münch. tierärztl. Wschr.*, **92**, 457 (1979).
17 BEAVER et al., *Amer. J. trop. Med. Hyg.*, N.S. **28**, 819 (1979).
18 BUNYARATVEJ et al., *Amer. J. trop. Med. Hyg.*, N.S. **31**, 36 (1982).
19 ROMMEL, M., in DUNSMORE, J. D. (Ed.), *Tropical Parasitoses and Parasitic Zoonoses*, World Association for the Advancement of Veterinary Parasitology, Perth, 1983, page 9.
20 MEHLHORN and HEYDORN, *Advanc. Parasit.*, **16**, 43 (1978).

No.	Protozoa *Synonyms*	Characteristics	Habitat Host Transmission	Associated disease
359	**Toxoplasma gondii** NICOLLE and MANCEAUX	Sickle-shaped intracellular tachyzoites (length 3.5–7 µm) seen in acute infection. Chronic stage: cysts in tissues, up to 200 µm in diameter, contain thousands of bradyzoites	Probably most widespread of all protozoal infections with very little intermediate host specificity. The domestic cat is the normal definitive host with the coccidial stages in the intestine. Oocysts are passed in the feces of the cat and infect a wide range of animals including rodents, domestic animals and man	Toxoplasmosis. Worldwide distribution. See text below

Toxoplasmosis

Toxoplasmosis is a zoonosis of worldwide distribution. In many populations, such as in Tahiti, El Salvador and France, infection rates based on serological tests are more than 90% by the 4th decade of life[1]. Serologic surveys indicate that 3–70% of healthy adults in the USA have been infected with *Toxoplasma*[1]. In general, the incidence of the infection varies with the population group and geographic location.

Although toxoplasmosis is probably the most prevalent of all human infections, the life cycle has only been worked out in the past 25 years[2–5]. The primary host is the domestic cat with the sexual stages of the parasite in the intestine. Oocysts are passed in the feces and develop in the external environment to produce infective sporozoites. When the sporozoites are ingested by a wide range of intermediate hosts, including man, they undergo asexual development first as intracellular parasites in the reticuloendothelial tissues and then as cysts in many parts of the body, including the brain. Infection is normally acquired by ingestion of the cysts in undercooked meat and transplacentally. The parasite is usually nonpathogenic, but clinical illness is seen in a few infected individuals, and it can have fatal consequences, especially in infants and increasingly in immunocom promised persons (including patients with AIDS). Toxoplasmosis is greatly underdiagnosed because of the diverse clinical features and the need to confirm the diagnosis by laboratory tests which are not universally available.

The principal clinical forms of toxoplasmosis are as follows:

- *Neonatal (congenitally acquired) toxoplasmosis*

  Congenital toxoplasmosis is acquired when the mother suffers from acute toxoplasmosis during pregnancy. It may lead to stillbirth, abortion or prematurity, but many infants infected in utero are normal at birth but later develop a generalized illness with involvement of the reticuloendothelial and central nervous systems[5–7]. The common complications are:

  (a) Lymphadenopathy, hepatomegaly, splenomegaly, fever and jaundice
  (b) Convulsions, choroidoretinitis, hydrocephaly, microcephaly, palsies, deafness and mental retardation

- *Acquired (postnatal) toxoplasmosis*

  This is usually seen following the ingestion of infected inadequately cooked meat or in laboratory workers who have been exposed to infection. The incubation period is 7–17 days[7]. The signs and symptoms include fever which may be influenza-like persisting for several weeks, headache, lymphadenopathy (usually the cervical glands), myalgia, anorexia, arthralgia and occasionally hepatitis[7, 8].

- *Ocular toxoplasmosis*

  Choroidoretinitis may be a complication of both neonatal and acquired toxoplasmosis. It is usually a unilateral chronic infection[9] and may be a presenting feature in patients with AIDS[7].

- *Opportunistic toxoplasmosis*

  In immunocompromised persons (including patients with AIDS), toxoplasmosis is usually the result of a recrudescence of a primary infection or a newly acquired acute infection[7, 10, 11].

Diagnosis

Infection is confirmed directly by demonstrating the parasite in tissues or by culture, or by animal inoculation, or indirectly by detecting antibodies or antigens[12].

(a) *Demonstration of the parasites.* The tachyzoites or bradyzoites can be seen in smears from infected tissues after staining with GIEMSA, or they can be seen in histological preparations stained with hematoxylin and eosin or by the use of antibody labelled with fluorescein or enzymes. Material from suspected tissues can be inoculated into the peritoneal cavity of athymic or nude mice or hamsters, and in positive cases tachyzoites can be demon-

Guidelines for interpretation of results of serological tests for antibodies against Toxoplasma gondii*[17]

	Positive titer	Titer in acute infection	Titer in chronic infection	Duration of elevated titer
SABIN–FELDMAN dye test (DT)	1:4; undiluted◊	⩾ 1:1000	1:4 to 1:2000	Years
Indirect fluorescent antibody test (conventional IFA)	1:10	⩾ 1:1000	1:4 to 1:2000	Years
Indirect hemagglutination test (IHA)†	1:16	⩾ 1:1000	1:16 to 1:256	Years
Complement-fixation test	1:4	Varies among laboratories	Negative to 1:8	Years
Agglutination test§	1:20	1:20 to ⩾ 1:1000	⩽ 1:12000 to 1:64000	Years
Indirect fluorescent antibody test for IgM antibodies (IgM-IFA)**				
– Infants	1:2	⩾ 1:2	Negative	Weeks to months
– Adults◊◊	1:16	⩾ 1:64	1:20	Weeks to months
Double sandwich ELISA for IgM (IgM-ELISA)††				
– Infants	1.0	⩾ 1.4	Unknown	Unknown
– Adults	1.7	⩾ 1.7	Negative to 3	Months to years

* Exceptions to these generalizations may occur. Also, values obtained in different laboratories may differ significantly.
◊ In toxoplasma chororoidoretinitis, the DT may be positive in undiluted serum only.
† The IHA may give false-negative results early in infection. Therefore, IHA should not be used to detect congenital infection or infection during pregnancy.
§ The agglutination test titers agree closely with DT titers.
** The IgM-IFA and the conventional IgM-ELISA (but not the double sandwich IgM-ELISA as described by NAOT and REMINGTON[18]), may give false-positive results in sera containing rheumatoid factor or antinuclear antibody.
◊◊ 'Natural' IgM antibodies occur in older children and adults but not in the neonate. This is the reason for difference in titers considered positive between infants and adults.
†† Titers are expressed as numerical values.

No.	**Protozoa** *Synonyms*	Characteristics	Habitat Host Transmission	Associated disease
360	**Plasmodium (Plasmodium) vivax** GRASSI and FELETTI *Haemamoeba vivax* *Plasmodium tertianae* Strains: *Plasmodium vivax hibernaus* *Plasmodium vivax multinucleatum*	Illustrations on pages 114, 115. Interval between asexual cycles 48 hours (tertian). Hypnozoites responsible for true relapses	Transmitted by *Anopheles* spp. female mosquitos. In the tropics the prepatent period is usually 15 days. Strains in northern latitudes (e.g. *P. vivax hibernaus*) have a very long prepatent period of more than 9 months For life cycle of *Plasmodium* spp., see text on next page	Benign tertian malaria. Widespread in tropical and subtropical regions; especially common in India and other parts of Asia, but very rarely fatal. Absent from pure Negroes of West African origin due to genetic insusceptibility For diagnosis and treatment, see text on pages 112, 113
361	**Plasmodium (Plasmodium) malariae** (GRASSI and FELETTI) *Haemamoeba malariae* *Plasmodium quartanae*	Illustrations on pages 114, 115. Interval between asexual cycles 72 hours (quartan). Infection persists for many years, but no hypnozoites	Transmitted by *Anopheles* spp. female mosquitos. Identical parasite (*P. rhodaini*) in African apes and in South American monkeys (*P. brazilianum*), but most human infections due to interhuman transmission For life cycle of *Plasmodium* spp., see text on next page	Quartan malaria (also malaria nephrotic syndrome). Widespread in all tropical regions For diagnosis and treatment, see text on pages 112, 113
362	**Plasmodium (Plasmodium) ovale** STEPHENS	Illustrations on pages 114, 115. Similar to *P. vivax*. Interval between asexual cycle 50 hours	Transmitted by *Anopheles* spp. female mosquitos For life cycle of *Plasmodium* spp., see text on next page	Ovale malaria (similar to benign tertian malaria). Largely confined to tropical Africa For diagnosis and treatment, see text on pages 112, 113
363	**Plasmodium (Laverania) falciparum** WELCH *Laverania malariae* *Haemamoeba praecox*	Illustrations on pages 114, 115. Interval between asexual cycles 48 hours. No relapse forms. Different subgenus with characteristic gametocytes	Transmitted by *Anopheles* spp. female mosquitos. Resistance of the parasite to chemotherapy and resistance of the *Anopheles* vectors to insecticides are increasing problems For life cycle of *Plasmodium* spp., see text on next page	Malignant tertian malaria (subtertian quotidian); also malaria encephalitis and blackwater fever. Widespread in the tropics, where it is a major cause of morbidity. Genetic abnormalities in the erythrocytes affect susceptibility and may reduce morbidity For diagnosis and treatment, see text on pages 112, 113

strated after 4–8 days. The parasites can also be grown in a variety of cell culture systems.

(b) *Immunodiagnosis*. Serological diagnosis depends on the demonstration of a rise in antibody titer between two or more specimens. IgM antibody develops early in the infection, but disappears to be replaced by IgG in the chronic stages. In some laboratories the SABIN-FELDMAN dye test is still used. This requires living *Toxoplasma* organisms; it is highly specific but does not separate IgG and IgM. Many other serological tests are available, including complement-fixation test and indirect hemagglutination, but they have been mainly replaced by enzyme-linked immunosorbent assay (ELISA) for the detection of either antibodies or antigens. Antibody levels are usually low in patients with AIDS[13].

A delayed hypersensitivity skin test is useful for epidemiological studies.

Treatment

The acute stage of the disease is best treated with a combination of pyrimethamine plus sulfadiazine – supplemented with folinic acid if there is evidence of decreased platelet or leukocyte counts[14, 15]. Spiramycin has been recommended as an alternative for the treatment of pregnant women and patients with AIDS[14]. Clindamycin may be of value for treatment of acute toxoplasmosis of the central nervous system[15, 19–21]. Corticosteroids can be given with a sulfonamide and pyrimethamine in patients with choroidoretinitis[14], but they must not be given alone because of the dangers of increasing parasite densities due to immunosuppression. It is doubtful if existing drugs have any effect on chronic infections; and most cases of postnatally acquired toxoplasmosis are self-limiting and need no treatment[16].

Control

The control of toxoplasmosis depends on limiting the cat population to prevent the dissemination of the oocysts. As this is an insurmountable problem and as most human infections are acquired from meat, the best method of limiting transmission to man is by ensuring that all meat is cooked to 60 °C.

References

1 MCCABE and REMINGTON, in MANDELL et al. (Eds.), *Principles and Practice of Infectious Diseases*, 3rd ed., Churchill Livingstone, New York, 1990, page 2090.
2 JACKSON and HUTCHINSON, *Advanc. Parasit.*, **28**, 55 (1989).
3 FRENKEL and RUIZ, *Amer. J. Epidem.*, **113**, 254 (1981).
4 BEVERLEY, J. K., *Vet. Rec.*, **99**, 123 (1976).
5 FRENKEL, J. K., *Parasit. Today*, **4**, 273 (1988).
6 WILSON et al., *Paediatrics*, **66**, 767 (1980).
7 COOK, G. C., *Quart. J. Med.*, N.S. **74**, 3 (1990).
8 KEAN et al., *J. Amer. med. Ass.*, **208**, 1002 (1969).
9 RAO and FONT, *Arch. Ophthal.*, **95**, 273 (1977).
10 RUSKIN and REMINGTON, *Ann. intern. Med.*, **84**, 193 (1976).
11 HOLLIMAN, R. E., *J. Infect.*, **16**, 121 (1988).
12 WELCH et al., *J. infect. Dis.*, **142**, 256 (1980).
13 LUFT, B. J., in WALZER and GENTA (Eds.), *Parasitic Infections in the Compromised Host*, Dekker, New York, 1989, page 179.
14 WHO Model Prescribing Information, *Drugs Used in Parasitic Diseases*, World Health Organization, Geneva, 1990.
15 *Med. Lett. Drug. Ther.*, **34**, No. 365 (1992).
16 FRENKEL, J. K., in STICKLAND, G. T. (Ed.), *Hunter's Tropical Medicine*, 7th ed., Saunders, Philadelphia, 1991, page 658.
17 MCCABE and REMINGTON, in WARREN and MAHMOUD (Eds.), *Tropical and Geographical Medicine*, 2nd ed., McGraw-Hill, New York, 1990, page 309.
18 NAOT and REMINGTON, *J. infect. Dis.*, **142**, 757 (1980).
19 RUF and POHLE, *Europ. J. Microbiol. infect. Dis.*, **10**, 183 (1991).
20 UBERTI FOPPA et al., *Europ. J. Microbiol. infect. Dis.*, **10**, 187 (1991).
21 KATLAMA, C., *Europ. J. Microbiol. infect. Dis.*, **10**, 189 (1991).

Malaria

Malaria is the most important parasitic disease affecting man. It is caused by 4 species of the genus *Plasmodium* (*P. vivax*, *P. malariae*, *P. ovale*, *P. falciparum*). The parasites are transmitted by female anopheline mosquitoes or by inoculation of infected blood (e.g. transfusion malaria, congenital malaria). Malaria associated with complications or a fatal outcome is almost always caused by *P. falciparum*.

In 1990, the World Health Organization estimated that 2073 million people are exposed to the risk of malaria, that about 270 million of these are infected with malaria parasites, 110 million develop clinical malaria every year – of which 90 million are in tropical Africa – and at least 1 million die with malaria every year[1]. As a result of increased travel to the tropics, cases of imported malaria are seen in Europe and North America with many thousands of cases requiring treatment every year[2]. Cases of congenital malaria in Europe and the USA in children born to mothers who have left the endemic areas have been reported[3], and 'airport' malaria has occurred in Britain, Belgium, France, Holland and Switzerland due to infected mosquitoes being transported accidentally in aircraft travelling from endemic areas[4].

The discovery of residual insecticides and highly effective drugs, such as chloroquine, led the World Health Organization in 1955 to declare a policy of global eradication, but more recently it has been recognized that the worldwide eradication of malaria is not an attainable goal in the foreseeable future[5]:
- In 1990 there are still no commercially available vaccines
- There have been very few advances in chemotherapy, and *Plasmodium falciparum* is becoming increasingly resistant to antimalarial drugs (see map on page 119 for chloroquine resistance)
- There have been no major advances in control of the *Anopheles* vectors

Life cycle of Plasmodium *in man*

First phase; tissue phase (preerythrocytic development)

The sporozoites are inoculated into man when infected female anopheline mosquitoes take a blood meal. The sporozoites remain in the blood stream for less than an hour. Initial development takes place in the hepatocytes either as the single-celled dormant hypnozoites in *P. vivax* or *P. ovale* malaria or as a rapidly multiplying tissue schizont of *P. falciparum* or *P. malariae*. There are no symptoms of malaria during this incubation period. The primary hypnozoite may remain dormant for long periods, for example in China *P. vivax* (*P. vivax multinucleatum*) remains dormant for nearly a year after the initial mosquito bite, and in all cases of *P. vivax* and *P. ovale* malaria the hypnozoites are responsible for relapses for several years after the first attack[6]. The hypnozoites eventually develop into preerythrocytic schizonts which may be 30–70 µm in diameter and produce thousands of merozoites that eventually rupture from the liver cell and invade the erythrocytes.

Second phase; blood phase

(a) *Asexual blood phase.* The merozoites enter the erythrocytes and undergo the stages of development illustrated on pages 114, 115. The early ring forms of trophozoites are similar with all four species, but they then develop into schizonts with morphological characteristics which distinguish the different species. The mature schizonts of *P. falciparum* are very rarely seen in the peripheral blood; they are sequestered in the internal capillaries including the capillaries of the brain, where they are responsible for the pathology resulting in cerebral malaria.

The rupture of the mature schizonts at regular intervals results in the characteristic tertian or quartan fever.

(b) *Sexual blood phase.* Some of the merozoites differentiate into male and female gametocytes which again have distinctive morphological characteristics. They are not pathogenic, and their persistence in the blood for several days after treatment with schizontocidal drugs often gives rise to unnecessary concern.

Life cycle of Plasmodium *in mosquitoes*

Following their ingestion by the mosquito, the male gametocyte produces microgametes which fertilize the female gametocyte to form an ookinete which penetrates the cells of the midgut of the mosquito to form an oocyst. The oocysts produce thousands of sporozoites which migrate to the salivary glands of the mosquito to complete the life cycle when the mosquito takes its next blood meal.

Clinical aspects

Several important advances in relation to the clinical aspects of malaria, and in particular the studies in Gambia and Thailand on *P. falciparum* malaria, have advanced our understanding of the pathogenesis and management of severe malaria[7–10]. Some of the more significant observations include the demonstration that in cerebral malaria
- Retinal hemorrhages are common
- Cerebral edema is not a constant feature
- Hypoglucosemia can occur within 2–3 days of treatment with quinine
- Septicemia is a common complication requiring urgent treatment
- Neurological complications are transient, and complete recovery is the rule after successful treatment even when the patient has been in deep coma
- Acute renal failure is an important complication

Ideally patients with severe malaria should be treated in an intensive care unit, and steroids should not be used in cerebral malaria. With malaria anemia, exchange transfusions may be life-saving if 25% of the erythrocytes are parasitized[11]. Pregnant women, especially primigravidae, are particularly at risk of developing severe malaria. The tropical splenomegaly syndrome is thought to be due to overactivity of B lymphocytes stimulated by malaria antigens; splenectomy in these cases is associated with a very high postoperative mortality[12]. Both riboflavin deficiency and iron deficiency anemia may have some protective effect against malaria in infants[13].

Human genetic factors are of fundamental importance in relation to susceptibility to malaria, e.g. the absence of Duffy blood group on the erythrocytes of Negroes is associated with their total insusceptibility to *P. vivax* infections, hemoglobin S heterozygotes are protected against the lethal effect of *P. falciparum*, and ovalocytosis, common in coastal New Guinea, also protects against *P. falciparum*[14].

Diagnosis

Assessment of clinical symptoms is an imprecise means of diagnosis in malaria[15]. Symptoms may precede a detectable level of parasitemia by a few days, so smears should be examined at least twice daily until parasites are detected. A diagnosis of malaria can only be excluded by obtaining negative blood smears on several successive days.

Microscopical examination of thick blood smears, dehemoglobinized and GIEMSA-stained, allows for the differentiation of the *Plasmodium* species responsible for a malaria infection. The examination of thin blood smears, fixed and GIEMSA-stained, permits better species differentiation and provides information on hematological parameters, but is much less sensitive and may miss low-grade infections.

Chemotherapeutic agents for malaria prophylaxis and treatment

Antimalarial drugs act on different stages of the life cycle:
- Tissue schizontocides act on the hypnozoites and prevent relapses
- Blood schizontocides destroy the asexual parasites in the blood stream; they are also clinical prophylactics in preventing disease
- Gametocytocidal drugs kill the sexual stages, or they can be causal prophylactics and prevent the development of the initial infection

As a general rule individuals with a marked degree of naturally acquired immunity require less drug than nonimmunes. The most important factor determining efficacy is the sensitivity of the local organism to the drug selected. In many regions *P. falciparum* is resistant to a wide range of antimalarials and resistant strains are spreading into most endemic areas[16,17]. For chloroquine resistance, see map on page 119.

The following classes of chemical compounds are in use against malaria:
- Chinchona derivatives: quinine, quinidine
- 4-Aminoquinolines: chloroquine, mefloquine
- 8-Aminoquinolines: primaquine, pamaquine
- Diaminopyrimidines: pyrimethamine
- Phenanthrenemethanols: halofantrine
- Biguanides: proguanil (chlorguanide), chlorproguanil, cycloguanil
- Sulfonamides and sulfones: sulfadoxine, sulfalene, dapsone
- Tetracyclines: tetracycline, doxycycline, minocycline
- Clindamycin
- Sesquiterpene lactones (qinghaosu) are still undergoing clinical trials

Prophylaxis and Treatment

It is essential in all cases to be aware of the species of malaria parasite and if possible the geographical origin of the infection. *P. vivax*, *P. ovale* and *P. malariae* infection are all susceptible to schizontocidal drugs and can be treated with chloroquine or mefloquine, but it is necessary to give primaquine to prevent relapses in *P. vivax* and *P. ovale* infections. Because *P. falciparum* resistant to chloroquine has extended its range to include many parts of Asia, South America and now Africa, and because the parasite may be resistant to other antimalarial drugs, it is not possible to lay down firm rules for either treatment or prophylaxis. When in doubt it is best to assume that resistance does occur.

Chemoprophylaxis. At present, no drug regimen guarantees protection against malaria in any endemic area; the range of drugs available for malaria suppression includes chloroquine, mefloquine, halofantrine, sulfones, sulfonamides, pyrimethamine and proguanil, as well as doxycycline[15, 18–20]. Pregnancy is not a contraindication against malaria prophylaxis with chloroquine; mefloquine is not indicated for pregnant women or children[18, 19].

Treatment. The priorities in the chemotherapy of uncomplicated malaria are clearly different from those in severe or complicated forms. The main objective in an uncomplicated *P. falciparum* infection is generally to provide a schizontocide that will lower parasite density and relieve illness; however, some patients at special risk may require chemotherapy that provides a radical cure, even though they may not have severe malaria (e.g. pregnant women, patients who have had repeated malaria attacks, patients with concurrent diseases, such as severe anemia, pneumonia or malnutrition)[15]. Complicated *P. falciparum* malaria demands the highest level of treatment available, preferably in an intensive care unit; therapy must be instituted early, without waiting for the laboratory to determine whether the parasite is resistant, with optimal doses of the appropriate drug administered by the parenteral route[15].

The following antimalarial drugs have been recommended (including dose schedules) by *The Medical Letter on Drugs and Therapeutics* in 1992[18]

- All *Plasmodium* species except chloroquine-resistant *P. falciparum*: oral chloroquine phosphate; parenteral quinidine gluconate or quinine dihydrochloride
- Chloroquine-resistant *P. falciparum*: oral quinine sulfate combined with pyrimethamine–sulfadoxine or with a tetracycline or with clindamycin; oral mefloquine or halofantrine are alternatives; parenteral quinidine gluconate or quinine dihydrochloride
- *P. vivax* and *P. ovale*: to prevent relapse, usual antimalarial therapy must be followed by primaquine for 14 days, or at a low dose for 8 weeks if glucose-6-phosphate deficiency is known or suspected

There are very few alternative antimalarial drugs to combat the increasing levels of parasite resistance. Excellent results have been obtained with qinghaosu (artemisinin) – a Chinese herbal remedy – and its derivatives[27].

Vaccine development

Experiments on the development of protective vaccines have been greatly facilitated by advances in molecular biology and the discovery that *P. falciparum* can be cultured *in vitro*[21]. Attempts are being made to produce 4 types of anti-malaria vaccine for different stages in the life cycle[22, 23]:

- An antisporozoite vaccine, as a true prophylactic, to prevent infection
- An antimerozoite vaccine which will prevent schizogony and therefore prevent the destruction of erythrocytes
- An antigametocyte vaccine which will inhibit the sexual cycle of the parasite in the mosquito – the so-called 'altruistic' vaccine because it will prevent transmission by the mosquitoes, but it will have no protective effect in the individual who is vaccinated
- An antipathology 'vaccine' which will prevent sequestration of the infected erythrocytes in the brain; this and other forms of immunotherapy could be useful adjuncts to treatment of cerebral malaria

Remark

A review on clinical malaria research was published by Gilles et al. in 1984[24]; for an overview of all aspects of malariology, see Bruce-Chwatt[25] and Wernsdorfer and McGregor[26].

References

[1] World Health Organization, *Wkly epidem. Rec.*, **65**, 189 (1990).
[2] Bruce-Chwatt, L. J., *Brit. med. Bull.*, **38**, 179 (1982).
[3] Quinn et al., *J. Pediat.*, **101**, 229 (1982).
[4] Saliou et al., *Bull. Soc. Path. exot.*, **71**, 342 (1978).
[5] WHO Scientific Group on the Biology of Malaria Parasites, *Wld Hlth Org. techn. Rep. Ser.*, No. 743 (1987).
[6] Krotoski, W. A., *Trans. roy. Soc. trop. Med. Hyg.*, **79**, 1 (1985).
[7] McGregor, I. A., *Brit. med. Bull.*, **38**, 115 (1982); *Trans. roy. Soc. trop. Med. Hyg.*, **78**, 1 (1984).
[8] Warrell et al., *New Engl. J. Med.*, **306**, 313 (1982); Warrell, D. A., *Quart. J. Med.*, N.S. **71**, 369 (1989).
[9] Phillips and Solomon, *Lancet*, **336**, 1355 (1990).
[10] WHO Malaria Action Programme. Severe and Complicated Malaria, *Trans. roy. Soc. trop. Med. Hyg.*, **84**, Suppl. 2, 1 (1990).
[11] Phillips et al., *Rev. infect. Dis.*, **12**, 1100 (1990).
[12] Greenwood and Fakunle, *The Role of the Spleen in the Immunology of Parasitic Diseases*, Schwabe, Basel, 1979.
[13] Oppenheimer et al., *Rev. clin. Nutr.*, Ser. A, **53**, 583 (1983).
[14] Nagel and Roth, *Blood*, **74**, 1213 (1989).
[15] WHO Scientific Group on Practical Chemotherapy of Malaria, *Wld Hlth Org. techn. Rep. Ser.*, No. 805 (1990).
[16] Peters, W., *Chemotherapy and Drug Resistance in Malaria*, Academic Press, London, 1987.
[17] Björkman and Phillips-Howard, *Trans. roy. Soc. trop. Med. Hyg.*, **84**, 177 (1990).
[18] *Med. Lett. Drug. Ther.*, **34**, No. 865 (1992).
[19] WHO Model Prescribing Information, *Drugs Used in Parasitic Diseases*, World Health Organization, Geneva, 1990.
[20] *Morb. Mort. wkly Rep.*, **39**, RR–3 (1990).
[21] Trager, W., *Brit. med. Bull.*, **38**, 129 (1982).
[22] Liew, F. Y. (Ed.), *Vaccination Strategies of Tropical Diseases*, CRC Press, Boca Raton, FA, 1989.
[23] Playfair et al., *Lancet*, **335**, 1263 (1990); Editorial, *Lancet*, **336**, 586 (1992).
[24] Gilles, H. M. (Ed.), *Recent Advances in Tropical Medicine*, Vol. 1, Churchill Livingstone, Edinburgh, 1984.
[25] Bruce-Chwatt, L. J., *Essential Malariology*, 2nd ed., Heinemann, London, 1985.
[26] Wernsdorfer and McGregor (Eds.), *Malaria: Principles and Practice of Malariology*, 2 vols, Churchill Livingstone, Edinburgh, 1988.
[27] White et al., *Lancet*, **339**, 317 (1992).

Important characteristics of human plasmodia (Giemsa stain)

	Infected erythrocyte	Young trophozoite Ring form	Older trophozoite	Mature schizont
Plasmodium vivax	Larger than normal Deformed Multiple infection fairly common Schüffner's dots common, but only in semi-mature trophozoites onwards	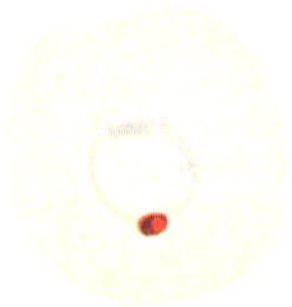	Pseudopodia 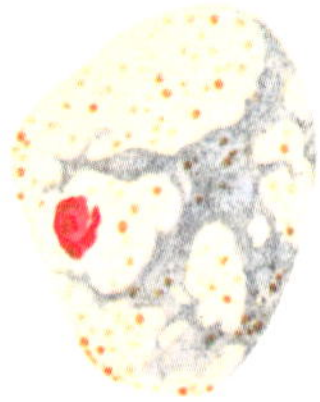 Pigment yellowish-brown	12–24 merozoites 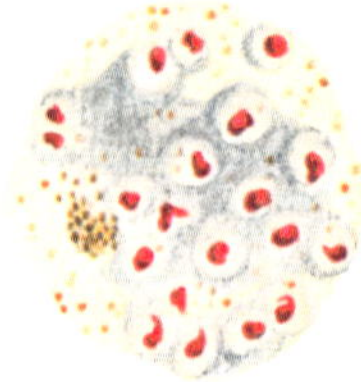 1–2 peripheral or central clumps of pigment
Plasmodium malariae	Normal or smaller than normal Multiple infection rare (Ziemann's stippling rare)		No pseudopodia Round or band form Vacuoles small or absent 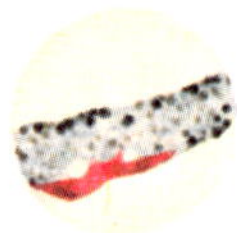 Pigment dark brown	6–12 (usually 8–10) merozoites, often in rosette arrangement 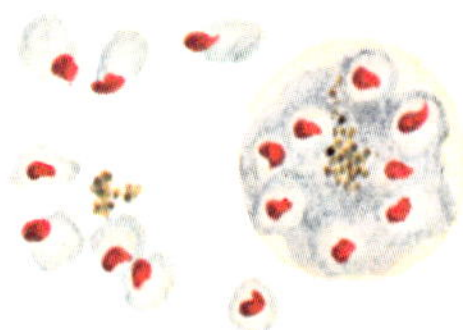 Pigment mainly centrally located
Plasmodium ovale	Rather larger than normal, often oval with ragged or irregular edges Schüffner's dots more marked than in *P. vivax* and seen even in young trophozoites	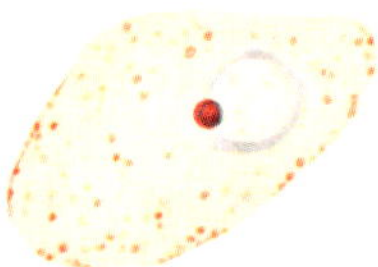	Roundish, mostly without pseudopodia Vacuoles small or absent 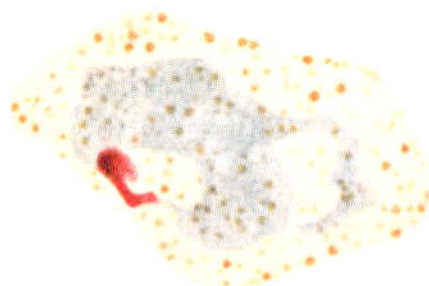 Pigment light brown, inconspicuous	8 merozoites 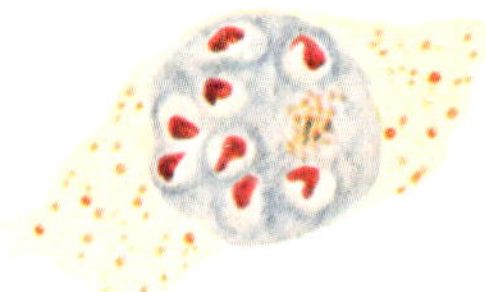 Pigment mainly centrally located
Plasmodium falciparum	Size and shape normal Multiple infection commoner than with *P. vivax* and *P. malariae* Maurer's dots rare	In young rings: plasma ring narrow vacuole small 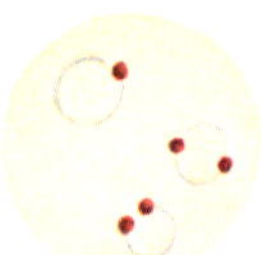 Nuclei small Double nuclei common	Vacuoles small or absent 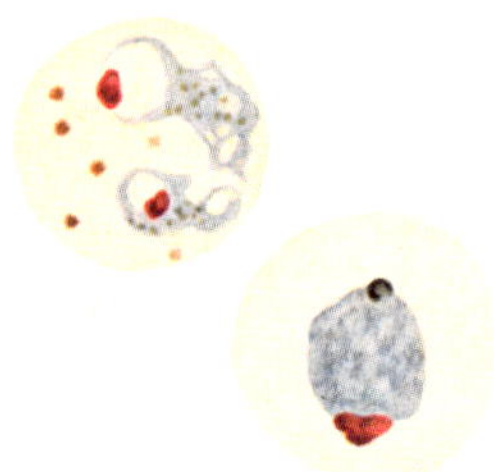 Pigment scattered and in light to very dark brown clumps	8–24 merozoites, sometimes more, very variable 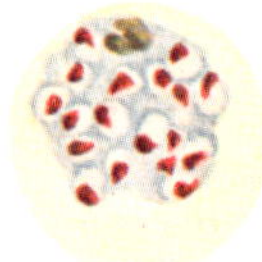 Pigment usually peripherally located

From GEIGY and HERBIG, *Erreger und Überträger tropischer Krankheiten*, Acta Tropica, Supplementum 6, Verlag für Recht und Gesellschaft, Basel, 1955.

Macrogametocyte mature	Microgametocyte mature	Duration of asexual cycle	Phases in peripheral blood
Round to ovoid 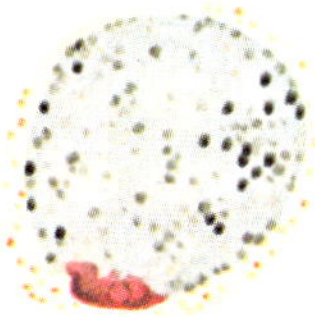 Nucleus small, eccentric, dark red Plasma uniformly blue with no vacuoles Pigment widely scattered	Round to ovoid 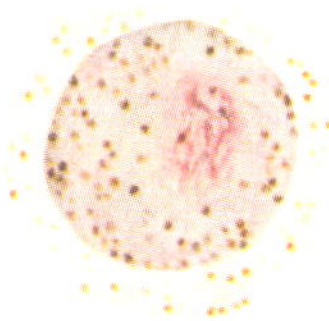 Nucleus larger than that of macrogametocytes, eccentric or central, diffuse, bright red Plasma bright blue to pink Pigment more finely granular than in macrogametocytes, diffuse	48 hours	All
Similar to *P. vivax* but smaller 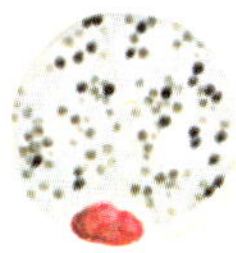	Similar to *P. vivax* but smaller 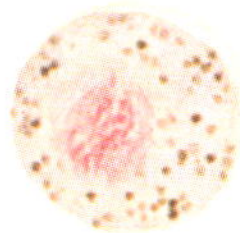	72 hours	All
Similar to *P. vivax*, very rare in oval erythrocytes 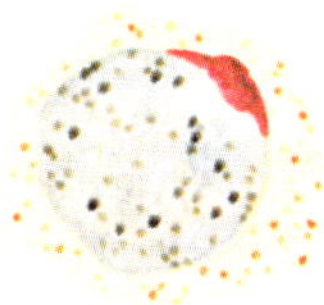	Similar to *P. vivax*, very rare in oval erythrocytes 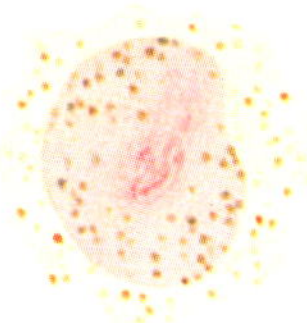	48 hours	All
Sickle-shaped 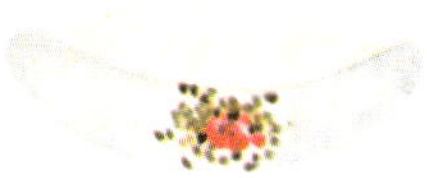 Nucleus central, compact, dark red Plasma uniformly blue to violet Pigment concentrated round the nucleus	Slightly sickle-shaped, wider and shorter than macrogametocyte 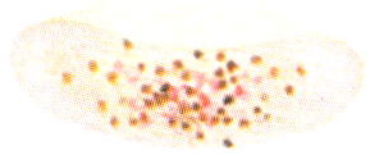 Nucleus larger than in macrogametocytes and diffuse; light red, scattered chromatin fragments and filaments Plasma pale violet to pink, always more reddish than in macrogametocytes Pigment scattered	48 hours (periodicity less marked)	Usually ring forms and gametocytes, rarely other phases except in severe cases

No.	Protozoa *Synonyms*	Characteristics	Habitat Host Transmission	Associated disease
364	**Babesia spp.** STARCOVICI *Haematococcus* *Pyrosoma* *Piroplasma*	Species infecting man: *B. divergens, B. bigemina* and *B. bovis* of cattle, *B. microti* of rodents. Intraerythrocytic pear-shaped or ovoid organisms, 1.5–5 μm in length. Trophozoites multiply by binary fission, forming tetrads of merozoites located marginally (*B. divergens*) or centrally (*B. microti*) in the erythrocytes[1] Difficult to distinguish from the 'ring' forms of *Plasmodium falciparum* in blood films, but *Babesia* have no pigment, no schizonts, no gametocytes and no stippling	Zoonoses transmitted to man by *Ixodes* ticks. In the USA, the main vector of *B. microti* is *I. dammini*, which also transmits *Borrelia burgdorferi* (*No. 6*) from the same rodent reservoir hosts[2]	Babesiosis[3,4]. In Europe *B. divergens* is a rare cause of usually fatal infections in splenectomized persons. *B. microti* is widespread in the northeastern region of the USA. It is less virulent than *B. divergens*, causing febrile illness in immunocompromised and elderly persons. Incubation period usually 1–3 weeks, occasionally 6 weeks. Probably most infections are mild and rarely diagnosed Diagnosis: detection of parasites in blood smears; by the presence of specific antibodies, by DNA probes, or by the isolation of the organism in inoculated hamsters[3,5] *Remark*. For treatment, clindamycin plus quinine are the drugs of choice[6]
365	**Enterocytozoon bieneusi** DESPORTES et al.	Obligate intracellular organisms. Ovoid, multinucleated meronts, 1–3 μm by 2–6 μm; repeated division by binary fission. Uninucleated sporoblasts. Ellipsoidal spores (1.5 μm by 2.5 μm) with a thick endospore, 4–7 coils of the polar tubules, and often a polar vacuole[7]	Duodenal and jejunal enterocytes in man. Whether the organism has a reservoir host is unknown[7,8]	Microsporidiosis with chronic diarrhea in patients with AIDS[8-12] Diagnosis: electron microscopy of small intestine biopsy specimens or finding of spores in fecal concentrates or duodenal fluid[12-14] *Remark*. For treatment, albendazole or mebendazole may be effective in patients with severe diarrhea[6,12]
365a	Other *Microsporidia* of clinical importance[7,9,15]: **Encephalitozoon cuniculi** **Encephalitozoon hellem** **Nosema connori** **Nosema corneum** **Pleistophora spp.**			*E. hellem* has been isolated from conjunctival scrapings and corneal tissue of AIDS patients with keratoconjunctivitis[12]
366	**Balantidium coli** (MALMSTEN) STEIN	Large, ovoid, ciliate trophozoites, 50–200 μm in length. Round or ovoid cysts, 45–75 μm in length	Colon of man and animals. Zoonosis. Widespread, especially in pigs and monkeys. Transmission to man by ingestion of cysts. Particularly common in Papua New Guinea where there is a close association with pigs[16]	Balantidiasis[17,18]. Asymptomatic to acute or chronic diarrhea and occasionally fatal dysentery Diagnosis: finding of ciliates or cysts in feces *Remark*. For treatment, a tetracycline is the drug of choice, iodoquinol or metronidazole are effective alternatives[6]

1 MEHLHORN and SCHEIN, *Advanc. Parasit.*, **23**, 37 (1984).
2 SPIELMAN et al., *Ann. Rev. Entom.*, **30**, 439 (1985).
3 GELFAND, J. A., in MANDELL et al. (Eds.), *Principles and Practice of Infectious Diseases*, 3rd ed., Churchill Livingstone, New York, 1990, page 2119.
4 RUEBUSH et al., *Amer. J. trop. Med. Hyg.*, N.S. **30**, 937 (1981).
5 REITER and WEILAND, *Trans. roy. Soc. trop. Med. Hyg.*, **83**, Suppl. 1, 21 (1989).
6 *Med. Lett. Drug. Ther.*, **34**, No. 865 (1992).
7 SHADDUCK and GREELEY, *Clin. Microbiol. Rev.*, **2**, 158 (1989).
8 MUSCAT, I., *J. Infect.*, **21**, 125 (1990).
9 BRYAN, R. T., in MANDELL et al. (Eds.), *Principles and Practice of Infectious Diseases*, 3rd ed., Churchill Livingstone, New York, 1990, page 2130.
10 ORENSTEIN et al., *Hum. Path.*, **21**, 475 (1990).
11 CANNING and HOLLISTER, *Trans. roy. Soc. trop. Med.*, **84**, 181 (1990).
12 ORENSTEIN, J. M., *J. Parasit.*, **77**, 843 (1991).
13 VAN GOOL et al., *Lancet*, **336**, 697 (1990).
14 ORENSTEIN et al., *Lancet*, **336**, 1127 (1990).
15 DIDIER et al., *J. infect. Dis.*, **163**, 617 (1991).
16 RADFORD, A. J., *Med. J. Aust.*, **1**, 238 (1973).
17 ZIERDT, C. H., *Publ. Hlth Lab.*, **36**, 147 (1978).
18 CROSS, J. H., in WARREN and MAHMOUD (Eds.), *Tropical and Geographic Medicine*, 2nd ed., McGraw-Hill, New York, 1990, page 349.

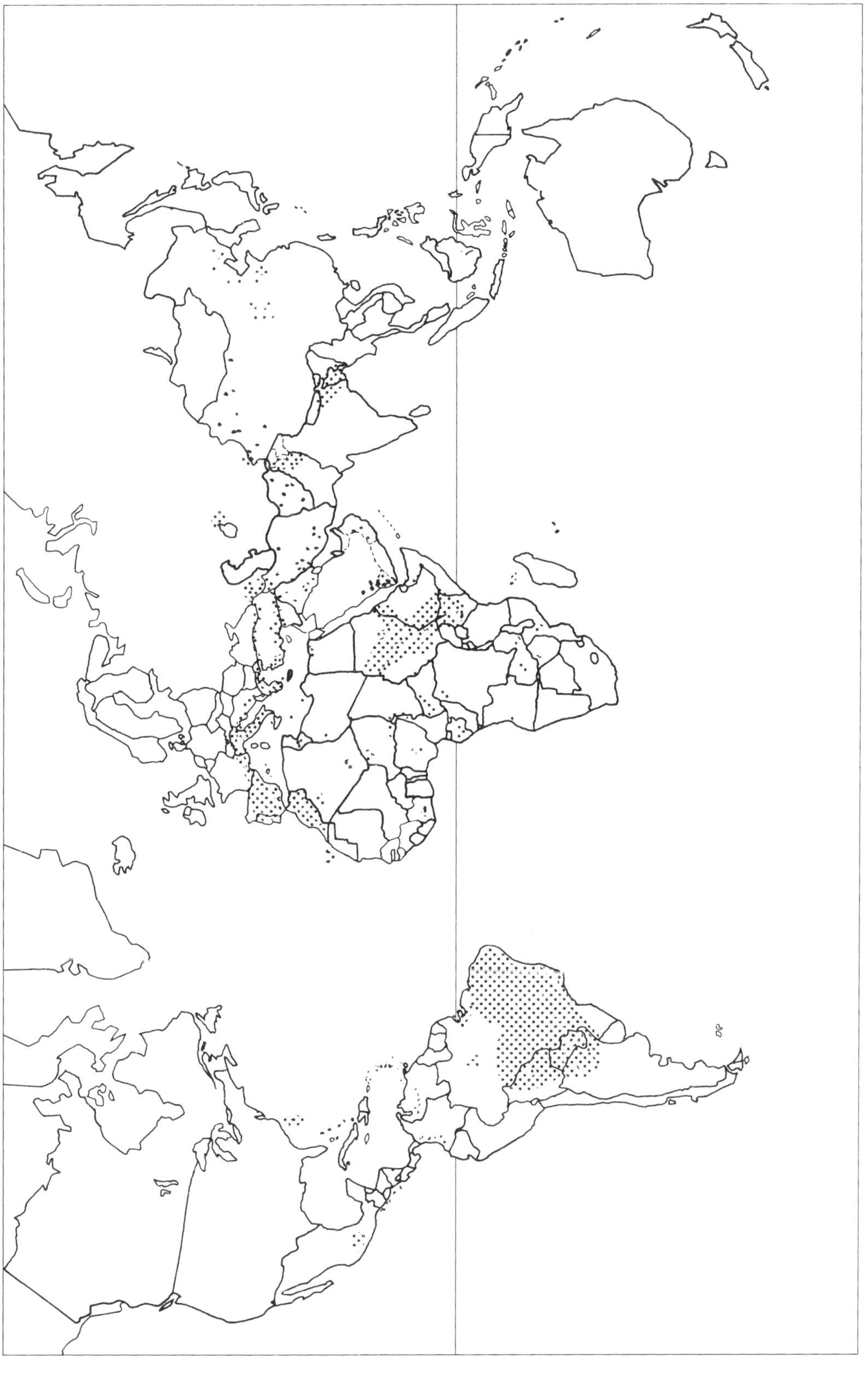

Global distribution of visceral leishmaniasis

(Reproduced, by permission, from: Control of the Leishmaniases. Report of a WHO Expert Committee, *Wld Hlth Org. techn. Rep. Ser.*, No. 793 [1990].)

Distribution of Old World cutaneous leishmaniasis due to Leishmania tropica *and* Leishmania aethiopica

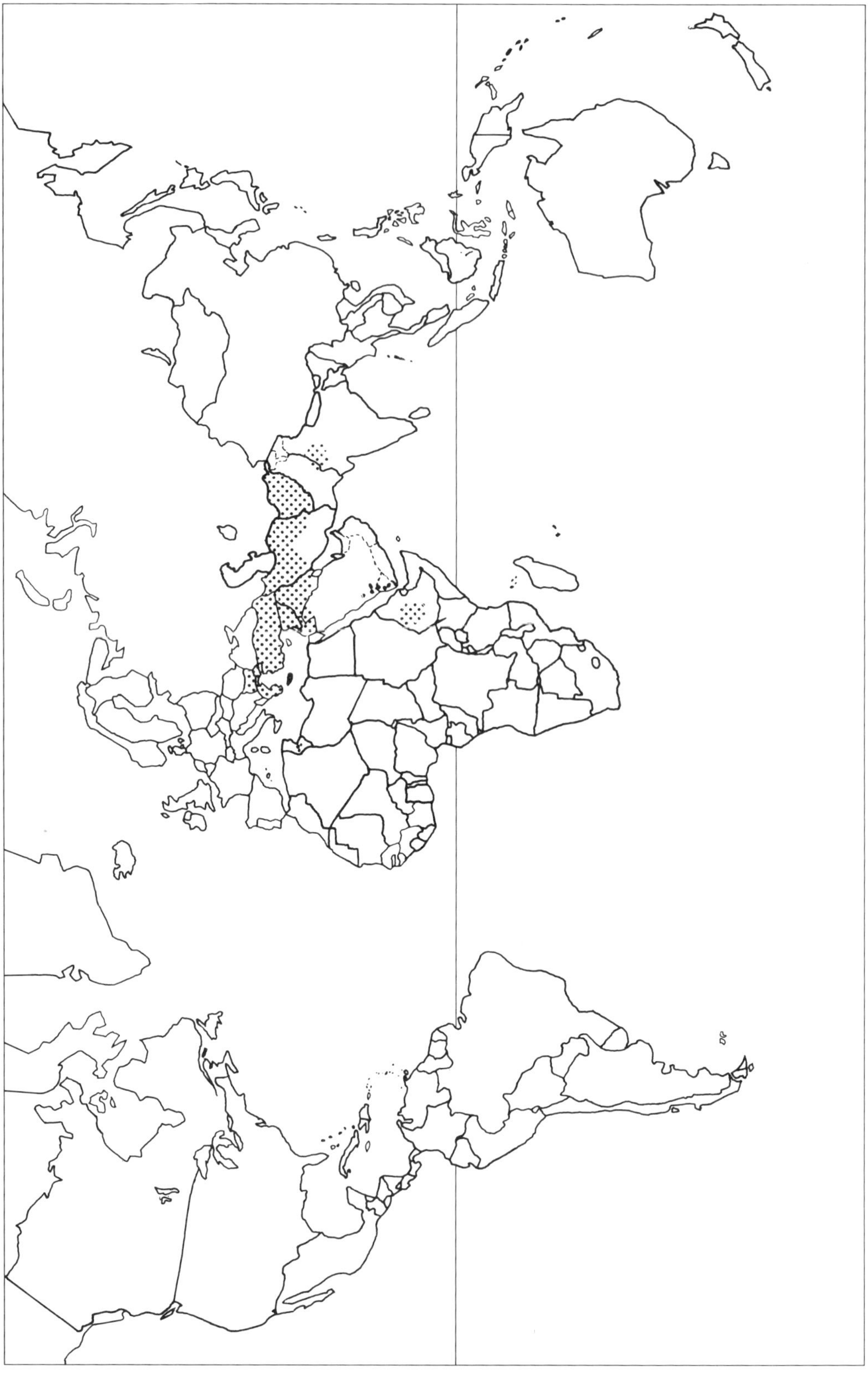

(Reproduced, by permission, from: Control of the Leishmaniases. Report of a WHO Expert Committee, *Wld Hlth Org. techn. Rep. Ser.*, No. 793 [1990].)

Areas with Plasmodium falciparum *resistant and sensitive to chloroquine (1990)*

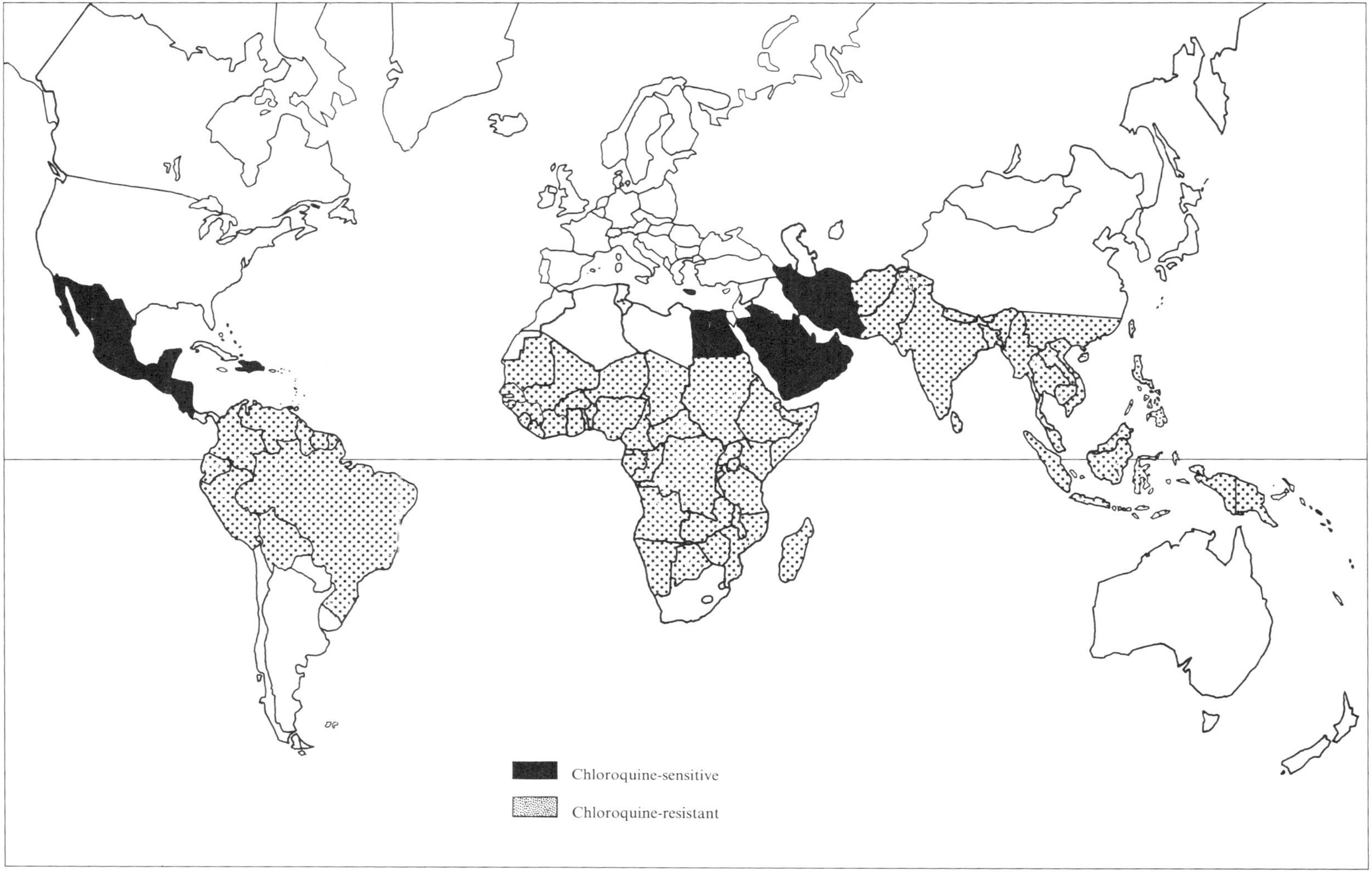

(Reproduced, by permission, from: Recommendations for the Prevention of Malaria among Travelers, *Morb. Mort. wkly Rep.*, **39**, RR-3 [1990].)

Distribution of sleeping sickness foci in Africa
(Shaded areas to the left of the dotted line are foci of *Trypanosoma brucei gambiense*, those to the right are of *Trypanosoma brucei rhodesiense*.)

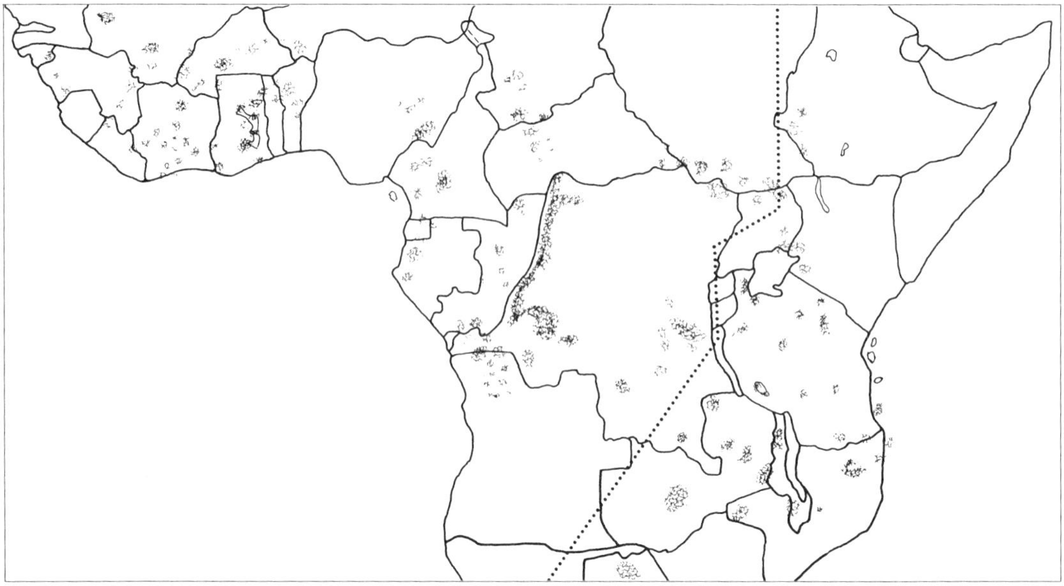

(Reproduced, by permission, from: Epidemiology and Control of African Trypanosomiasis. Report of a WHO Expert Committee, *Wld Hlth Org. techn. Rep. Ser.*, No. 739 [1986].)

Introduction

Helminths of medical importance include flatworms in the phylum Platyhelminthes and roundworms in the phylum Nemathelminthes. The flatworms include flukes in the class Trematoda and tapeworms in the class Cestoidea (see the Classification of helminths on next page). The parasitic worms differ from the protozoa of medical importance in that they are multinucleated metazoan parasites, either hermaphroditic (for example the flukes and cestodes with characteristic sex organs in the same individual) or dioecious with separate male and female worms (for example the nematodes and schistosomes). They usually produce eggs or larvae, which escape from the host to complete the life cycle in the external environment, often through an intermediate host. They undergo several metamorphoses with the various life cycle stages so distinct that they have sometimes been classified by mistake in different families. Unlike the protozoa the helminths usually do not multiply in man (a rare exception is *Strongyloides stercoralis* in immunosuppressed individuals). The severity of helminthic disease is therefore proportional to the worm load, and this depends on the intensity of transmission and the extent to which there is an accumulation of parasites in the body. Many helminths live for long periods; hence the severity of the disease is also proportional to the duration of the infection. Immune responses are relatively weak, and resistance to reinfection is manifested by a reduction in the worm load or as an amelioration of the disease, but rarely as complete protection, such as is seen with other infective agents.

Helminths are not uniform species and variants occur with marked differences in their infectivity, pathogenicity and epidemiology. For example, the strain of *Schistosoma japonicum* in Taiwan is prevalent in wild animals but will not infect man, whereas *S. japonicum* on the mainland of China is highly infective to man and animals. Another example of subspecific variation can be seen with *Wuchereria bancrofti*, the parasite causing elephantiasis. In the eastern Pacific, *W. bancrofti* has microfilariae in the blood during the day to ensure transmission by day-biting mosquitoes, whereas the most prevalent form of *W. bancrofti* in India and Africa produces microfilariae with marked nocturnal periodicity as an adaptation for transmission by night-biting mosquitoes.

In most of the developing countries in the tropics, whole communities are infected with several different species of worms. The extent of man's worm burden was first estimated by STOLL in 1947 in a publication entitled *The Wormy World*[1]. He calculated that there were more than 2200 million infections in man, and because of simultaneous infections with different species of worms the total number of infections was more than the total world population. More recent estimates suggest that there has been very little change and that with the increase in the world population the number of people with helminth infections is more than double the 1947 estimate[2]. Many of these infections are relatively harmless, and some parasites could be indirectly beneficial by stimulating defense mechanisms against other disorders[3], but even if only 5% of the people infected with worms have demonstrable ill effects, this amounts to an enormous burden of morbidity in the world. Helminths are particularly important causes of morbidity where there is concomitant malnutrition[4].

Although a great deal is known about the transmission of helminths and although there are many effective anthelminthic drugs, the control of helminths has proved difficult especially in developing countries where the effect of poor sanitation and the biotic potential of the worms combine to produce formidable public health problems. Many helminth infections are zoonoses defined by a Joint WHO/FAO Expert Committee as 'those diseases and infections which are naturally transmitted between vertebrate animals and man'[5]. For example, the tapeworms *Taenia saginata* and *Taenia solium* have obligatory life cycles depending on transmission between man and cattle and man and pigs. Other helminth infections, such as hydatid disease and trichinosis, are also zoonoses, so that the control of these and many other parasitic infections depends on close collaboration between the medical and veterinary professions[6]. Many of the advances in the treatment and control of the helminths of medical importance have resulted from research aimed at controlling helminths of livestock.

Because helminth infections are a major cause of morbidity in farm animals there has been a great deal of research on anthelminthics by veterinarians.

Drugs such as praziquantel, ivermectin and the benzimidazoles (e.g. flubendazole), which were first used in veterinary practice, are now being used extensively for controlling helminth infection in man. So far there have been no reports of drug resistance with antinematode drugs in man, although this is a major problem in the livestock industry. On the other hand, drug resistance has been reported in man with the antischistosome drugs hycanthone and oxamniquine, but there are no reports of drug resistance in trematodes of veterinary importance.

Recent advances have been made in the maintenance of helminths by cryopreservation or by culture, and there have been important advances made in understanding immune mechanisms in helminth infections, but as yet there are no vaccines for controlling the parasites in man, although some antihelminth vaccines are available for the control of nematode and cestode infections in cattle and sheep[7,8].

The tables on pages 123–141 list the most important species of helminths infecting man. The species are ordered on the basis of the classification on next page.

For a detailed description of the helminths and the diseases caused by them, the reader is referred to more extensive publications on parasitology and tropical diseases (see General References).

References

1 STOLL, N. R., *J. Parasit.*, **33**, 1 (1947).

2 PETERS, W., in TAYLOR and MULLER (Eds.), *The Relevance of Parasitology to Human Welfare Today*, Blackwell, Oxford, 1978, page 25.

3 NELSON, G. S., in DONALDSON, R. J. (Ed.), *Parasites and Western Man*, MTP Press, Lancaster, 1979, page 1.

4 STEPHENSON, L. S., *Impact of Helminth Infections on Human Nutrition*, Taylor & Francis, London, 1987.

5 Joint FAO/WHO Expert Committee on Zoonoses, *Wld Hlth Org. techn. Rep. Ser.*, No. 378 (1967).

6 SCHWABE, C. W., *Veterinary Medicine and Human Health*, 3rd ed., Williams & Wilkins, Baltimore, 1984.

7 COHEN and WARREN (Eds.), *Immunology of Parasitic Infections*, 2nd ed., Blackwell, Oxford, 1982.

8 RICKARD, M. D., in MCADAM, K. P. (Ed.), *New Strategies in Parasitology*, Churchill Livingstone, London, 1989, page 3.

General References

ASH and ORIHEL, *Atlas of Human Parasitology*, 3rd ed., Raven, New York, 1990.

TAYLOR and MULLER (Eds.), *Problems in the Identification of Parasites and Their Vectors*, Blackwell, Oxford, 1979.

BINFORD and CONNOR (Eds.), *Pathology of Tropical and Extraordinary Diseases*, 2 vols, US Armed Forces Institute of Pathology, Washington, 1976.

DONALDSON, R. J. (Ed.), *Parasites and Western Man*, MTP Press, Lancaster, 1979.

MULLER, R., *Worms and Disease. A Manual of Medical Helminthology*, Heinemann, London, 1975.

PETERS and GILLES, *A Colour Atlas of Tropical Medicine and Parasitology*, 3rd ed., Wolfe, London, 1989.

VON BRAND, T., *Biochemistry and Physiology of Endoparasites*, Elsevier, Amsterdam, 1979.

World Health Organization, *The 'In Vitro' Cultivation of the Pathogens of Tropical Diseases*, Tropical Diseases Research Series, No. 3, Schwabe, Basel, 1980.

World Health Organization, *New Approaches to the Identification of Parasites and Their Vectors*, Tropical Diseases Research Series, No. 5, Schwabe, Basel, 1984.

BEAVER et al., *Clinical Parasitology*, 9th ed., Lea & Febiger, Philadelphia, 1984.

STRICKLAND, G. T. (Ed.), *Hunter's Tropical Medicine*, 7th ed., Saunders, Philadelphia, 1991.

MANSON-BAHR and BELL, *Manson's Tropical Diseases*, 19th ed., Baillière Tindall, London, 1987.

WARREN and MAHMOUD, *Tropical and Geographical Medicine*, 2nd ed., McGraw-Hill, New York, 1990.

ZAMAN, V., *Atlas of Medical Parasitology*, 2nd eds., ADIS Health Science Press, Sydney, 1985.

HUBBERT et al. (Eds.), *Diseases Transmitted from Animals to Man*, 6th ed., Thomas, Springfield, 1975.

BAER, J. G., *Ecology of Animal Parasites*, University of Illinois Press, Urbana, 1951.

GILLES, H. M. (Ed.), *Recent Advances in Tropical Medicine*, Vol. 1, Churchill Livingstone, London, 1984.

TAYLOR and BAKER, *The Cultivation of Parasites 'In Vitro'*, Blackwell, Oxford, 1968.

GENTILINI et al., *Médecine tropicale*, 2nd ed., Flammarion, Paris, 1977.

KEAN et al. (Eds.), *Tropical Medicine and Parasitology: Classic Investigations*, 2 vols, Cornell University Press, Ithaca, 1978.

GEIGY and HERBIG, *Erreger und Überträger tropischer Krankheiten*, Verlag für Recht und Gesellschaft, Basel, 1955.

BEHNKE, J. M. (Ed.), *Parasites: Immunity and Pathology*, Taylor & Francis, London, 1990.

PIEKARSKI, G., *Medizinische Parasitologie in Tafeln*, 3rd ed., Springer, Berlin, 1987.

Classification of helminths (modified from Beaver et al., *Clinical Parasitology*, 9th ed., Lea & Febiger, Philadelphia, 1984)

The italic numbers are the serial numbers appearing in column 1 of the tables.

Phylum	Platyhelminthes (flatworms)	
Class	Trematoda (flukes)	
Subclass	Digenea	
Order	Prosostomata	
Superfamily	Schistosomatoidea Stiles and Hassall	
Family	Schistosomatidae Looss	
	Schistosoma	*367–369*
Superfamily	Paramphistomatoidea Stiles and Goldberger	
Family	Gastrodiscoididae Stiles and Goldberger	
	Gastrodiscoides	*370*
Superfamily	Echinostomatoidea Faust	
Family	Echinostomatidae Looss	
	Echinostoma	*371*
Family	Fasciolidae Railliet	
	Fasciolopsis, Fasciola	*372, 373*
Superfamily	Plagiorchioidea Dollfus	
Family	Dicrocoeliidae Odhner	
	Dicrocoelium	*374*
Family	Troglotrematidae Odhner	
	Paragonimus	*375*
Superfamily	Opisthorchioidea Vogel	
Family	Opisthorchiidae Braun	
	Opisthorchis (*Clonorchis*)	*376–378*
Family	Heterophyidae Odhner	
	Metagonimus, Heterophyes	*379, 380*
Class	Cestoidea (tapeworms)	
Subclass	Cestoda	
Order	Pseudophylloidea	
Superfamily	Bothriocephaloidea Braun	
Family	Diphyllobothriidae Lühe	
	Diphyllobothrium, Spirometra (*Sparganum*)	*381, 382*
Order	Cyclophyllidea	
Superfamily	Taenioidea Zwicke	
Family	Hymenolepididae Railliet and Henry	
	Hymenolepis	*383, 384*
Family	Dilepididae Fuhrmann	
	Dipylidium	*385*
Family	Taeniidae Ludwig	
	Taenia	*386–387a*
	Multiceps	*388, 389*
	Echinococcus	*390, 391*

Phylum	Nemathelminthes (roundworms)	
Class	Nematoda	
Subclass	Adenophorea (Aphasmidia)	
Order	Enoplida Chitwood	
Superfamily	Trichuroidea Railliet	
Family	Trichuridae Railliet	
	Trichuris	*392*
Family	Trichinellidae Ward	
	Trichinella	*393*
Family	Capillaridae	
	Capillaria	*394*
Subclass	Secernentea (Phasmidia)	
Order	Rhabditida Chitwood	
Superfamily	Rhabdiasoidea Railliet	
	Strongyloides	*395, 396*
Order	Strongylida Diesing	
Superfamily	Ancylostomatoidea Nicoll	
	Ancylostoma	*397*
	Necator	*398*
Superfamily	Strongyloidea Hall	
	Ternidens	*399*
Superfamily	Trichostrongyloidea Cram	
	Trichostrongylus	*400*
Superfamily	Metastrongyloidea Cram	
	Angiostrongylus	*401, 401a*
Order	Oxyurida Weinland	
Superfamily	Oxyuroidea Railliet	
	Enterobius	*402*
Order	Ascaridida Yamaguti	
Superfamily	Ascaridoidea Railliet and Henry	
	Ascaris	*403*
	Toxocara	*404, 404a*
	Anisakis	*405*
Order	Spirurida Chitwood	
Superfamily	Dracunculoidea Cameron	
	Dracunculus	*406*
Suborder	Spirurina Railliet and Henry	
Superfamily	Gnathostomatoidea Lane	
	Gnathostoma	*407*
Superfamily	Filarioidea Stiles	
	Wuchereria, Brugia, Onchocerca, Loa, Mansonella	*408–414*

No.	Flatworm (Platyhelminthes) *Synonyms* Common names	Characteristics	Host Transmission	Associated disease
367	**Schistosoma haematobium** (BILHARZ) WEINLAND *Bilharzia capensis* *Bilharzia haematobia* Vesical blood fluke	Male: length 10–15 mm, width 0.5–1 mm. Carries longer female in gynecophoral canal. Eggs with terminal spine, 115–170 µm by 45–65 µm Differentiation of different schistosomes: the larger terminally spined eggs of *S. mattheei* are frequently found in the urine and feces of man in Central and Southern Africa. This is probably not pathogenic, but *S. intercalatum*, a parasite very similar to *S. mattheei* which can cause intestinal disturbances, is often seen with a high prevalence rate in Zaire	Intermediate host: snails *Bulinus* spp. Interhuman transmission	Schistosomiasis (bilharziasis). Almost every country in Africa from Libya and Egypt in the North to the Republic of South Africa in the South and from Senegal and Gambia in the West to Ethiopia and Tanzania in the East. Also in the Middle East, Iraq, Iran, Saudi Arabia, Yemen, and small focus in India. In many countries infection rate as high as 60–90%, especially in children For distribution, see map on page 125. For diagnosis and treatment, see text below
368	**Schistosoma japonicum** KATSURADA *Schistosoma cattoi* *Sinobilharzia japonica*	Male: length 12–20 mm. Female: length 15–30 mm. Eggs rounded with residual spine, 70–100 µm by 50–65 µm	Intermediate host: snails *Oncomelania* spp. Zoonosis; maintenance host: numerous wild and domestic animals, and also man	Schistosomiasis. Common in China, Philippines, Indonesia. Eradicated from Japan. Similar species: *S. mekongi* in Cambodia, Laos and Malaysia For distribution, see map on page 125. For diagnosis and treatment, see text below
369	**Schistosoma mansoni** SAMBON *Schistosoma americanum* *Afrobilharzia mansoni*	Male: length 7–12 mm. Female: length 8–18 mm. Eggs with lateral spine, 115–175 µm by 45 to 68 µm	Intermediate host: snails *Biomphalaria* spp. Interhuman transmission, but wild animal hosts include rodents and baboons in Africa, and numerous animals in South America	Schistosomiasis. Most countries in Africa, except hot coastal plains (very high infection rates in the Nile delta and eastern Central Africa); also found in Saudi Arabia, the Caribbean and South America, especially Brazil For distribution, see map on page 126. For diagnosis and treatment, see text below
370	**Gastrodiscoides hominis** (LEWIS and MACCONNELL) LEIPER *Amphistomum hominis* *Gastrodiscus hominis*	Length 5–12 mm. Width 5 mm. Eggs operculated, 127–160 µm by 62–75 µm	Intermediate host: planorbid snails[1]. Prevalent in pigs and rodents	Gastrodisciasis[2]. Inhabits cecum and may cause diarrhea. Common in India (especially Assam), also reported from Burma, Thailand, Malaysia, Vietnam Diagnosis: operculate eggs in feces *Remark*. Treatment with praziquantel may be effective[2]

[1] DUTT and SRIVASTAVA, *J. Helminth.*, **46**, 35 (1972).

[2] BUNNAG, D., in WARREN and MAHMOUD (Eds.), *Tropical and Geographical Medicine*, 2nd ed., McGraw-Hill, New York, 1990, page 473.

Schistosomiasis (bilharziasis)

Schistosomiasis is regarded by the World Health Organization as second only to malaria as a parasitic disease problem in developing countries. The estimated number of people infected is at least 200 million, but this is probably an underestimate because of inadequate data from many of the worst affected areas (see maps on pages 125, 126). Schistosomiasis has been given priority by the WHO Special Programme for Research and Training in Tropical Diseases because, in areas where there are suitable snail hosts, schistosomiasis is an increasing problem due to water resource developments for agriculture and hydroelectricity. For example, *Schistosoma mansoni* has greatly increased in Egypt as a result of building the Aswan High Dam, and *S. haematobium* has become a major problem around the Volta Lake in Ghana, which is the largest man-made lake in the world[1]. The severity of the disease is proportional to the number of eggs of the parasite accumulating in the tissues, and this is related to the degree of exposure to water containing the infective cercariae.

The snails are infected by the miracidia escaping from the eggs when they enter the water. The parasite undergoes development inside the snail to produce sporocysts, which in turn produce the cercariae. Thousands of *S. mansoni* cercariae can be produced from a single *Biomphalaria* snail every day for many months; fewer cercariae of *S. haematobium* and *S. japonicum* are produced by *Bulinus* and *Oncomelania* snails, but these snails are often present in enormous numbers[2].

The cercariae swim freely in the water for 24–48 hours, and by the use of proteolytic enzyme secretions they penetrate the human skin within a few minutes of attachment, which may cause a cercarial dermatitis, but this is often much more severe following exposure to 'nonhuman' cercariae, e.g. *Trichobilharzia* from birds, *Schistosoma spindale* from water buffalo, and *S. bovis* and *S. mattheei* from cattle and sheep. These heterologous infections may confer some degree of protection against infection with the human parasites[3]. After penetrating the skin the cercaria is transformed into a schistosomule, which migrates first to the lungs and then to the liver. All three of the human schistosomes mature and pair in the liver before migrating to their egg-laying sites, which are predominantly in the inferior mesenteric veins for *S. mansoni* and *S. japonicum*, and in the systemic veins of the pelvis for *S. haematobium*. The prepatent period from the time of contracting the infection to the passing of eggs in the urine or feces is between 4 and 7 weeks and is often symptomless, but when the excretion of eggs begins there may be a follicular colitis with blood and mucus in the feces following *S. mansoni* and *S. japonicum* infections, or a follicular cystitis with hematuria in the case of *S. haematobium* infections. In the early stages of the infection allergic manifesta-

(Continued on next page)

tion occurs, referred to as the Katayama disease, this may resemble serum sickness possibly due to excess of antigen over antibody. In the main endemic areas almost all the children are infected before the age of 12 years.

The early signs and symptoms are usually well tolerated, but not all the eggs are excreted in the urine or feces, and many accumulate in the tissues, where they provoke a granulomatous reaction followed by fibrosis. This leads to the chronic manifestations which cause a high level of morbidity, and in long-standing untreated cases the complications may be fatal. There is epidemiological evidence suggesting that man develops some degree of immunity to reinfection with schistosomes, but most individuals are susceptible to reinfection after treatment[4,5].

S. haematobium, the pathogen of urogenital schistosomiasis, inhabits the vesical venous plexus, the urethral veins, the inferior mesenteric and rectal veins and the veins around the male and female genital organs. The eggs are excreted in the urine and vaginal secretions, but many eggs accumulate in the tissues and cause pseudopapilloma in the bladder with chronic hematuria. In some countries these chronic lesions develop into squamous cell cancers of the bladder[6]. Eggs accumulating in the bladder wall become calcified and lead to contraction of the bladder. Involvement of the urethra causes hydroureter and hydronephrosis, often with secondary infections. Schistosomal granuloma occurs in all the pelvic organs including the fallopian tubes, ovaries, cervix, vagina and vulva in the female, and the prostate and seminal vesicles in males.

S. mansoni inhabits the mesenteric veins, particularly the inferior mesenteric. Most of the eggs escape through the intestinal mucosa into the feces or accumulate as pseudopapilloma in the wall of the large intestine, but some are swept back along the portal venous system to accumulate in the liver as emboli provoking a granulomatous reaction which can develop into periportal fibrosis and portal hypertension with splenomegaly, hepatomegaly, esophageal varices and death from hematemesis. Eggs reach the lungs through anastomoses between the portal and systemic veins, and this can result in pulmonary fibrosis and cor pulmonale. Eggs may be deposited in the spinal cord and cause paraplegia[7].

S. japonicum, like *S. mansoni*, causes intestinal and splenohepatic schistosomiasis. The female worms produce approximately 1500 eggs per day compared with an average of less than 250 per day for *S. mansoni* and *S. haematobium*. The complications are similar to those seen with *S. mansoni* infections. *S. japonicum* may also 'metastasize' to the brain with the development of space-occupying lesions which may be mistaken clinically for tumors[8].

S. intercalatum is restricted in distribution to the western part of Central Africa. It is only mildly pathogenic. The terminally spined eggs, which resemble those of *S. haematobium*, are excreted in the feces and cause intestinal disturbances. Man develops a strong immunity to reinfection[9].

Diagnosis

S. haematobium. The characteristic eggs are easily demonstrated by simple sedimentation or by centrifugation or filtration of the urine through Nucleopore® filters[10]. Cystoscopy is rarely necessary and may result in secondary infections which can be fatal.

S. mansoni and *S. japonicum*. The characteristic eggs are found in simple fecal smears in all heavy infections, but concentration techniques, for example the acid-ether or KATO techniques or the miracidial hatching technique, are necessary for detecting light infections[11]. Rectal snips will also reveal eggs in the mucosa (including eggs of *S. haematobium* which accumulate in the rectal mucosa, but rarely appear in the feces).

Numerous immunological techniques have been developed for schistosomiasis diagnosis, but false positive reactions often occur, especially with cercarial and adult worm antigens and with skin tests. The most sensitive and specific tests depend on the detection of anti-egg antibodies or circulating egg antigens. The circumoval precipitation test has shown itself to be particularly valuable in detecting *S. japonicum* infections, and an enzyme-linked immunosorbent assay using *S. mansoni* egg antigens is highly specific[12-14]. Many other immunological tests have been developed, but they are rarely available in the endemic areas; detection of the parasite eggs remains the most reliable method of diagnosis.

Treatment

All the schistosomes infecting man are susceptible to treatment, but success depends on making a diagnosis before severe chronic lesions have developed. Following treatment schedules have been published in 1990 and 1992[15]:

S. haematobium. Drug of choice: praziquantel (related to body mass) 40 mg/kg, administered in a single oral dose or in 2 doses in one day. Possible alternative: metrifonate.

S. japonicum. Drug of choice: praziquantel (related to body mass) 60 mg/kg, administered in 3 oral doses in one day.

S. mansoni. Drug of choice: praziquantel (related to body mass) 40 mg/kg, administered in a single oral dose or in 2 doses in one day. Alternative: oxamniquine (related to body mass) 15 mg/kg, administered in a single oral dose. This has proved to be effective in Brazil, except in cases where the parasite has shown a marked degree of resistance[16]. Higher doses of oxamniquine are required in North and East Africa.

S. mekongi. Drug of choice: praziquantel (related to body mass) 60 mg/kg, administered in 3 oral doses in one day.

Control

Control of the disease depends on the following:

- Killing the parasites in man; this has now become possible on a large scale with the introduction of praziquantel as a safe and effective single-dose treatment
- Killing the snails with molluscicides or modifying the habitat to prevent the snail host from breeding; this has proved difficult because of the enormous biotic potential of the snails, but there has been some success with niclosamide, especially against the snail host of *S. haematobium*
- Avoiding exposure; this is best achieved through health education and by providing safe water for domestic use[17]

The presence of animal reservoirs of *S. japonicum* in wild and domestic animals and of *S. mansoni* in baboons and rodents makes reinfection of the community likely unless all three masures are used simultaneously[18].

There have been some successful control campaigns particularly in Japan and China. Also *S. haematobium* was eliminated from the Fayoum oasis in Egypt by the combined use of molluscicides and mass chemotherapy, but in most of the endemic areas the main emphasis is on reducing morbidity rather than the elimination of transmission[19]. The paradox remains that, despite excellent tools for controlling the disease, schistosomiasis is still an increasing problem in many developing areas, mainly due to improved agricultural development[20]. This has been well illustrated in a study of newly introduced rice-farming methods in Liberia[19], but similar examples of 'man-made' schistosomiasis can be seen in many parts of the world[21,22].

References

1 JORDAN, P., in STANLEY and ALPERS (Eds.), *Man Made Lakes and Human Health*, Academic Press, London, 1975, page 35.
2 JORDAN and WEBBE (Eds.), *Schistosomiasis: Epidemiology, Treatment and Control*, Heinemann, London, 1982.
3 NELSON, G. S., in SOULSBY, E. J. (Ed.), *Parasitic Zoonoses: Clinical and Experimental Studies*, Academic Press, New York, 1974, page 273.
4 SMITHERS and DOENHOFF, in COHEN and WARREN (Eds.), *Immunology of Parasitic Infections*, 2nd ed., Blackwell, Oxford, 1982, page 527.
5 BUTTERWORTH et al., in MCADAM, K. P. (Ed.), *New Strategies in Parasitology*, Churchill Livingstone, London, 1989, page 193; BUTTERWORTH, A. E., in ENGLUND and SHER (Eds.), *The Biology of Parasitism*, Wiley, New York, 1988, page 43.
6 HICKS, R. M., *J. roy. Soc. Med.*, **76**, 16 (1983).
7 Editorial, *J. Amer. med. Ass.*, **252**, 1116 (1984).
8 BROWN and VOGE, *Neuropathology of Parasitic Infections*, Oxford University Press, Oxford, 1982.
9 FISHER, A. C., *Trans. roy. Soc. trop. Med. Hyg.*, **28**, 277 (1934).
10 WEBBE, G., *Trop. Doct.*, **14**, 144 (1984).
11 BARTHOLOMEW et al., *Ann. trop. Med. Parasit.*, **75**, 401 (1981).
12 CABRERA et al., *Acta med. philipp.*, **4**, 168 (1968).
13 MCLAREN et al., *Trans. roy. Soc. trop. Med. Hyg.*, **75**, 72 (1981).
14 DUNNE et al., *Trans. roy. Soc. trop. Med. Hyg.*, **78**, 460 (1984).
15 WHO Model Prescribing Information, *Drugs Used in Parasitic Diseases*, World Health Organization, Geneva, 1990; *Med. Lett. Drug. Ther.*, **34**, No. 865 (1992).
16 PEDRO et al., *Rev. Inst. Med. trop. S. Paulo*, **22**, Suppl. 4, 32 (1980).
17 JORDAN, P., *Schistosomiasis*, The St. Lucia Project, Cambridge University Press, Cambridge, 1985.
18 NELSON, G. S., *Trans. roy. Soc. trop. Med. Hyg.*, **84**, 3 (1990).
19 MAHMOUD et al., *Lancet*, **1**, 849 (1983); CLINE, B. L., *Amer. J. trop. Med. Hyg.*, N.S. **31**, 75 (1982).
20 KAZURA et al., *Amer. J. trop. Med. Hyg.*, N.S. **34**, 107 (1985).
21 WHO Expert Committee on The Control of Schistosomiasis, *Wld Hlth Org. techn. Rep. Ser.*, No. 728 (1985).
22 ROLLINSON and SIMPSON, *The Biology of Schistosomes from Genes to Latrines*, Academic Press, London, 1987.

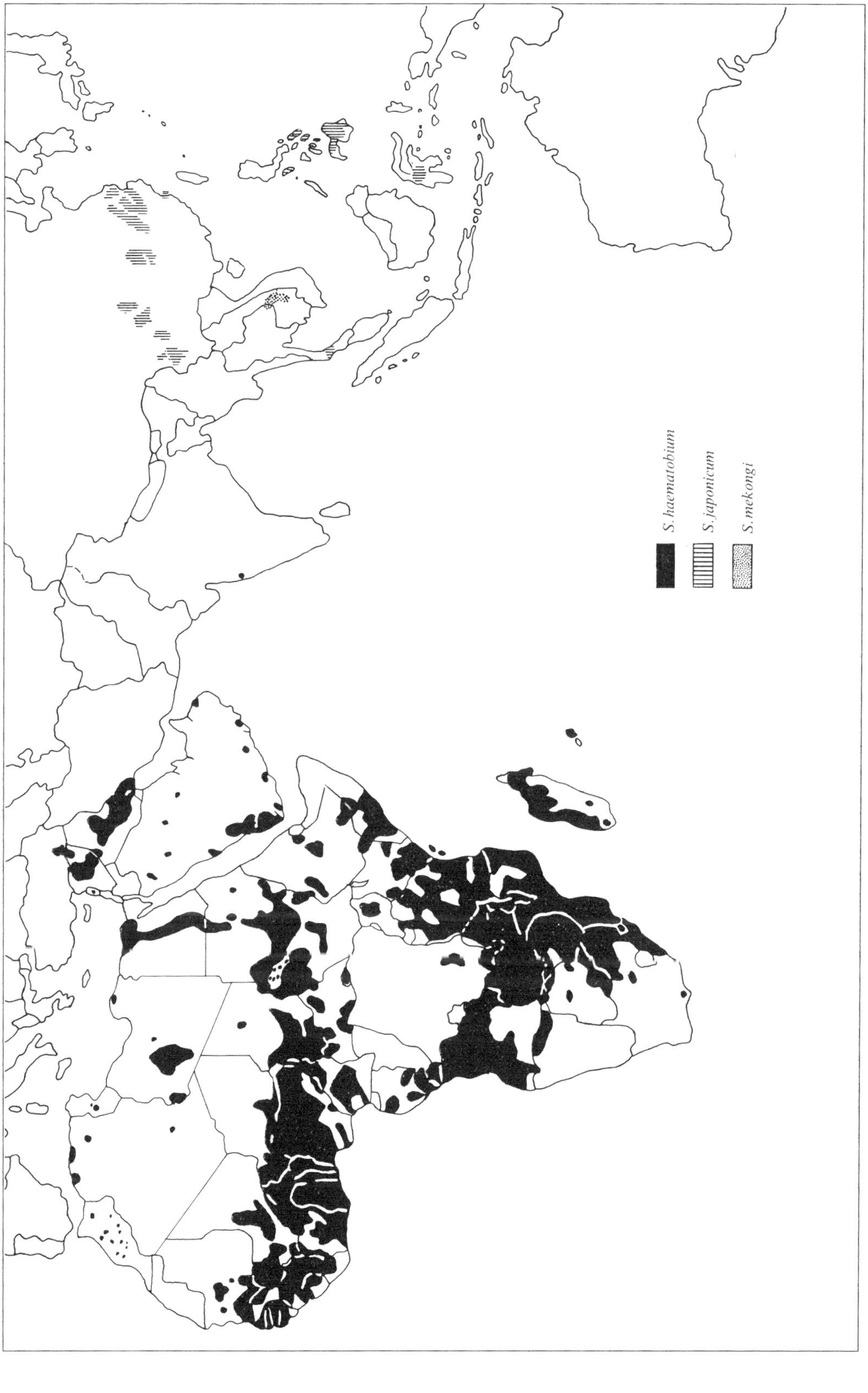

Global distribution of schistosomiasis due to Schistosoma haematobium, Schistosoma japonicum *and* Schistosoma mekongi

(Reproduced, by permission, from: Control of Schistosomiasis. Report of a WHO Expert Committee, *Wld Hlth Org. techn. Rep. Ser.*, No. 728 [1985].)

Global distribution of schistosomiasis due to Schistosoma mansoni *and* Schistosoma intercalatum

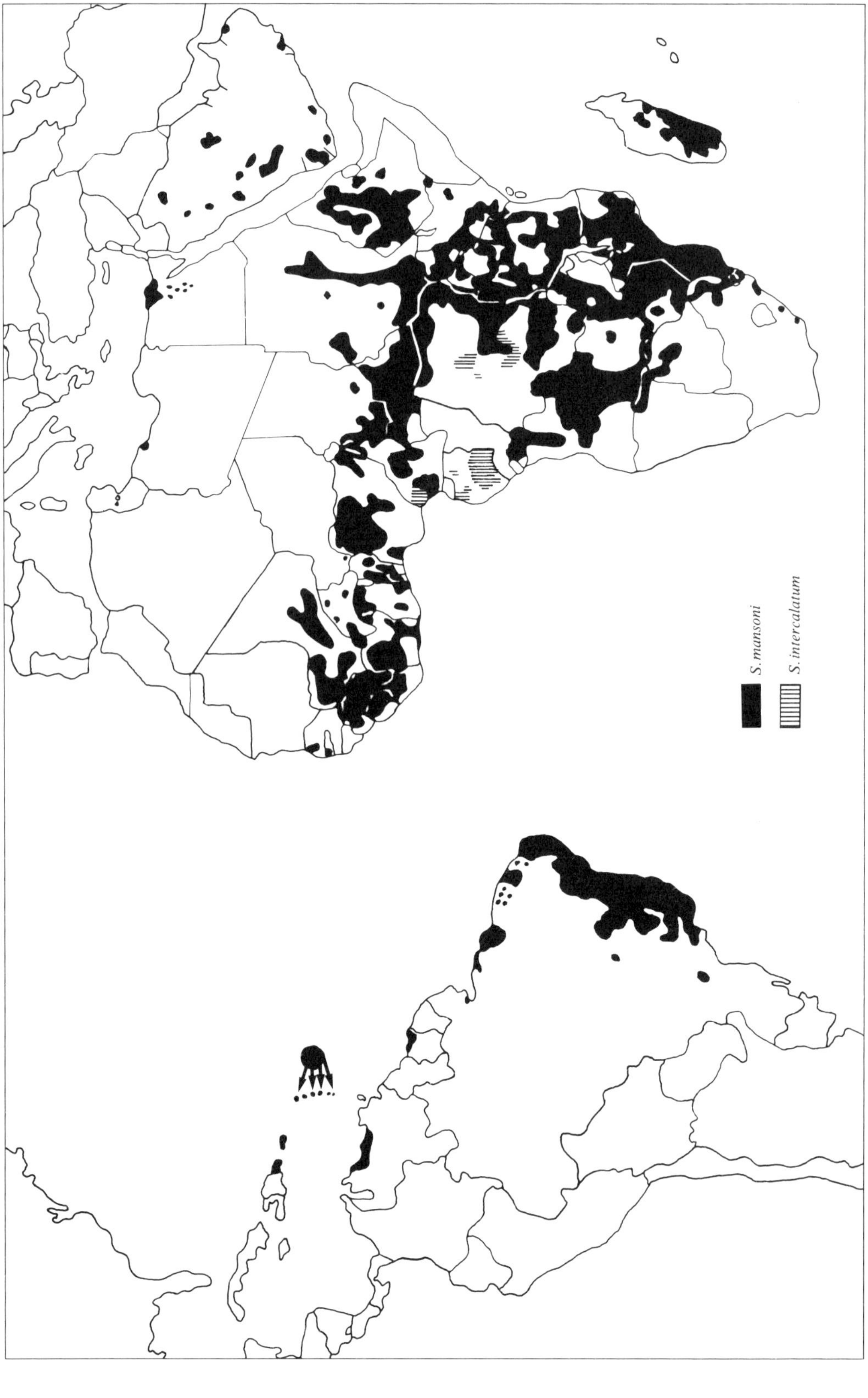

(Reproduced, by permission, from: Control of Schistosomiasis. Report of a WHO Expert Committee. *Wld Hlth Org. techn. Rep. Ser.*, No. 728 [1985].)

No.	**Flatworm** (Platyhelminthes) *Synonyms* Common names	Characteristics	Host Transmission	Associated disease
371	**Echinostoma ilocanum** (GARRISON) ODHNER *Euparyphium ilocanum* GARRISON's fluke	Length 2.5–6 mm, width 0.5 to 1.5 mm. Several other echinostomes reported from man include *E. lindoense*, *E. revolutum*, *E. cinetorchis* together with many other related species	First intermediate host: planorbid snails. Second intermediate host: numerous species of freshwater molluscs including large edible species such as *Pila* and *Vivaparus*. Zoonosis with many wild animal hosts; man infected by eating second intermediate snail host	Echinostomiasis[1]. Adult worms in small intestine may cause diarrhea. Common in Indonesia, Philippines, Thailand and Taiwan Diagnosis: operculate eggs in feces *Remark*. Treatment with praziquantel is effective[2]
372	**Fasciolopsis buski** (LANKESTER) ODHNER *Fasciolopsis fülleborni* BUSK's fluke	Length 20–75 mm, width 8 to 20 mm. Eggs operculated, 130 to 140 µm by 80–85 µm	Intermediate host: mainly planorbid snails of genus *Segmentina*; cercariae encyst on water plants. Maintenance host: man and pigs. Man infected from ingestion of metacercariae on water chestnut (*Eleocharis tuberosa*), water caltrop (*Trapa natans*) or other water plants	Fasciolopsiasis[1]. Fluke inhabits small intestine, causes diarrhea; in a few cases, severe infection causes anemia and edema. Prevalent in Thailand and other southeastern Asian countries. Control depends on health education and better pig husbandry[3,4] Diagnosis: operculate eggs in feces *Remark*. For treatment, praziquantel or niclosamide are the drugs of choice[5]
373	**Fasciola hepatica** LINNÉ *Distoma hepaticum* *Fasciola californica* *Fasciola halli* Sheep-liver fluke	Length 10–30 mm, width 8 to 15 mm. Eggs operculated, similar to those of *F. buski*	Intermediate host: snails *Lymnae* spp. Zoonosis; maintenance host: sheep and other herbivores. Metacercariae on aquatic vegetation. Transmission to man mainly by eating contaminated watercress (*Nasturtium officinale*)[6,14]	Fascioliasis[1]. Hepatitis due to migrating flukes; in chronic cases inflammation of the bile ducts and cholelithiasis with some ectopic lesions[7]. Prevalent in domestic herbivores worldwide[8]. Epidemics in Brazil, Japan[9], England[10], France[11], depending on climatic conditions[12], and occasionally other parts of Europe; sporadic in sheep in most areas, particularly common in the Andes region of South America Diagnosis: operculate eggs in feces. Spurious infections common due to passage of eggs in feces following ingestion of infected liver. Serology helpful when no eggs in feces[9] *Remarks*. For treatment, bithionol is the drug of choice[5]. The action of praziquantel has been discussed[13]. Triclabendazole may be effective[14]
374	**Dicrocoelium dendriticum** (RUDOLPHI) LOOSS *Dicrocoelium lanceolatum* *Fasciola dendritica* Lanceolate fluke	Length 5–15 mm, width 1.5 to 2.5 mm. Eggs operculated, 35 to 45 µm by 20–30 µm	First intermediate host: land snails, *Helicella*, *Zebrina*, *Codilicella*. Second intermediate host: ants of the genus *Formica*. Zoonosis: worldwide in herbivores (man incidental host)	Rare infection of liver and bile duct, usually symptomless. Most infections are spurious due to passage of eggs in feces following ingestion of infected sheep liver, but hepatitis with infection of *D. hospes* in Sierra Leone reported[15] Diagnosis: operculate eggs in feces *Remark*. Treatment possibly as for *Fasciola hepatica*

[1] BUNNAG, D., in WARREN and MAHMOUD (Eds.), *Tropical and Geographical Medicine*, 2nd ed., McGraw-Hill, New York, 1990, page 473.
[2] RADOMYOS et al., *S.E. Asian J. trop. Med. publ. Hlth*, **13**, 265 (1982).
[3] MANNING and RATANARAT, *Amer. J. trop. Med. Hyg.*, N.S. **19**, 613 (1970).
[4] WENG et al., *Chin. J. parasit. Dis.*, **7**, 108 (1989).
[5] *Med. Lett. Drug. Ther.*, **34**, No. 865 (1992).
[6] DESCHIENS et al., *Ann. Inst. Pasteur*, **10**, 5 (1961).
[7] CHEN and MOTT, *Trop. Dis. Bull.*, **87**, No. 4, R 1 (1990).
[8] PANTELOURIS, E. M., *The Common Liver Fluke, Fasciola hepatica*, Pergamon, Oxford, 1965.
[9] AMARAL and BUSETTI, *Rev. Inst. Med. trop. S. Paulo*, **21**, 141 (1979).
[10] ASHTON et al., *Brit. med. J.*, **3**, 500 (1970).
[11] RONDELAND, D., *Ann. Parasit. hum. comp.*, **55**, 393 (1980).
[12] OLLERENSHAW, C. B., in TAYLOR and MULLER (Eds.), *The Effects of Meteorological Factors Upon Parasites*, Blackwell, Oxford, 1974.
[13] FARID et al., *Trans. roy. Soc. trop. Med. Hyg.*, **83**, 813 (1989).
[14] LOUTAN et al., *Lancet*, **2**, 383 (1989).
[15] KING, E. V., *J. Parasit.*, **57**, 989 (1971).

No.	Flatworm (Platyhelminthes) *Synonyms* Common names	Characteristics	Host Transmission	Associated disease
375	**Paragonimus westermani** (KERBERT) BRAUN *Distoma westermani* *Distoma ringeri* Oriental lung fluke	Ovoid, 7–12 mm by 4–6 mm. Other species of *Paragonimus* infesting man, include *P. skrjabini*, *P. heterotremus* and *P. philippinensis* in South East Asia, *P. ecuadoriensis* and *P. mexicanus* in Central and South America[1–3], and *P. africanus* and *P. uterobilateralis* in West Africa[4]	First intermediate host: pleurocerid and thiarid snails. Second intermediate host: freshwater crustaceans including crabs, crayfish and shrimps. Zoonosis; maintenance host: mainly carnivores and crab-eating mongooses. Man infected by ingestion of metacercariae in inadequately cooked second intermediate hosts	Paragonimiasis[5]. Different species produce different pathology with involvement of almost all organs. *P. westermani*, endemic in Southeast Asia and the Far East, usually affects lungs (confusion with tuberculosis). Similar clinical feature with species of *Paragonimus* in West Africa (brain also affected with epilepsy and other signs of space-occupying lesion) Diagnosis: characteristic eggs in feces or sputum or by finding adult worms in biopsy specimens. Serology is useful in cryptic infections. Differentiation of species usually depends on finding the adult worms *Remark*. For treatment, praziquantel is the drug of choice, bithionol an effective alternative[6]
376	**Opisthorchis sinensis** (COBBOLD) DAWES *Clonorchis sinensis* Chinese liver fluke	Length 10–25 mm, width 3.5 mm. Eggs operculated, 25–35 µm by 12–20 µm	First intermediate host: snails *Parafossarulus* and *Bulimus* spp. Second intermediate host: freshwater fish (*Cyprinidae*)[7]. Zoonosis; maintenance host: fish-eating mammals and man. Man infected by ingesting metacercariae in undercooked fish. For review, see KOMIYA[8]	Opisthorchiasis (clonorchiasis)[5]. Adult worms in bile duct and occasionally pancreatic duct; many infections asymptomatic but can cause cholangitis, pancreatitis and in some chronic cases adenocarcinoma of the bile ducts[9, 10]. Common in China, Japan, Korea, Vietnam Diagnosis: eggs in feces *Remark*. For treatment, praziquantel is the drug of choice[6, 11]
377	**Opisthorchis felineus** (RIVOLTA) BLANCHARD *Opisthorchis tenuicollis* Cat-liver fluke Siberian liver fluke	Length 7–12 mm, width 2–3 mm. Eggs similar to those of *O. sinensis*	Life cycle similar to *O. sinensis*, with many wild animals naturally infected[12]	Opisthorchiasis[5]. Similar to *O. sinensis*, but less pathogenic. Reported from the CIS and Europe Diagnosis: eggs in feces *Remark*. Treatment as for *O. sinensis*
378	**Opisthorchis viverrini** (PORIER) STILES and HASSALL	Similar to *O. sinensis*, but eggs smaller, 20–30 µm by 10–18 µm	Life cycle similar to *O. sinensis*	Opisthorchiasis[5]. Usually asymptomatic, but can lead to same complications as *O. sinensis* and especially cholangiocarcinoma[13]. Very common in Thailand, also in Laos and Cambodia Diagnosis: eggs in feces *Remark*. Treatment as for *O. sinensis*
379	**Metagonimus yokogawai** KATSURADA *Heterophyes yokogawai* *Yokogawa yokogawai* YOKOGAWA's fluke	Length 1–2.5 mm, width 0.4 to 0.7 mm. Eggs 26–28 µm by 15 to 17 µm	First intermediate host: freshwater snails of genus *Semisulcospira*. Second intermediate host: freshwater fish, especially oriental trout (*Plectoglossus* and *Salmo*). Normal final hosts are fish-eating mammals and birds	Metagonimiasis[5, 14]. Usually symptomless, but can cause intestinal disturbances. Very common in China, Japan, Korea and Taiwan, also reported from the CIS and the Balkans Diagnosis: small, operculate eggs in feces *Remark*. For treatment, praziquantel is the drug of choice[6]

[1] YOKOGAWA, M., *Advanc. Parasit.*, **3**, 99 (1965), and **7**, 375 (1969).
[2] YOKOGAWA, M., *J. Formosan med. Ass.*, **81**, 774 (1982).
[3] MIYAZAKI et al., *Taxonomic and Biological Studies on the Lung Flukes of Central America*, Fukuoka University, Fukuoka, 1980.
[4] SACHS and VOELKER, *Tropenmed. Parasit.*, **33**, 15 (1982).
[5] BUNNAG, D., in WARREN and MAHMOUD (Eds.), *Tropical and Geographical Medicine*, 2nd ed., McGraw-Hill, New York, 1990, page 473.
[6] *Med. Lett. Drug. Ther.*, **34**, No. 865 (1992).
[7] YOSHIMURA, H., *J. Parasit.*, **51**, 961 (1965).
[8] KOMIYA, Y., *Advanc. Parasit.*, **4**, 53 (1966).
[9] EVANS et al., *Amer. J. trop. Med. Hyg.*, N.S. **20**, 667 (1971).
[10] FLAVELL, D. J., *Trans. roy. Soc. trop. Med. Hyg.*, **75**, 814 (1981).
[11] VIRAVAN et al., *S.E. Asian J. trop. Med. Publ. Hlth*, **17**, 63 (1986).
[12] ERHARDT et al., *Parasit. Schriftenreihe*, No. 15, 1 (1962).
[13] WYKOFF et al., *Amer. J. trop. Med. Hyg.*, N.S. **15**, 914 (1966).
[14] ZUBOV et al., *Med. Parazit. (Mosk.)*, **39**, 392 (1970).

No.	**Flatworm** (Platyhelminthes) *Synonyms* Common names	Characteristics	Host Transmission	Associated disease
380	**Heterophyes heterophyes** (VON SIEBOLD) STILES and HASSALL	Length 1–2 mm, width 0.3 to 0.6 mm. Eggs 28–30 µm by 15 to 17 µm	First intermediate host: brackish-water snails of the genus *Pironella*. Second intermediate host: fish, especially mullet (*Mugil* spp.) and *Tilapia* spp. Zoonosis; common parasite of fish-eating mammals and birds (man incidental host)	Heterophyiasis[1]. Usually symptomless, but can cause diarrhea, myocarditis[2] and neurological complications[3]. Common in Egypt, the Middle and Far East Diagnosis: small, operculate eggs in feces *Remark*. For treatment, praziquantel is the drug of choice[4]
381	**Diphyllobothrium latum** (LINNÉ) LÜHE *Dibothriocephalus latus* Broad tapeworm Fish tapeworm	The largest tapeworm infecting man. Length 2–10 m, width 10 to 20 mm; segments wider than long. Eggs operculated, 55 to 75 µm by 40–50 µm. For review, see VON BONSDORFF[5] *Diphyllobothrium pacificum*[6], a parasite with a life cycle involving seals and sea fish, is not uncommon in man in Peru and Chile. Eggs 50–60 µm by 36 to 40 µm	First intermediate host: small crustaceans (copepods). Second intermediate host: numerous species of freshwater fish including many edible species. Zoonosis; final host: domestic and wild carnivores and man	Diphyllobothriasis[7]. Often asymptomatic, but some intestinal disturbances. A small proportion of patients develop macrocytic, megaloblastic anemia due to absorption of vitamin B_{12} by worms. Mainly in temperate regions, e.g. eastern Europe, Finland, Canada and Alaska Diagnosis: operculate eggs in feces *Remarks*. For treatment, praziquantel or niclosamide are the drugs of choice[4,8]. Gastrografin® can also expel this and other large tapeworms[9]
382	**Spirometra** spp. (Sparganum)	The plerocercoid larvae of several species of *Spirometra* including *S. mansonoides*, *S. theileri*, *S. mansoni* and *S. proliferum*. White, rounded larvae, length 1 mm to 20 cm, some branching	Life cycle similar to *Diphyllobothrium latum* except second intermediate hosts usually amphibians, reptiles or mammals. Final hosts are usually carnivores. Man is a secondary host either due to ingesting infected copepods or by direct application of infected secondary hosts such as frogs as poultices to the eye and superficial wounds[10]	Sparganosis[7]. Human infection can involve skin, muscle, viscera and brain. Most commonly seen in Southeast Asia, but sporadic cases reported from East Africa and North America. *S. theileri* in East Africa may be mistaken for Guinea worms[11] Diagnosis: examination of extracted larvae *Remarks*. Surgery is the usual treatment for localized infections. Praziquantel may be effective[12]
383	**Hymenolepis nana** (VON SIEBOLD) BLANCHARD *Hymenolepis fraterna* Dwarf tapeworm	Length up to 40 mm, width 1 mm. Characteristic eggs, 50 µm by 40 µm (with polar filaments)	Host: man. Can develop in the jejunum without an intermediate host, but also develops in fleas and beetles. Interhuman transmission common, especially in children living under insanitary conditions	Hymenolepiasis. Usually well tolerated but internal autoinfection can produce heavy infection with gastrointestinal disorders[13]. In experimental infections aberrant tumor-like metastases occur in the brain after immunosuppression[14]. Cosmopolitan, but most prevalent in the tropics Diagnosis: characteristic eggs in feces; must be distinguished from *Hymenolepis diminuta* *Remark*. For treatment, praziquantel is the drug of choice, niclosamide an alternative[4]
384	**Hymenolepis diminuta** (RUDOLPHI) BLANCHARD *Taenia diminuta* Rat tapeworm	Length up to 60 cm, width 4 mm. Eggs 75 µm by 45 µm (no polar filaments)	Host: wild and semidomestic rodents. Transmitted to man by ingestion of infected fleas; no interhuman transmission	Hymenolepiasis. Cosmopolitan, but rare infection in man Diagnosis: characteristic eggs in feces *Remark*. Treatment as for *H. nana*

[1] BUNNAG, D., in WARREN and MAHMOUD (Eds.), *Tropical and Geographical Medicine*, 2nd ed., McGraw-Hill, New York, 1990, page 473.
[2] KEAN and BRESLAU, *Parasites of the Human Heart*, Grune & Stratton, New York, 1964.
[3] CHAI et al., *Seoul J. Med.*, **26**, 319 (1985).
[4] *Med. Lett. Drug. Ther.*, **34**, No. 865 (1992).
[5] VON BONSDORFF, B., *Diphyllobothriasis in Man*, Academic Press, London, 1977.
[6] BAER, J. G., *J. Fish. Res. Bd. Canada*, **26**, 717 (1969).
[7] PAWLOWSKI, Z. S., in WARREN and MAHMOUD (Eds.), *Tropical and Geographical Medicine*, 2nd ed., McGraw-Hill, New York, 1990, page 490.
[8] WHO Model Prescription Information, *Drugs Used in Parasitic Diseases*, World Health Organization, Geneva, 1990.
[9] NISHIYAMA et al., *Jap. J. trop. Med. Hyg.*, **17**, 197 (1989).
[10] DALY, J. J., in STEELE et al. (Eds.), *CRC Handbook Series in Zoonoses*, Section C, Vol. 1, Part 2, CRC Press, Boca Raton FA, 1982, page 293.
[11] NELSON et al., *Trans. roy. Soc. trop. Med. Hyg.*, **59**, 507 (1965).
[12] NORMAN and KREUTNER, *Sth. med. J. (Bgham, Ala.)*, **73**, 297 (1980).
[13] DONCKASTER and HABIBE, *Bol. chil. Parasit.*, **13**, 9 (1958).
[14] LUCAS et al., *J. Helminth.*, **54**, 75 (1980).

No.	**Flatworm** (Platyhelminthes) *Synonyms* Common names	Characteristics	Host Transmission	Associated disease
385	**Dipylidium caninum** (LINNÉ) RAILLIET *Taenia canina* Dog tapeworm	Length 15–40 cm, width 3 mm. Mature segments reddish colored	Intermediate host: fleas (*Ctenocephalides* spp.) and dog lice (*Trichodectes canis*). Zoonosis; normal host: domestic and wild carnivores. Man incidental host, especially children who swallow infected fleas	Dipylidiasis. Human infections are rare and asymptomatic, but cause distress when tapeworm segments are passed through the anus. The parasite is cosmopolitan in dogs and cats Diagnosis: usually by finding of 'rice-grain' egg clusters in feces, but must be distinguished from other rare infections such as *Inermicapsifer* and *Raillietina* *Remark*. For treatment, praziquantel or niclosamide are the drugs of choice[1]
386	**Taenia solium** LINNÉ *Taenia curbitina* *Taenia africana* Pork tapeworm	Length 2–3 m, sometimes up to 8 m. Scolex armed with double row of hooks. Proglottides square or elongated; less than 13 lateral uterine branches. Characteristic eggs: thickwalled, brown staining, containing embryo with 3 pairs of hooks	Zoonosis with man as obligatory final host and pigs as obligatory intermediate host with hooked larval cysticerci ('measles') in muscles throughout the body. Adult worms develop in man following ingestion of undercooked infected meat. Man can also act as an intermediate host developing cysticerci in the muscles and brain after swallowing the eggs of *T. solium*	Taeniasis[2,3] and cysticercosis[2–5]. Intestinal infections with the adult worms are usually asymptomatic, but cysticercosis is a common cause of epilepsy and other neurological syndromes[5,6]. The parasite also produces multiple cysts in the muscles and subcutaneous tissues and occurs in the eye. Widespread in areas where there are poor standards of meat hygiene and where pork meat is not adequately cooked. It is particularly common in Mexico and Chile and parts of India. There is an ongoing epidemic of human cysticercosis in West Irian in Indonesia following the importation of infected pigs[7]
			Diagnosis: adult worm infections usually by examining proglottides passed through the anus or by finding eggs in the feces. Cysticercosis is diagnosed by biopsy or by the characteristic appearance seen by radiology, sonography, or by scanning techniques. Serology is also of value[8] *Remarks*. For elimination of adult worms, praziquantel or niclosamide are the drugs of choice[1,9]. Praziquantel is also effective against living cysts in the muscle and subcutaneous tissue, and it can be life-saving and curative in many cases of neurocysticercosis[9–13]; albendazole is also effective when administered daily for several weeks[9,14]. Surgery may be necessary in intractable cases[15]	
387	**Taenia saginata** GOEZE *Taenia confusa* *Taenia mediocanellata* *Taeniorhynchus saginatus* Beef tapeworm	Length 4–10 m; no hooks on scolex. Proglottides elongated; more than 13 lateral uterine branches. Eggs morphologically identical to *T. solium*	Zoonosis with man as obligatory final host and cattle as obligatory intermediate host with unhooked cysticerci in muscles. Adult worms develop in man following ingestion of undercooked (often barbecued) beef. The cysticercus of *T. saginata* does not develop in man. An unusual form with pigs as intermediate hosts occurs in remote areas in Taiwan and the Philippines[17]	Taeniasis[2,3,16]. Usually asymptomatic except for distress caused by proglottides actively migrating past the anal sphincter. Cosmopolitan in beef-eating communities, but prevalence low where there are high standards of meat hygiene Diagnosis: usually by finding the proglottides; eggs indistinguishable from those of *T. solium* and rarely found in feces *Remark*. For elimination of adult worms, praziquantel or niclosamide are the drugs of choice[1,9]
387a	**Taenia crassiceps** (ZEDER) RUDOLPHI	Ovoid larvae (*Cysticercus longicollis*), 2–3 mm long, with 32–34 hooks and retracted scolex	Host: fox, dogs. Intermediate host: rodents. Endemic in Europe, the USA and Canada	Cysticercosis reported in a patient with AIDS[18]

[1] *Med. Lett. Drug. Ther.*, **34**, No. 865 (1992).
[2] GEMMEL et al. (Eds.), *Guidelines for Surveillance, Prevention and Control of Taeniasis/Cysticercosis*, World Health Organization, Geneva, 1983.
[3] PAWLOWSKI, Z. S., in WARREN and MAHMOUD (Eds.), *Tropical and Geographical Medicine*, 2nd ed., McGraw-Hill, New York, 1990, page 490.
[4] FLISSER et al. (Eds.), *Cysticercosis*, Academic Press, New York, 1982.
[5] BROWN and VOGE, *Pediat. Clin. N. Amer.*, **32**, 953 (1985).
[6] COOK, G. C., *Quart. J. Med.*, N.S. **68**, 575 (1988).
[7] GAJDUSEK, D. C., *Papua N. Guinea med. J.*, **21**, 329 (1978).
[8] COKER-VANN et al., *Trans. roy. Soc. trop. Med. Hyg.*, **78**, 492 (1984).
[9] WHO Model Prescribing Information, *Drugs Used in Parasitic Disease*, World Health Organization, Geneva, 1990.
[10] SOTELO et al., *New Engl. J. Med.*, **310**, 1001 (1984).
[11] SPINA-FRANCA et al., *Tropenmed. Parasit.*, **33**, 1 (1982).
[12] BELL, D. R., *Brit. med. J.*, **289**, 857 (1984).
[13] BOTERO and CASTAÑO, *Amer. J. trop. Med. Hyg.*, N.S. **31**, 811 (1982).
[14] ZENGH et al., *Chin. J. Parasitol. Parasit. Dis.*, **7**, 67 (1989).
[15] MCCORMICK et al., *Arch. Neurol. (Chic.)*, **39**, 534 (1982).
[16] PAWLOWSKI and SCHULTZ, *Advanc. Parasit.*, **10**, 269 (1972).
[17] FAN et al., *J. Helminth.*, **64**, 223 (1990).
[18] KLINKER et al., *Dtsch. med. Wschr.*, **117**, 133 (1992).

No.	**Flatworm** (Platyhelminthes) *Synonyms* Common names	Characteristics	Host Transmission	Associated disease
388	**Multiceps multiceps** (LESKE) HALL *Taenia multiceps* *Coenurus cerebralis*	Length 0.5–1 m. The larval cystic stage (coenurus) develops several protoscolices. Distinguished from other species by different life cycle and different size of rostellar hooks	Host: dogs and other carnivores. Intermediate host: sheep and rarely man who is infected by ingesting eggs from dog feces. Coenurus develops in the brain	Coenurosis. Human infection usually presents as a space-occupying lesion of the brain. Widespread in sheep in Europe and the CIS, causing 'gid' or 'staggers', a cerebellar ataxia Diagnosis: scanning techniques, confirmed by examining cysts removed surgically or at autopsy *Remark.* Surgical treatment
389	**Multiceps brauni** (SEFFI) FAIN et al.	Smaller than *M. multiceps*	Host: dog, genet cat and other wild carnivores. Intermediate host: rodents with coenurus in the subcutaneous tissues	Coenurosis. Widespread in wild animals in Africa, with occasional infections in man particularly in Uganda, where more than 30 cases have been reported with the coenurus in the eye or subcutaneous tissues[1] *Remark.* Surgical treatment
390	**Echinococcus granulosus** (BATSCH) RUDOLPHI *Taenia echinococcus* *Hydatigena granulosa* Dwarf tapeworm Hydatid	Length 3–6 mm; only 3 or 4 proglottides. Several subspecies have been described mainly on the basis of differences in the life cycle and host specificity. Hydatid cysts uniocular with laminated membrane and typically with numerous endogenous daughter cysts containing brood capsules and thousands of protoscolices. The parasite has been cultured *in vitro*[2] For review on cestodes, see ARME and PAPPAS[3]	Host: adult worms often found in thousands in the intestine of dogs and other carnivores. Intermediate hosts which support the development of hydatid cysts include most of the domestic herbivores and many wild herbivores. Man is usually infected by ingesting eggs of *Echinococcus* from dog feces. The subspecies *E. granulosus equinus* which is common in dogs and horses in Europe is probably not infective to man[4]	Echinococcosis (cystic hydatid disease)[5–7]. In man more than 70% of cysts develop in the liver, but in some areas the lungs are commonly involved. Cysts may also be found in many other organs including the spleen, brain, kidney, bones and eye. In many cases the cysts are slow-growing and symptomless, but serious complications can occur due to pressure or occasionally due to rupture with anaphylaxis and dissemination with secondary cysts, especially in the peritoneal cavity. Worldwide distribution, but most prevalent in countries where man uses dogs to herd his domestic animals, especially sheep and camels, or where dogs have an intimate association with man, as in Turkana in Kenya where the heavily infected dogs are used to 'nurse' children[8,9]
			Diagnosis: based on clinical evidence supported by sonography, radiological and scanning techniques (ultrasound is particularly useful in detecting abdominal hydatids). Serology is useful for surveys and for confirming the diagnosis, but false positive and false negative results are common[10]. Immunoelectrophoresis for specific antibodies and tests for circulating antigens are the most reliable methods[11–13] *Remarks.* For treatment, albendazole is the drug of choice[14], but surgery is still necessary in many patients. Albendazole may also be useful preoperatively in case of spill during surgery[15]. There have been several successful control schemes, e.g. in New Zealand and Tasmania. The most effective methods depend on health education and treating all infected dogs with praziquantel to eliminate the adult worm, but praziquantel yields disappointing results when treating hydatid cysts in man and animals; it kills the protoscolices and it can be used together with albendazole to prevent recurrence of cysts after surgery[16,17]	

[1] TEMPLETON, A. C., *Trop. geogr. Med.*, **23**, 105 (1971).
[2] SMYTH, J. D., *Parasitology*, **52**, 441 (1962).
[3] ARME and PAPPAS (Eds.), *The Biology of Encestoda*, Vols 1 and 2, Academic Press, London, 1984.
[4] THOMPSON and SMYTH, *Vet. Parasit.*, **1**, 107 (1975).
[5] FAO/UNEP/WHO *Guidelines for Surveillance, Prevention and Control of Echinococcosis/Hydatidosis*, World Health Organization, Geneva, 1981.
[6] THOMPSON, R. C. (Ed.), *The Biology of Echinococcus and Hydatid Disease*, Allen & Unwin, London, 1986.
[7] SCHANZ and OKELO, in WARREN and MAHMOUD (Eds.), *Tropical and Geographical Medicine*, 2nd ed., McGraw-Hill, New York, 1990, page 505.
[8] NELSON and RAUSCH, *Ann. trop. Med. Parasit.*, **57**, 136 (1963).
[9] FRENCH et al., *Ann. trop. Med. Parasit.*, **76**, 425 (1982).
[10] KAGAN, I. G., *Parasit. Hungarica*, **11**, 31 (1978).
[11] MATOSSIAN et al., *J. Helminth.*, **53**, 287 (1979).
[12] CAPRON et al., *Path. et Biol.*, **16**, 121 (1968).
[13] CRAIG and NELSON, *Ann. trop. Med. Parasit.*, **78**, 219 (1984).
[14] *Med. Lett. Drug. Ther.*, **32**, No. 814 (1990).
[15] HORTON, R. J., *Trans. roy. Soc. trop. Med. Hyg.*, **83**, 97 (1989).
[16] GEMMELL et al., *Bull. Wld Hlth Org.*, **64**, 333 (1986).
[17] XIAO et al., *Acta pharmacol. sinica*, **10**, 285 (1989).

No.	**Flatworm** (Platyhelminthes) *Synonyms* Common names	Characteristics	Host Transmission	Associated disease
391	**Echinococcus multilocularis** LEUCKART *Alveococcus multilocularis* *Echinococcus alveolaris* *Echinococcus sibiricensis* Malignant hydatid	Length 1–3 mm	Host: fox, dogs, cats. Intermediate host: rodents. Man (rare incidental host) infected by ingesting eggs Other species with wild life cycles which may infect man in Central and South America are *E. oligarthrus* and *E. vogeli*[1]	Alveolar echinococcosis (malignant hydatid disease)[2-4]. Commonest site of development in the liver with infiltration and destruction of liver tissue and metastases. Widespread in Arctic and northern temperate regions (Alaska, Canada, Siberia, Alpine regions, Himalaya) Diagnosis: scanning techniques and histological examination of tissue removed at surgery *Remark*. Surgical excision is the only reliable means of treatment[5], use of albendazole or mebendazole limits the growth of the cyst in inoperable cases[6-8]

[1] D'ALESSANDRO et al., *Amer. J. trop. Med. Hyg.*, N.S. **28**, 303 (1979).
[2] SCHANZ and OKELO, in WARREN and MAHMOUD (Eds.), *Tropical and Geographical Medicine*, 2nd ed., McGraw-Hill, New York, 1990, page 505.
[3] VOGEL, H., *Dtsch. med. Wschr.*, **80**, 931 (1955).
[4] LUKASHENKO, N. P., *Alveococcos*, Medicina, Moskow, 1975.
[5] *Med. Lett. Drug. Ther.*, **34**, No. 865 (1992).
[6] WILSON et al., *Amer. J. trop. Med. Hyg.*, N.S. **37**, 162 (1987).
[7] DAVIES et al., *Bull. Wld Hlth Org.*, **64**, 383 (1986).
[8] ZHANG, J. Y., *Endem. Dis. Bull.*, **4**, 83 (1989).

No.	**Roundworm** (Nematoda) *Synonyms* Common names	Characteristics	Host Transmission	Associated disease
392	**Trichuris trichiura** (LINNÉ) STILES *Trichocephalus trichiuris* *Trichocephalus dispar* Whipworm	Length 30–50 mm; long attenuated anterior end (the whip). Male coiled up tail with single spicule. Eggs 50 µm by 22 µm, dark staining, with characteristic polar plugs	Interhuman transmission; adult worms usually in cecum, but heavy infections in children may involve colon and rectum. Infection acquired by ingesting embryonated eggs Often associated with *Ascaris lumbricoides*	Trichuriasis (trichocephaliasis)[1–3]. Symptoms usually mild abdominal disturbances. Heavy infections especially in children cause loss of appetite, diarrhea, anemia, prolapse of the rectum and growth stunting. Worldwide distribution, but most prevalent in subtropical and tropical regions with low standards of sanitation or where human feces used as fertilizer Diagnosis: eggs in feces *Remark.* For treatment, mebendazole or albendazole are the drugs of choice[4,5]. Repeated treatment may be necessary due to rapidity of reinfection[3]
393	**Trichinella spiralis** (OWEN) RAILLIET *Trichina spiralis* Trichina Porkworm	Length: males 1–1.5 mm, females 2–3 mm. Cysts in muscle 0.4 mm by 0.25 mm Species which are morphologically similar but differ in their biological characteristics have been separated by genetic and isoenzyme techniques into *T. spiralis*, *T. nativa*, *T. nelsoni* and *T. pseudospiralis*[6]	Maintenance in nature in cannibalistic or carrion-feeding carnivores, e.g. bears in the Arctic, foxes in temperate regions, hyenas in Africa with secondary infections in omnivorous wild pigs and rodents[7]; artificial domestic cycle maintained by feeding pigs with garbage containing pig meat. Most human infection acquired by eating undercooked pork products, e.g. ham and sausages, also horsemeat[8], occasionally from eating wild animals such as bears and bush pigs. Ingested cysts develop into adult worms in the intestine and then produce larvae which encyst in muscles	Trichinosis (trichinellosis)[9–11]. Mild infections (rarely diagnosed) resemble pyrexial illnesses, such as influenza and typhoid. Heavy infection characterized by myalgia, pyrexia, edema of the eyelids, eosinophilia and occasionally splinter hemorrhages under the fingernails. Death due to myocarditis or the generalized inflammation associated with the developing larvae[12]. Worldwide except for Australasia. Declining incidence of trichinosis due to improved meat hygiene and domestic refrigeration of pork products[8] Diagnosis: usually based on clinical and epidemiological evidence with confirmation by serology or muscle biopsy to demonstrate the parasite[13] *Remarks.* Mild disease may be treated with salicylates or mild analgesics. For severe symptoms, mebendazole plus a corticosteroid (to prevent severe reactions around dead larvae in tissue) are the drugs of choice[5]
394	**Capillaria philippinensis** CHITWOOD, VALESQUEZ and SALAZAR	Length: males 2–3 mm, females 2.5–4 mm. Eggs with polar plugs, superficially similar to *Trichuris*	Host: fish-eating birds. Intermediate host: brackish-water fish. Man infected by eating undercooked or raw fish. Internal autoinfection results in massive worm loads[14]	Capillariasis[15]. Intestinal malabsorption, chronic diarrhea, rapid loss of body mass resembling sprue or even cholera; often fatal if untreated. Widespread in Luzon area of Philippines; also reported from Thailand Diagnosis: eggs in feces *Remarks.* For treatment, mebendazole is the drug of choice, albendazole or thiabendazole are effective alternatives[5]. Relapse should be prevented with long course of treatment

[1] JUNG and BEAVER, *Pediatrics*, **8**, 548 (1951).
[2] BUNDY, D. A. P., *Trans. roy. Soc. trop. Med. Hyg.*, **80**, 706 (1986).
[3] BUNDY and COOPER, in WARREN and MAHMOUD (Eds.), *Tropical and Geographical Medicine*, 2nd ed., McGraw-Hill, New York, 1990, page 399.
[4] WHO Model Prescribing Information, *Drugs Used in Parasitic Diseases*, World Health Organization, Geneva, 1990.
[5] *Med. Lett. Drug. Ther.*, **34**, No. 865 (1992).
[6] POZIO et al., in TANNER, C. E. (Ed.), *Trichinellosis*, ICT 7, CSIC Press, Madrid, 1989, page 76.
[7] NELSON, G. S., *Symp. zool. Soc. Lond.*, **50**, 181 (1982).
[8] VAN KNAPEN, F., *Ann. Méd. vét.*, **132**, 441 (1988).
[9] GOULD, S. E. (Ed.), *Trichinosis in Man and Animals*, Thomas, Springfield (1970).
[10] CAMPBELL, W. C., *Trichinella and Trichinellosis*, Plenum Press, New York, 1983.
[11] KAZURA, J. W., in WARREN and MAHMOUD (Eds.), *Tropical and Geographical Medicine*, 2nd ed., McGraw-Hill, New York, 1990, page 442.
[12] BESSOUDO et al., *Chest*, **79**, 698 (1981).
[13] KAZURA, J. W., in COHEN and WARREN (Eds.), *Immunology of Parasitic Infections*, 2nd ed., Blackwell, Oxford, 1982, page 654.
[14] CROSS et al., in *Health Policies in Developing Countries*, Roy. Soc. Med., Symposium 24, Academic Press, London, 1980, page 81.
[15] WATTEN et al., *Trans. roy. Soc. trop. Med. Hyg.*, **66**, 828 (1972).

No.	**Roundworm** (Nematoda) *Synonyms* Common names	Characteristics	Host Transmission	Associated disease
395	**Strongyloides stercoralis** (BAVAY) STILES and HASSALL *Anguillula intestinalis* *Anguillula stercoralis* *Strongyloides intestinalis*	Length: parasitic (parthenogenetic) females 2.2 mm; free-living females 1 mm, males 0.7 mm. First stage rhabditiform larvae up to 250 µm in length are found in the feces	Host: man, occasionally cats and dogs. Mainly interhuman transmission (a) by direct development of infective larvae penetrating the skin from soil contaminated by human feces, (b) indirectly after development through a free-living generation of males and females in the soil, (c) by autoinfection either through the perianal region or from larvae in the intestine. Autoinfection is often fatal in immunosuppressed individuals. The larvae migrate through the circulation to the lungs, up the trachea and down the esophagus to their final site of development in the small intestine, where they can persist for years	Strongyloidiasis[1,2]. Often asymptomatic, but a variety of intestinal disorders occur which may resemble peptic ulcer, and in long-standing cases larva currens can be a problem due to rapidly migrating larvae in the dermis especially in the anal region[3]. Hyperinfections which occur in immunosuppressed individuals can be fatal with larvae migrating to all parts of the body, especially the lungs[4,5]. It is surprising that hyperinfections are not a feature of immunosuppression in AIDS[6]. Widespread, with up to 20% infection rate in the tropics and subtropics; endemic foci have been reported in many temperate countries[7]
			Diagnosis: demonstration of the rhabditiform larvae in feces, or the different larval stages or adult worms in tissues or following culture of feces[8] *Remarks*. For treatment, thiabendazole or ivermectin or albendazole are the drugs of choice[9]. It is essential to diagnose and treat all cases of *Strongyloides* in patients on immunosuppressive drugs, especially transplant patients[10]	
396	**Strongyloides fülleborni** VON LINSTOW	Similar to *S. stercoralis*, but with distinct postvulvar constriction in the female. Eggs, not larvae, found in feces (50 µm by 35 µm)	Host: a widespread parasite of monkeys. Life cycle similar to *S. stercoralis*, but transmammary infection also reported[11]	Strongyloidiasis. Prevalent in man in rural areas of Central Africa, especially Zaire[12]. A similar if not identical parasite responsible for 'swollen belly sickness' in infants in Papua New Guinea[13,14]. In Africa, infections are usually asymptomatic, but in Papua New Guinea hyperinfection occurs with severe diarrhea which is fatal unless treated[15] Diagnosis: small, hookworm-like eggs in the feces *Remark*. Treatment with thiabendazole or mebendazole is highly effective[15,16]
397	**Ancylostoma duodenale** (DUBINI) CREPLIN *Uncinaria duodenalis* Assassin worm 'Old World' hookworm	Males: 10 mm long, 0.5 mm thick. Females: 12–15 mm long, 1 mm thick. Buccal capsule with two pairs of teeth. Broad bursa with divided spicules at posterior tip of male. Eggs thin-shelled, 60 µm by 40 µm The smaller species *Ancylostoma ceylanicum* is occasionally found in man in South East Asia	Host: man, occasionally dogs. Mainly interhuman transmission, acquired either through the skin with migration through the lungs or by mouth with direct development in the intestine. Larvae may remain dormant (hypobiosis) and develop several months after exposure to infection. For life cycle, see text on next page	Ancylostomiasis (hookworm disease). See text on next page. Most prevalent in subtropical regions (Mediterranean, North India, China, Japan, Peru, Chile), but spreading to tropical areas and now found in Southeast Asia and Africa (in these areas much less prevalent than *Necator americanus*). *Ancylostoma braziliense*: main cause of creeping eruption Diagnosis: eggs in feces morphologically identical to those of *N. americanus*; fecal cultures to produce infective larvae or examination of adult worms necessary to distinguish species For treatment and control, see text on next page

[1] GROVE, D. I. (Ed.), *Strongyloidiasis: A Major Roundworm Infection in Man*, Taylor & Francis, London, 1989.
[2] GROVE, D. I., in WARREN and MAHMOUD (Eds.), *Tropical and Geographical Medicine*, 2nd ed., McGraw-Hill, New York, 1990, page 393.
[3] GILL and BELL, *Lancet*, **1**, 958 (1982).
[4] CRUZ et al., *New Engl. J. Med.*, **275**, 1093 (1966).
[5] BATONI et al., *Rev. Inst. Med. trop. S. Paulo*, **18**, 283 (1976).
[6] LUCAS, S. B., *Trans. roy. Soc. trop. Med. Hyg.*, **84**, Suppl. 1, 34 (1990).
[7] GENTA et al., *Quart. J. Med.*, N.S. **68**, 679 (1988).
[8] WHO Scientific Group on Intestinal Protozoan and Helminthic Infections, *Wld Hlth Org. techn. Rep. Ser.*, No. 666 (1981).
[9] *Med. Lett. Drug. Ther.*, **34**, No. 865 (1992).
[10] DEVAULT et al., *Rev. infect. Dis.*, **12**, 653 (1990).
[11] BROWN and GIRARDEAU, *Amer. J. trop. Med. Hyg.*, N.S. **26**, 215 (1977).
[12] PAMPIGLIONE and RICCIARDI, *Bull. Soc. Path. exot.*, **65**, 112 (1972).
[13] KELLY et al., *Amer. J. trop. Med. Hyg.*, N.S. **25**, 694 (1976).
[14] BARNISH and ASHFORD, *Trans. roy. Soc. trop. Med. Hyg.*, **83**, 684 (1989).
[15] ASHFORD et al., *Papua N. Guinea med. J.*, **22**, 128 (1979).
[16] VINCE et al., *Papua N. Guinea med. J.*, **22**, 120 (1979).

No.	**Roundworm** (Nematoda) *Synonyms* Common names	Characteristics	Host Transmission	Associated disease
398	**Necator americanus** (STILES) STILES *Uncinaria americana* 'New World' hookworm (a misnomer, since it was introduced from Africa)	Smaller than *Ancylostoma duodenale*. Males: 8 mm long, 0.3 mm thick. Females: 10 mm long, 0.4 mm thick. Buccal capsule with cutting plates, no teeth. Long bursa with fused spicule at posterior tip of male. Eggs indistinguishable from those of *A. duodenale*	Host: man, but similar species recorded from apes and monkeys. Mainly interhuman transmission by the intradermal route. No development of ingested larvae	Necatoriasis (hookworm disease). See text below. Prevalent throughout tropical and many subtropical regions, probably infecting more than 600 million people Diagnosis: as for *A. duodenale* For treatment and control, see text below
399	**Ternidens deminutus** RAILLIET and HENRY 'False hookworm'	Males: 9 mm long, 0.5 mm thick. Females: 14 mm long, 0.7 mm thick. Buccal capsule, forked teeth. Bursa with long, equal spicules at posterior tip of male. Eggs similar to those of *A. duodenale*, but larger	Host: old-world monkeys. Life cycle unknown	'False hookworm' infection. Most prevalent in Zimbabwe, but also in other African countries. Usually not pathogenic; hence essential to distinguish from pathogenic hookworms Diagnosis: eggs in feces must be measured so as to distinguish from *Necator* and *Ancylostoma*; fecal culture for infective larvae *Remark*. Treatment as for hookworm infections. See text below

Hookworm disease

The hookworms, *Ancylostoma duodenale* and *Necator americanus*, are responsible for a great deal of morbidity in the world[1,2]. The prevalence and intensity of hookworm infections have decreased to some extent in parts of the world which have seen general improvements in sanitation and where there have been intensive health campaigns, for example in the Southern States of the USA and in southern regions of the CIS, as well as in Cuba, Japan and China, but hookworm disease is still a major problem in most of the rural areas of the tropics.

The life cycle of the human hookworms was first described by LOOSS in Egypt in 1896. Eggs hatch in the soil and then rhabditiform larvae go through two stages of development – separated by one molt – to become infective third stage filariform larvae. When man contacts contaminated soil, the infective larvae penetrate the skin. The larvae are carried with the circulation to the lungs, penetrate the alveolar walls, and make their way up the trachea to be swallowed and carried to their final habitat in the small intestine. More recent studies, particularly in Japan[3], suggest that although this is true for *N. americanus*, it is not true for the main method of infection with *A. duodenale*, which is by the oral route with direct development in the small intestine. Another major difference between the two species is that *A. duodenale* larvae can undergo a long period of dormancy (hypobiosis) in man as an adaptation to seasonal transmission. This was first observed in India, where the parasites reached their peak of development just before the monsoon period to ensure ideal conditions in the moist soil for development of the egg to the infective stage[4]. These differences in the life cycle together with differences in pathogenicity and response to treatment suggest that the term 'ancylostomiasis' should be reserved for infection with *A. duodenale* and that infection with *N. americanus* should be referred to as 'necatoriasis'.

Clinical features

Penetration of the skin by the infective larvae causes pruritis (ground itch), and in some cases dermal larva migrans, although this is much more likely to be caused when man is infected with the larvae of *Ancylostoma braziliense*, the common hookworm of cats and dogs[5]. In infections with *A. duodenale* or *N. americanus* the first symptoms may be associated with the larvae in the lungs, i.e. pneumonitis or allergic manifestations[6], but usually the first sign of infection occurs when the worms are developing from larvae to adult worms in the small intestine (mainly the jejunum and not the duodenum). A variety of gastrointestinal disorders occur which may be mistaken for peptic ulceration or other chronic disorders.

The commonest manifestation of hookworm disease is iron deficiency anemia, the severity being directly related to the duration of

(Continued on next page)

Diagnostic features of Strongyloides and hookworm filariform larvae found in human coprocultures

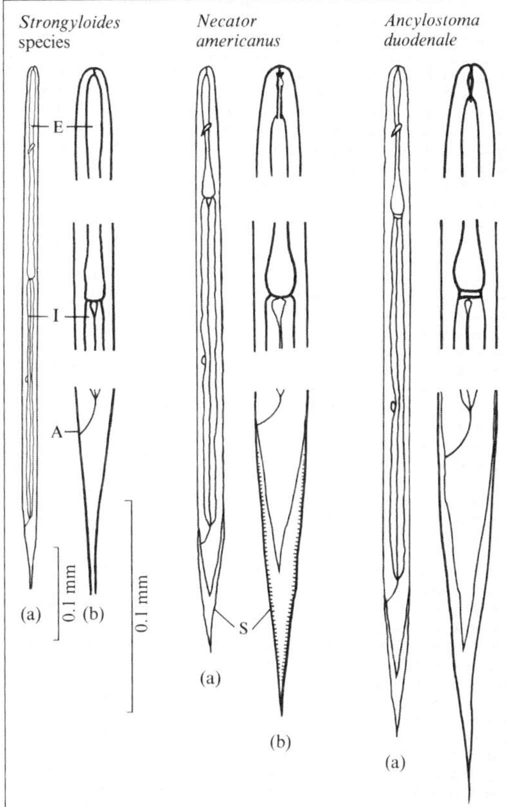

(a) Intact larvae, (b) portions of larvae.
A: anus, E: esophagus, I: intestine, S: sheath. (b)

(Reproduced, by permission, from: Intestinal Protozoan and Helminthic Infections. Report of a WHO Expert Committee, *Wld Hlth Org. techn. Rep. Ser.*, No. 666 [1981].)

No.	**Roundworm** (Nematoda) *Synonyms* Common names	Characteristics	Host Transmission	Associated disease
400	**Trichostrongylus** spp. Looss Wireworms (in livestock)	Length: male 5–8 mm, female 5 to 12 mm. Eggs similar to those of hookworms, but longer and thinner (85 µm by 35 µm). Species may be distinguished on male bursa	Host: domestic livestock (e.g. sheep, cattle, camels). 8 species infect man following ingestion of infective larvae on contaminated food	Trichostrongyliasis[1]. Usually asymptomatic, but heavy infections cause diarrhea and bleeding from intestine. Widespread in Asia with high prevalence in Iran Diagnosis: need to distinguish from hookworms by measuring eggs in feces or by culturing feces and examining the infective larvae *Remarks.* For treatment, pyrantel pamoate is the drug of choice, mebendazole or albendazole are effective alternatives[2]

[1] Ghadirian and Arfaa, *Amer. J. trop. Med. Hyg.*, NS **24**, 935 (1975).
[2] *Med. Lett. Drug. Ther.*, **34**, No. 865 (1992).

infection and to blood loss as a result of the worms browsing in the small intestine[7]. The disease is most severe in heavily infected individuals and in pregnant women and children, especially in areas where there is inadequate iron in the diet or where there is blood loss or failure of absorption of iron from other causes. The daily blood loss caused by *Necator* can be as much as 0.1 mL per worm, and *Ancylostoma* can cause a loss of 0.3 mL per worm, so that the severity is usually proportional to the worm load. The anemia may take many weeks to develop, depending on the level of the preexisting iron stores, but in infants extensive hemorrhages can occur in the bowel even before the worms reach full maturity[8]. The loss of blood results in a loss of protein from the bowel, and this can cause hypoproteinemia and precipitate kwashiorkor. In many individuals with only a few worms or those on a good diet there are no symptoms or signs of infection other than the presence of eggs in the feces.

It is essential to exclude the possibility of infection with the 'false hookworm' (*Ternidens deminutus*) especially in Central Africa, where it is highly prevalent but not usually pathogenic[9].

Diagnosis

The worm load can be determined by estimating the number of eggs in the feces by the dilution method of Stoll or by a modified Kato technique. In epidemiological studies and in assessing the efficacy of treatment it is necessary to differentiate the species of hookworms and separate them from other nematodes with similar eggs and from *Strongyloides*. This can be done by the simple Harada–Mori coproculture method, which produces infective larvae with their characteristic morphology[2] (see figure on page 135). It is also necessary to obtain adult material for detailed study, especially where *A. ceylanicum* occurs, because this parasite of dogs can reach maturity in man and cause anemia[10,11].

Treatment

Tetrachlorethylene is still extensively used in poorer countries because of low cost, although it does have toxicity. Several anthelminthics have been recommended to eliminate hookworms from the bowel in 1990 and 1992[12,13]:

- Mebendazole, albendazole and levamisole are equally effective against *Ancylostoma* and *Necator*.
- Pyrantel pamoate is more effective against *Ancylostoma* than against *Necator*.

In patients with anemia it is necessary to give supplementary iron, but intramuscular iron should be avoided because of the danger of precipitating other infections[14].

Control

The prevalence of hookworm infection and hookworm disease can be achieved by combining the following measures[15]:

- Mass chemotherapy, preferably with a drug which can be given in a single oral dose, e.g. pyrantel pamoate, levamisole or albendazole. These compounds have the advantage that they are also highly effective against many of the other intestinal nematodes, especially *Ascaris lumbricoides*. In China, mass chemotherapy has been initiated by incorporating albendazole in cooking salt
- Improved sanitation with emphasis on provision of 'safe' latrines and the composting or sterilization of human feces used as fertilizer
- The use of protective footwear by agricultural workers to prevent the invasion of infective larvae
- Improved diet with particular reference to the iron intake
- Health education and community participation to ensure that the community has the will and knowledge to control the disease

There has been a recent renewed interest in hookworm disease, and all aspects of the subject are reviewed in the proceedings of a meeting organized by the Rockefeller Foundation in 1988[16]. The special problems of hookworms in Africa have been discussed by Goldsmid[17].

References

1 Banwell and Schad, *Clin. Gastroent.*, **7**, 129 (1978). Schad and Banwell, in Warren and Mahmoud (Eds.), *Tropical and Geographical Medicine*, 2nd ed., McGraw-Hill, New York, 1990, page 379.
2 WHO Scientific Group on Intestinal Protozoan and Helminthic Infections, *Wld Hlth Org. techn. Rep. Ser.*, No. 666 (1981).
3 Mizuno and Yanagisawa, *Jap. J. Hyg.*, **13**, 311 (1963).
4 Nawalinsky and Schad, *Amer. J. trop. Med. Hyg.*, N.S. **23**, 895 (1974).
5 Beaver, P. C., *Industr. Med. Surg.*, **33**, 319 (1964).
6 Yoshida and Nakanishi, *Jap. J. Parasit.*, **7**, 442 (1958).
7 Roche and Layrisse, *Amer. J. trop. Med. Hyg.*, N.S. **15**, 1030 (1966).
8 Nwosu, A. B., *Trop. geogr. Med.*, **33**, 105 (1981); Wang Cheng-i, *Parasit. today*, **4**, 284 (1988).
9 Goldsmid, J. M., *Cent. Afr. J. Med.*, **18**, Suppl. (1972).
10 Anten and Zuidema, *Ned. T. Geneesk.*, **108**, 1664 (1964).
11 Zuidema et al., *Trop. geogr. Med.*, **24**, 68 (1972).
12 WHO Model Prescribing Information, *Drugs Used in Parasitic Diseases*, World Health Organization, Geneva, 1990.
13 *Med. Lett. Drug. Ther.*, **34**, No. 865 (1992).
14 Oppenheimer et al., *Trans. roy. Soc. trop. Med. Hyg.*, **80**, 603 (1986).
15 WHO Expert Committee on Prevention and Control of Intestinal Parasitic Infections, *Wld Hlth Org. techn. Rep. Ser.*, No. 749 (1987).
16 Schad and Warren (Eds.), *Hookworm Disease: Current Status and New Directions*, Taylor & Francis, London, 1990.
17 Goldsmid, J. M., in MacPherson and Craig (Eds.), *Parasitic Helminths and Zoonoses in Africa*, Unwin Hyam, London, 1991, page 101.

No.	Roundworm (Nematoda) *Synonyms* Common names	Characteristics	Host Transmission	Associated disease
401	**Angiostrongylus cantonensis** (CHEN) DOUGHERTY *Pulmonema cantonensis* Rodent lung worm	Infective larvae in man about 0.5 mm long	Host: rodents, with adult worms in pulmonary arteries. Intermediate host: land snails and slugs. Man is infected following ingestion of infective larvae in snails	Angiostrongyliasis[1,2]. In man eosinophilic meningitis due to migration of infective larvae and developing worms in the CNS, with headache, neckstiffness, vomiting, vertigo, hyperesthesia of the skin and sometimes ocular signs with photophobia. Widespread in Southeast Asia and Pacific Islands, with numerous cases in Thailand and Taiwan[3,4] Diagnosis: based on clinical finding, but developing worms can be found in CSF and sometimes in the eye *Remarks*. Usually self-limiting, headache relieved by withdrawal of CSF. Anthelminthics usually not recommended, but mebendazole may be effective[5]
401a	**Angiostrongylus costaricensis** MORERA and CESPEDES *Morerastrongylus costaricensis*	Length of adult worms (in rodents): male up to 22 mm, female up to 42 mm. Ovoid eggs, ~90 µm long. In man, adult worms and eggs seen in granulomas removed at surgery	Lifecycle in rodents similar to that of *A. cantonensis*, but adult worms in mesenteric blood vessels. Intermediate host: slugs. Man is infected following ingestion of infective larvae in slugs	Abdominal angiostrongyliasis[6,7]. Clinical picture often resembles appendicitis with pain, tenderness and palpable mass in lower abdomen, fever and leucocytosis with eosinophilia up to 60%. Widespread in Central and South America Diagnosis: confirmed histologically by examining specimens removed surgically for worms and eggs *Remarks*. Usually self-limiting, but surgery may be necessary. Anthelminthics usually not recommended[8], but thiabendazole may be effective[5]
402	**Enterobius vermicularis** (LINNÉ) LEACH *Oxyuris vermicularis* Pin worm Seat worm Threadworm	Males: 2–5 mm long, 0.1–0.2 mm thick. Females: 8–13 mm long, 0.3–0.5 mm thick. Ovoid eggs, 50–60 µm by 20–30 µm, flattened on one side	Host: man and apes. Transmission within families and institutions by ingestion of embryonated eggs which are deposited in the perianal region by the female worm. Autoinfection can occur following scratching of the irritated anus. The infective eggs are also present in clothing and in the environment, in bed linen and house dust	Enterobiasis (oxyuriasis). The male and female worms mate in the cecal region of the large intestine, and there may be involvement of the appendix. Most cases asymptomatic (especially in adults), but *Enterobius* is probably the commonest cause of pruritis ani and pruritis vulvae in children[9,10] and it seems to be a common cause of lower abdominal pain, especially in females[11]. Worldwide distribution; the commonest helminthic parasite of temperate, well-sanitized areas, e.g. in Europe, where the infection rate in schoolchildren may reach 100%[12]
			Diagnosis: by perianal swab or the simple scotch-tape egg adhesion technique; eggs are rarely found in the feces *Remarks*. For treatment, pyrantel pamoate or mebendazole or albendazole are the drugs of choice[5]. All stages of worm development are killed by these drugs[13]. Piperazine is also effective if taken regularly for 7 consecutive days[14]. All family members should be treated simultaneously[15]	

[1] ROSEN et al., *J. Amer. med. Ass.*, **179**, 620 (1962).
[2] ALICATA, J. E., *J. trop. Med. Hyg.*, **72**, 53 (1969).
[3] PUNYAGUPTA et al., *Amer. J. trop. Med. Hyg.*, NS **24**, 921 (1975).
[4] CHEN, E. R., in CROSS, J. H. (Ed.), *Studies on Angiostrongyliasis in Eastern Asia and Australia*, Special Publication US Naval Medical Research Unit No. 2, Taipei, 1979, page 57.
[5] *Med. Lett. Drug. Ther.*, **34**, No. 865 (1992).
[6] LORIA-CORTÉS and LOBO-SANAHUJA, *Amer. J. trop. Med. Hyg.*, NS **29**, 538 (1980).
[7] MORERA, P., *Clin. trop. Med. comm. Dis.*, **2**, 747 (1987).
[8] MORERA, P., in STICKLAND, G. T. (Ed.), *Hunter's Tropical Medicine*, 7th ed., Saunders, Philadelphia, 1991, page 771.
[9] BROADBENT, V., *Brit. med. J.*, **1**, 89 (1975).
[10] SIMON, R. D., *Amer. J. Dis. Child.*, **128**, 21 (1974).
[11] NUTTING et al., *Canad. J. Surg.*, **23**, 286 (1980).
[12] SCHUFFNER, W., *Münch. med. Wschr.*, **31/32**, 411 (1944).
[13] CHO et al., *Korean J. Parasit.*, **18**, 45 (1980).
[14] WHO Model Prescribing Information, *Drugs Used in Parasitic Diseases*, World Health Organization, Geneva, 1990.
[15] WHO Scientific Group on Intestinal Protozoan and Helminthic Infections, *Wld Hlth Org. techn. Rep. Ser.*, No. 666 (1981).

No.	Roundworm (Nematoda) *Synonyms* Common names	Characteristics	Host Transmission	Associated disease
403	**Ascaris lumbricoides** LINNÉ Large intestinal roundworm	Males: 14–25 cm long, 3 mm thick. Females: 20–40 cm long, 5 mm thick. Eggs thick-shelled, 60 μm by 45 μm	Host: man (small intestine). Transmission by consumption of food, especially raw vegetables contaminated with embryonated eggs when human feces used as a fertilizer[1]. Freshly passed eggs are not infective; they must remain in moist, warm, shady conditions for more than 20 days to develop to the infective stage. Eggs can survive in the soil for many months or possibly years[2]	Ascariasis[2–5]. Often associated with *Trichuris trichiura* (*No. 392*). The larvae liberated from the eggs in the stomach pass via the liver, heart, lungs and trachea up to the pharynx and down into the small intestine. The migration causes seasonal pneumonitis with eosinophilia (LOEFFLER's syndrome)[6]. The adult worms sometimes migrate and can obstruct the bile ducts and cause liver abscess[7]. Less often the pancreatic duct is obstructed, and the worms will perforate the bowel, especially after abdominal surgery. In heavy infections, and sometimes following anthelminthic treatment, they can cause obstruction of the bowel. Individuals with light infections are usually asymptomatic and show resistance to reinfection[8,9], but heavy infections in children cause impairment of growth[10]. Worldwide distribution infecting more than 1 billion people[11] Diagnosis: finding of eggs in feces; a single female worm can produce 200 000 eggs per day *Remarks*. For treatment, mebendazole or pyrantel pamoate or albendazole are the drugs of choice[12]. Piperazine is effective, but less well tolerated[13]
404	**Toxocara canis** (WERNER) JOHNSTON Dog ascarid	Adult worms rarely reach maturity in man. Larvae 0.4–0.5 mm long, 20 μm thick	Host: dogs. Adult worms and larvae in dogs can be transmitted transplacentally or by the transmammary route to pups[14]. Transmission to man through ingestion of embryonated eggs. Main cause of visceral larva migrans in children, the larvae failing to reach maturity, but persisting in the tissues	Toxocariasis[15]. Larvae produce eosinophilic granulomas in the liver, lungs and other tissues including the brain and eye, where the granuloma may be mistaken for a malignant tumor[16]. Severity depends on number of eggs ingested. Often asymptomatic, but causes hypereosinophilia, hepatomegaly, pneumonitis and endophthalmitis[17]. Universal where dogs are in association with man Diagnosis: persistent eosinophilia; serology[18] and occasionally biopsy *Remarks*. For treatment, diethylcarbamazine is the drug of choice, thiabendazole or mebendazole are effective alternatives[12]. Ivermectin or albendazole may also be effective[19]

[1] SHEPHARD, M. R. N., *Helminth. Abstr.*, **40**, 1 (1971).
[2] PAWLOWSKI, Z. S., in WARREN and MAHMOUD (Eds.), *Tropical and Geographical Medicine*, 2nd ed., McGraw-Hill, New York, 1990, page 369.
[3] PAWLOWSKI, Z. S., *Clin. Gastroent.*, **7**, 157 (1978).
[4] CROMPTON et al. (Eds.), *Ascariasis and its Public Health Significance*, Taylor & Francis, London, 1985.
[5] CROMPTON et al. (Eds.), *Ascariasis and its Prevention and Control*, Taylor & Francis, London, 1989.
[6] GELPI and MUSTAPHA, *Amer. J. trop. Med. Hyg.*, N.S. **16**, 646 (1967).
[7] JAMES, T., *Med. Proc.*, **16**, 127 (1970).
[8] CHEN, E. R., *Formosan Sci.*, **25**, 27 (1971).
[9] OGILVIE and SAVIGNY, in COHEN and WARREN (Eds.), *Immunology of Parasitic Infections*, 2nd ed., Blackwell, Oxford, 1982, page 715.
[10] STEPHENSON, L. S., *Impact of Helminth Infections on Human Nutrition*, Taylor & Francis, London, 1987.
[11] WHO Scientific Group, Intestinal Protozoan and Helminthic Infections, *Wld Hlth Org. techn. Rep. Ser.*, No. 666 (1981).
[12] *Med. Lett. Drug. Ther.*, **34**, No. 865 (1992).
[13] WHO Model Prescribing Information, *Drugs Used in Parasitic Diseases*, World Health Organization, Geneva, 1990.
[14] BEAVER, P. J., *J. Parasit.*, **55**, 3 (1969).
[15] GLICKMAN, L. T., in WARREN and MAHMOUD (Eds.), *Tropical and Geographical Medicine*, 2nd ed., McGraw-Hill, New York, 1990, page 446.
[16] BEAVER et al., *Pediatrics*, **9**, 7 (1952).
[17] SCHANTZ and GLICKMAN, *New Engl. J. Med.*, **298**, 436 (1978).
[18] WOODRUFF et al., *Brit. med. J.*, **284**, 309 (1982).
[19] STÜRCHLER et al., *Ann. trop. Med. Parasit.*, **83**, 473 (1989).

No.	**Roundworm** (Nematoda) *Synonyms* Common names	Characteristics	Host Transmission	Associated disease
404a	**Toxocara cati** (Schrank) Brumpt Cat ascarid	Similar to *T. canis*	Host: cats. Transmission as for *T. canis*. Rare cause of visceral larva migrans in children	Toxocariasis
405	**Anisakis simplex**	Larvae removed from tissues in man about 20 mm long and 0.4 mm thick, with characteristic hook at anterior end	Host: saltwater fish and squid. Man is infected by eating raw, salted, pickled, smoked or undercooked fish	Anisakiasis[1]. Man is an accidental host. Larvae penetrate into the stomach or small intestine, cause upper and/or lower abdominal symptoms. Rare cause of visceral larva migrans[2]. Common in Japan *Remark*. Surgical treatment or endoscopic removal usually necessary[3,4]
406	**Dracunculus medinensis** (Linné) Gallandant *Filaria medinensis* Guinea worm Medina worm Serpent worm Dragon worm	Males: 12–30 mm long, 0.3 to 0.4 mm thick. Females: 70 to 120 cm long, 0.7–1.7 mm thick. Larvae 500–750 µm by 15–25 µm	Host: man and carnivores. Transmission by ingestion of infective stage in crustaceans (*Cyclops* spp.) from contaminated drinking water, especially step wells. Long incubation period of approximately 1 year and no evidence of acquired immunity; annual epidemics occur in the most heavily infected areas	Dracunculiasis (dracontiasis, Guinea worm disease)[5-7]. In man the worms live in the subcutaneous tissues, where the male fertilizes the female. The female migrates usually to the lower limbs, and when fully gravid produces a blister in the skin which ruptures to allow thousands of larvae to escape every time the affected area is immersed in water. At this time the patient may develop allergic reactions, which may be anaphylactic in nature. Sterile abscesses develop if the worm is ruptured in the tissues. Secondary complications include arthritis, synovitis, ankylosis and occasionally tetanus. Dead calcified worms are frequently detected radiologically. The disease is most prevalent in the dry areas of India and Africa, a few remaining endemic areas in the Middle East, with an annual incidence of 5 million[8]. The method of eradication of dracunculiasis is by supplying safe drinking water[9] Diagnosis: usually obvious from the appearance of the blister and the presence of the adult worm in the tissues *Remarks*. Slow extraction of the worm by winding it around a small stick. Treatment with metronidazole or thiabendazole not curative, but decreases inflammation and facilitates removal of the worm[4]

[1] Ishikura and Kikuchi (Eds.), *Intestinal Anisakiasis in Japan*, Springer, Tokyo, 1990.
[2] Fujino et al., *Jap. J. Parasit.*, **33**, 73 (1984).
[3] Wittner et al., *New Engl. J. Med.*, **320**, 1124 (1989).
[4] *Med. Lett. Drug. Ther.*, **34**, No. 865 (1992).
[5] Muller, R., *Advanc. Parasit.*, **9**, 73 (1971).
[6] Hopkins, D. R., in Warren and Mahmoud (Eds.), *Tropical and Geographical Medicine*, 2nd ed., McGraw-Hill, New York, 1990, page 439.
[7] Muller, R., in MacPherson and Craig (Eds.), *Parasitic Helminths and Zoonoses in Africa*, Unwin Hyam, London, 1991, page 204.
[8] *Morb. Mort. wkly Rep.*, **40**, 245 (1991).
[9] *Morb. Mort. wkly Rep.*, **38**, 882 (1989).

No.	**Roundworm** (Nematoda) *Synonyms* Common names	Characteristics	Host Transmission	Associated disease
407	**Gnathostoma spinigerum** OWEN *Gnathostoma siamense*	Adult worms not seen in man. Larvae 0.3 mm long and 0.06 mm thick, with 4 anterior rows of hooklets	Zoonosis with wide range of carnivores as final hosts, including cats and dogs. First intermediate host: crustaceans (*Cyclops* spp.). Second intermediate host: freshwater fish, frogs and birds, which are the source of infective stage for the normal final host. Man is infected by eating undercooked food containing the infective larvae	Gnathostomiasis[1]. Man is an accidental host and develops hemorrhagic and granulomatous reactions along the migratory route of the larvae, which may be subcutaneous, subconjunctival or in any of the internal viscera, including the brain, with resulting eosinophilic myeloencephalitis. Occurs mainly in Southeast Asia, but sporadic cases elsewhere Diagnosis: difficult unless the larvae are obtained by exploratory surgery; serology may be of some help *Remark*. Surgical excision or treatment with mebendazole[2]
408	**Wuchereria bancrofti** (COBBOLD) SEURAT *Filaria nocturna* *Filaria sanguinis* BANCROFT's filaria	Males: 2–4 cm long, 0.2 mm thick. Females: 5–12 cm long, 0.5 to 1.5 mm thick. Female with double uterus containing thousands of microfilariae whose egg membranes are retained after the microfilariae have been discharged. Sheathed microfilariae in blood films. Microfilariae 300 µm long. Absence of caudal nuclei	Two forms of *W. bancrofti* are defined on the basis of the periodicity of circulating microfilariae. Host: man. Transmission by mosquitoes, which serve as intermediate hosts, with development of microfilariae to the infective stage in the flight muscles of the insect. *Culex quinquefasciatus* is the commonest vector of the nocturnal periodic type in the urban and semi-urban endemic areas and in the rural areas of India. In Africa and parts of South East Asia the *Anopheles* vectors of malaria also transmit filariasis. In the eastern Pacific the parasite has a subperiodic diurnal periodicity, and it is transmitted by day-biting mosquitoes	Bancroftian lymphatic filariasis. Widespread in hot humid parts of the tropics. See text on next page
409	**Brugia malayi** (BRUG) BUCKLEY *Wuchereria malayi*	Males: 1.3–2.3 cm long, 75 µm thick. Females: 4.3–5.5 cm long, 130–170 µm thick. Sheathed microfilariae in blood films. Distinguished from *W. bancrofti* by presence of caudal nuclei	Two forms of *B. malayi* are defined on the basis of physiological differences. Nocturnal periodic form: mainly parasitic to man; transmission by *Anopheles* and *Mansonia* mosquitoes. Subperiodic form: a zoonosis with reservoir in leaf monkeys (*Presbytis* spp.); transmission by *Mansonia* mosquitoes	Brugian lymphatic filariasis. Confined to Southeast and East Asia. See text on next page
410	**Onchocerca volvulus** (LEUCKART) RAILLIET and HENRY *Filaria volvulus* *Onchocerca caecutiens* Blinding filaria	Males: up to 4 cm long, 0.2 mm thick. Females: up to 50 cm long, 0.4 mm thick. Males and females live together in the subcutaneous tissues, often in nodules. Unsheathed microfilariae, 250 to 300 µm long; many in the skin and eye (but in blood and urine and other body fluids in heavy infection)	Several strains exist; the most pathogenic strains are found in the African savanna. Host: man. Transmission by riverine blackflies of the genus *Simulium*	Onchocerciasis ('river blindness'). See text on page 142
411	**Loa loa** (COBBOLD) CASTELLANI and CHALMERS *Microfilaria diurna* *Dracunculus loa* *Filaria oculi humanus* Eye worm	Males: 3–3.5 cm long, 0.4 mm thick. Females: 4–7 cm long, 0.5 mm thick. Microfilariae in blood sheathed, but sheath not stained by GIEMSA	Host: man; similar parasite in monkeys. Transmission by outside day-biting horse flies of the genus *Chrysops*. Microfilariae: diurnal periodicity	Loiasis. Confined to rain forest regions of West and Central Africa. See text on page 143

[1] DAENSVANG, S., *A Monograph on the Genus Gnasthostoma and Gnasthostomiasis in Thailand*, South East Asian Medical Information Centre, Tokyo, 1980.
[2] *Med. Lett. Drug. Ther.*, **34**, No. 865 (1992).

No.	**Roundworm** (Nematoda) *Synonyms* Common names	Characteristics	Host Transmission	Associated disease
412	**Mansonella perstans** (MANSON) ORIHEL and EBERHARD *Dipetalonema perstans* *Acanthocheilonema perstans* *Tetrapetalonema perstans*	Males: 4.5 cm long, 60 µm thick. Females: 7–8 cm long, 120 µm thick. Unsheathed microfilariae, 200 µm long, in blood	Host: man and African anthropoids. Microfilariae: no periodicity. Transmission by *Culicoides* spp.	Generally not pathogenic in man. Widely distributed in African rain forest regions and Central and South America. See text on page 143
413	**Mansonella streptocerca** (MACFIE and CORSON) ORIHEL and EBERHARD	Adult worms similar to *M. perstans*. Microfilariae in the skin unsheathed, 180–240 µm long, 2.5–5 µm thick	Host: man and anthropoid apes. Transmission by *Culicoides* spp.	Streptocerciasis, a mild skin disease. Confined to West and Central African rain forest regions. See text on page 143
414	**Mansonella ozzardi** (MANSON) ORIHEL and EBERHARD	Males: 2.5 cm long, 80 µm thick. Females: 7 cm long, 200 µm thick. Unsheathed microfilariae, 250 µm long, in skin and blood	Host: man. Transmission by *Culicoides* spp. and *Simulium* spp.	Mansonellosis, probably not pathogenic in man. Confined to the Caribbean, Central America and northern parts of South America. See text on page 143

Lymphatic filariasis

The most prevalent of the filarial parasites is *Wuchereria bancrofti*. At least 90 million people are infected, especially in India, Southeast Asia, along the east coast of Africa and on the Pacific Islands, but there are pockets of infection in the Caribbean, as well as in Egypt and South America[1]. The most important mosquito vector, *Culex quinquefasciatus* (*fatigans*), breeds in latrines and waste water and is resistant to most insecticides.

The other important lymphatic-dwelling parasites are *Brugia malayi* and *Brugia timori*, which are major causes of elephantiasis in some areas of South India, Malaysia and Indonesia.

Male and female filarial worms live in a state of permanent copula and produce enormous numbers of immature larval stages called 'microfilariae'. They are long-lived parasites surviving up to 15 years, so the infections persist long after the patients have left the endemic areas. The microfilariae have a characteristic morphology and are found in the blood, adapted for transmission by the appropriate vector.

Adult filarial worms (unlike malarial parasites) do not multiply in man, and the number of worms present in a patient and the severity of the disease are proportional to the amount of transmission. Filarial infections are cumulative; therefore, expatriates and tourists or indigenous people living under good social conditions rarely develop advanced lesions such as elephantiasis or blindness. Lightly infected people may have troublesome symptoms which are difficult to diagnose.

When the insect vectors bite, they ingest microfilariae with the blood meal. The microfilariae migrate from the midgut into the flight muscles of the insect, and they grow until they are infective – usually this takes about 12 days. Following a bite by an infective mosquito the larvae migrate from the skin to the lymphatics, where during the next 3 to 6 months, if male and female worms can find each other, they mate and produce microfilariae, which enter the bloodstream.

Pathogenesis and clinical features

The pathogenic changes and the resulting clinical features in bancroftian filariasis are due to the presence of the developing and mature worms in the lymphatics. The microfilariae are usually innocuous, though they may be present in the blood at densities exceeding 15000/mL. *W. bancrofti* has a predilection for the lymphatics of the leg and spermatic cord, and the commonest presenting features are lymphangitis, fever, funiculitis, epididymitis, or orchitis with tender swollen inguinal lymph nodes and eosinophilia.

The hydrocele rate in infected adult males may be more than 40%, though surgeons who spend a great deal of time treating these cases rarely recognize their filarial etiology. Elephantiasis is a relatively rare complication of filariasis – even in heavily infected communities, less than 5% of the people develop this complication –, and there is often confusion with nonfilarial elephantiasis, which is prevalent in red soil areas of the tropics[2]. The initial stage of filarial lymphedema is reversible by treatment.

The acute stages of infection with *B. malayi* and *B. timori* are often more pronounced than *W. bancrofti* – severe fever, lymphangitis and abscess formation in the affected lymph nodes –, but *Brugia* rarely affects the spermatic cord or scrotum.

In very heavily infected individuals the worms affect the main lymphatic trunk in the abdomen; the vessels become obstructed and grossly dilated, with numerous anastomoses, which sometimes rupture into the kidney or bladder, with subsequent chyluria or lymphuria.

Tropical pulmonary eosinophilia syndrome

An unusual host reaction to the lymphatic-dwelling parasites is the tropical pulmonary eosinophilia syndrome, which is characterized by chronic cough, asthmatic attack and a persistent eosinophilia sometimes reaching over 50×10^9/L. This may be due to infections with filarial worms of animal origin, but the usual cause is a hyperimmune response to *W. bancrofti* or *B. malayi*, with the elimination of microfilariae from the peripheral blood. There is a dramatic response to treatment with diethylcarbamazine[3, 4].

Diagnosis

The diagnosis of filariasis can be made with certainty by finding the parasites, but this may be very difficult, especially in early and chronic infections. The best way to confirm the diagnosis is to examine the blood for microfilariae at the time of their peak periodicity, that is, as near midnight as possible with nocturnal periodic strains of *W. bancrofti* and *B. malayi*, and during the day for the diurnal periodic parasites. Thick blood smears should be stained with GIEMSA. This method is of value in moderate or heavy infections with microfilarial density between 250 and 20000/mL, but for light infections concentration techniques are necessary. The best concentration method is to take 5 mL of hemolyzed blood and pass it through a 3 µm Nuclepore® membrane filter. This traps all the microfilariae, and they can be stained on the filter with GIEMSA after fixation with methanol.

In most lightly infected individuals – this includes most short-term visitors to endemic areas – and, even more importantly, in most patients with advanced stages of elephantiasis, there are no microfilariae in the circulation, and the diagnosis must be based on the clinical history and history of travel in endemic areas, together with supporting immunodiagnosis.

Treatment

Diethylcarbamazine is the drug of choice for treating lymphatic filariasis[5, 6]; it is usually effective in killing microfilariae and most of the adult worms. Many countries have developed their own specific treatment regimens. A total cumulative dose (related to body mass) of 72 mg/kg, administered at a daily rate of 6 mg/kg for 12 days, has been recommended[6]. Reactions to the death of the worms can be unpleasant with fever, lymphangitis and even abscess formation, but there is no danger of precipitating elephantiasis[7]. *Brugia* is more susceptible to diethylcarbamazine than *W. bancrofti*; to avoid severe reactions to dead worms, half the dose should be used[8]. A single dose of ivermectin has been reported to be effective for treatment of bancroftian filariasis[9].

(Continued on next page)

Control

Control of the disease in the community has proved difficult because of resistance of mosquitoes to insecticides and the difficulties in administering diethylcarbamazine. The main methods of control are:

- Avoidance of mosquito bites by the use of insecticide-impregnated bed nets
- Reduction of the vector population by killing adult mosquitoes in houses and by reducing mosquito breeding through simple sanitation and the use of larvicides or polystyrene beads in pit latrines[10]
- Removal of the parasite from the reservoir host, which in the case of *W. bancrofti* is man; mass treatment can be effective against *W. bancrofti*[11], but with *Brugia* the animal reservoir poses special problems

Lymphatic filariasis has been extensively reviewed by the WHO Expert Committee on Filariasis[1] and by SASA[12].

References

1 WHO Expert Committee on Filariasis, *Wld Hlth Org. techn. Rep. Ser.*, No. 702 (1984).
2 PRICE and HENDERSON, *Trans. roy. Soc. trop. Med. Hyg.*, **73**, 640 (1979).
3 BUCKLEY, J. J. C., *E. Afr. med. J.*, **35**, 493 (1958).
4 LIE, K. J., *Amer. J. trop. Med. Hyg.*, N.S. **11**, 646 (1962).
5 *Med. Lett. Drug. Ther.*, **34**, No. 865 (1992).
6 WHO Model Prescribing Information, *Drugs Used in Parasitic Diseases*, World Health Organization, Geneva, 1990.
7 DENHAM and McGREEVY, *Advanc. Parasit.*, **15**, 243 (1977).
8 MAK, J. W., *Filariasis*, Bull. No. 19, Institute for Medical Research, Kuala Lumpur, 1983.
9 KUMARASWAMI et al., *J. Amer. med. Ass.*, **259**, 3150 (1988).
10 MAXWELL et al., *Trans. roy. Soc. Med. Hyg.*, **84**, 709 (1990).
11 OTTESEN, E. A., *Rev. infect. Dis.*, **7**, 341 (1985).
12 SASA, M., *Human Filariasis: A Global Survey of Epidemiology and Control*, University Park Press, Baltimore, 1976.

Onchocerciasis

Onchocerciasis ('river blindness') affects more than 30 million people in the savanna and rain forest areas of Africa; it causes untold misery, with blindness rates as high as 30% in the worst affected villages, and whole communities suffer the unsightly and intolerable skin changes caused by the parasite *Onchocerca volvulus*[1]. Although it is mainly a parasite of Africa, there are a few isolated foci in Saudi Arabia, the Yemen, Mexico, Guatemala, Venezuela, Ecuador, Colombia and Brazil. In spite of its formidable symptomatology, it is a disease that is rarely diagnosed, except in special surveys.

There are several strains of *O. volvulus* with different vectors and with differences in pathogenesis and clinical features[2,3]. The most pathogenic forms, with high blindness rates, are found in the West African savanna and in Mexico and Guatemala. The disease in the Yemen is unusual in that there is very little blindness, but a characteristic clinical picture of 'sowda' or 'black disease' due to hyperimmune reactions[4].

Pathogenesis and clinical features

The severity of the disease is proportional to the worm load, which, like that of other helminths, is cumulative and depends on the duration and intensity of transmission, so that temporary visitors to endemic areas very rarely develop advanced lesions.

In contrast to *Wuchereria bancrofti* it is the microfilariae and not the developing and adult worms which produce the main pathology. In early and light infections the adult worms are usually impalpable, but they eventually become encapsulated in dense fibrous tissue and form the characteristic, smooth and rubbery *Onchocerca* nodules, 0.5–5 cm in diameter, which are easily removed under local anesthetic. In Africa the commonest site for the adult worms is around the pelvis and in the midaxillary line; in Central America the commonest site is around the head. Some of the worms lie around the capsule of the hip joint, where they can produce arthritis. The microfilariae, which are relatively large (300 μm long), migrate to the skin, where in heavy infections the microfilarial density may exceed 500/mg. When the microfilarial density reaches 10/mg in the skin of the face, the eyes are invaded.

The disease is due to reactions to dead microfilariae. The initial allergic reactions result in a rash with pigmentary changes, and in long-standing cases, there is loss of the elastic layer of the skin and production of presbydermia. The loss of elasticity often results in 'hanging groins' and hernias in Africa or pouches under the eyes, the so-called 'leonine facies' of Central America. Many of the affected people in the endemic areas look prematurely aged.

When there are microfilariae in the skin of the face they migrate through the sclera into the cornea. The first signs of ocular onchocerciasis are snowflake opacities, which are cellular accumulations around dead microfilariae. They may be associated with photophobia. These early lesions disappear spontaneously or progress to the development of a sclerosing keratitis with the formation of a dense pannus. This extends from the sides and bottom of the cornea, and after many years it may cause complete anterior blindness. The iris usually becomes involved, with distortion of the pupil, depigmentation and sometimes secondary glaucoma. Examination with the slit lamp confirms the presence of the microfilariae, which can be seen in the cornea and also swimming freely in the anterior chamber. The fundus may show a characteristic choroidoretinitis with patchy pigmentation and sclerosis. The optic nerve may be affected, and this can result in reduced visual fields and complete blindness.

Diagnosis

Diagnosis is easy in heavy infections – skin snips (2–3 mm in diameter) are taken from the areas of highest expected microfilarial counts, e.g. the thigh in Africa, the shoulder in Central America, or the ankle in the Yemen, by inserting a needle into the superficial layer of the skin and lifting up a bloodless cone. This cone is cut off against the needle point with a razor blade (without local anesthetic) and the skin snip is placed in a drop of saline and examined half an hour later for active microfilariae.

If no microfilariae have been found in several skin snips the next step is to perform a MAZZOTTI test by giving 50 mg diethylcarbamazine, which kills the microfilariae and exacerbates the skin lesions and itching. The test is positive within 30 minutes to 24 hours and can be quite dramatic. It is dangerous to perform the MAZZOTTI test in patients with heavy infections; therefore it is only used when skin snips are negative. In heavy infections microfilariae can be found in the blood, the urine, the tears, the sputum and the CSF, especially after treatment with diethylcarbamazine[5].

Treatment

Excision of nodules on the head, particularly in children, reduces the risk of blindness. For chemotherapy, ivermectin is the drug of choice[6,7]. It appears to kill microfilariae and to inhibit their expulsion from the uterus of the female worm[7]. Ivermectin is given in a single oral dose (related to body mass) of 150 μg/kg every 6 to 12 months[6,7]; no food should be taken for at least 2 hours before or after dosage. Diethylcarbamazine is no longer recommended for treatment, because of the frequency with which it induces severe host reactions (MAZZOTTI reaction)[7]. Suramin – a macrofilaricide – is nephrotoxic. It is given intravenously in repeated doses; its use should be restricted to persons with moderate to heavy infections who cannot take repeated doses of ivermectin[8].

Control

Control of onchocerciasis depends on the following:

- Suppressive mass chemotherapy with ivermectin, repeated every 6 to 12 months[6,7]. It fails to interrupt transmission, but reduces microfilarial load and clinical complications
- Reducing transmission by elimination of the *Simulium* vectors in the rivers with insecticides (successful in some areas of Africa[1,9–11]). Because of longevity of the worm, vector control should continue for more than 15 years

Onchocerciasis has been reviewed by NELSON[12], BIANCO[13] and the WHO Expert Committee on Onchocerciasis[1] (the ocular complications and their treatment by ANDERSON and FUGLSANG[14]).

References

1 WHO Expert Committee on Onchocerciasis, *Wld Hlth Org. techn. Rep. Ser.*, No. 752 (1987).
2 DUKE and ANDERSON, *Z. Tropenmed. Parasit.*, **23**, 354 (1972).
3 ANDERSON et al., *Trans. roy. Soc. trop. Med. Hyg.*, **68**, 190 (1974).
4 CONNOR et al., *Amer. J. trop. Med. Hyg.*, N.S. **32**, 207 (1983).
5 FUGLSANG and ANDERSON, *J. Helminth.*, **48**, 93 (1974).
6 *Med. Lett. Drug. Ther.*, **34**, No. 865 (1992).
7 WHO Model Prescribing Information, *Drugs Used in Parasitic Diseases*, World Health Organization, Geneva, 1990.
8 GREENE, B. M., in WARREN and MAHMOUD (Eds.), *Tropical and Geographical Medicine*, 2nd ed., McGraw-Hill, New York, 1990, page 429.
9 McMAHON et al., *Bull. Wld Hlth Org.*, **19**, 75 (1958).
10 PRENTICE, M. A., *PAHO Sci. Publ.*, **298**, 87 (1974).
11 WALSH et al., in LAIRD, M. (Ed.), *Blackflies*, Academic Press, London, 1981, page 85.
12 NELSON, G. S., *Advanc. Parasit.*, **8**, 173 (1970).
13 BIANCO, A. E., in MACPHERSON and CRAIG (Eds.), *Parasitic Helminths and Zoonoses in Africa*, Unwin Hyam, London, 1991, page 138.
14 ANDERSON and FUGLSANG, *Trop. Dis. Bull.*, **74**, 257 (1977).

Loiasis and filarial infections caused by *Mansonella* spp.

The parasite *Loa loa* is confined to the rain forest areas of West and Central Africa. The microfilariae have a diurnal periodicity, and transmission is by day-biting tabanid 'horse flies' of the genus *Chrysops*. The main symptoms are due to allergic reactions to the parasite with recurrent angioedema (Calabar swellings) around the adult worms, which migrate through the subcutaneous tissues. Loiasis is the most likely cause of high-level eosinophilia in people who have visited or worked in the rain forest areas in Africa. A dramatic sign of the disease is the presence of relatively large adult worms, 3–7 cm in length, migrating slowly under the conjunctiva. The diagnosis is confirmed by finding sheated microfilariae in the blood during the day, using the techniques recommended for the diagnosis of *W. bancrofti*. Diethylcarbamazine is the only drug of proven value[1,2] (effective against all forms of the parasite).

Mansonella streptocerca, like *Loa loa*, is confined to the rain forest regions of Africa. It is a small worm; both adult worms and microfilariae occur in the skin. It is usually nonpathogenic (no eye lesions), but it can produce a dermatitis similar to onchocerciasis. The microfilariae must be distinguished from *O. volvulus* in skin snips. It is susceptible to treatment with diethylcarbamazine[3,4].

Mansonella perstans is widespread in Africa, Central and South America. It may produce eosinophilia, but it is generally innocuous. The small microfilariae are present in the blood during the day and are transmitted by midges at night. Prolonged treatment with diethylcarbamazine, mebendazole or ivermectin may be effective[1,3,5].

Mansonella ozzardi is confined to the Caribbean and South America. The microfilariae are found in the blood and the skin, and it is transmitted by both midges and *Simulium*. It is generally nonpathogenic, but it has caused confusion in the diagnosis of *Wuchereria bancrofti* in the Caribbean and of onchocerciasis in Brazil[6].

For a general account of filarial infections, see Beaver et al.[7] and Stickland[8].

References

1 *Med. Lett. Drug. Ther.*, **34**, No. 865 (1992).
2 WHO Model Prescribing Information, *Drugs Used in Parasitic Diseases*, World Health Organization, Geneva, 1990.
3 Greene, B. M., in Warren and Mahmoud (Eds.), *Tropical and Geographical Medicine*, 2nd ed., McGraw-Hill, New York, 1990, page 429.
4 Meyers et al., *Amer. J. trop. Med. Hyg.*, N.S. **21**, 528 (1972); Meyers et al., *Amer. J. trop. Med. Hyg.*, N.S. **27**, 1137 (1978).
5 Wahlgren and Frolov, *Trans. roy. Soc. trop. Med. Hyg.*, **77**, 422 (1983).
6 Nelson and Davies, *Trans. roy. Soc. trop. Med. Hyg.*, **70**, 16 (1976).
7 Beaver et al., *Clinical Parasitology*, 9th ed., Lea & Febiger, Philadelphia, 1984.
8 Stickland, G. T. (Ed.), *Hunter's Tropical Medicine*, 7th ed., Saunders, Philadelphia, 1991.

Index

The italic numbers are the serial numbers of the organisms listed in the tables.

A

B

The italic numbers are the serial numbers of the organisms listed in the tables.

C

Index

The italic numbers are the serial numbers of the organisms listed in the tables.

The italic numbers are the serial numbers of the organisms listed in the tables.

Index

The italic numbers are the serial numbers of the organisms listed in the tables.

Index

The italic numbers are the serial numbers of the organisms listed in the tables.

The italic numbers are the serial numbers of the organisms listed in the tables.

The italic numbers are the serial numbers of the organisms listed in the tables.

Index

The italic numbers are the serial numbers of the organisms listed in the tables.

The italic numbers are the serial numbers of the organisms listed in the tables.

14679e XY / ST